The Positive Psychology of
Meaning & Spirituality

Selected Papers from Meaning Conferences

Edited by
Paul T. P. Wong
Lilian C. J. Wong
Marvin J. McDonald
Derrick W. Klaassen

Published by
Purpose Research, LLC, in cooperation with the
International Network on Personal Meaning

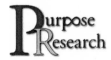

This edition published by Purpose Research, LLC, Birmingham, Alabama, USA with permission of the International Network on Personal Meaning. Originally published by INPM Press, Abbotsford BC, Canada, a division of the International Network on Personal Meaning. INPM on the web: http://meaning.ca and http://existentialpsychology.org

Cover design by Cailin Greene, Avalon Design, Vancouver, BC.

LC: BF463.M4

Printed in the United States of America.

First Purpose Research edition, July, 2012.

This edition has been newly typeset, with extensive copyediting and revision to tables and graphics. Because this book contains articles from authors around the world, both British and American (U.S.) spellings may be appropriate. For example, an academic department in Canada might call itself "Counselling Centre" while in the United States it might be "Counseling Center."

Soft cover edition
ISBN 978-0-982478-0-4

Printed in the United States of America

Contents

PART ONE
MEANING, SPIRITUALITY, & RELIGIOSITY

PART TWO
EXISTENTIAL, RELIGIOUS, & NARRATIVE THERAPIES

PART FOUR
POSITIVE PSYCHOLOGY OF GOOD WORK
AND OTHER VIRTUES

Acknowledgements

It has taken several years to produce this edited volume, much longer than anticipated. The delay is partially caused by two events that have disrupted the editorial process: first, a major change in the editorial team; second, the big move of Paul and Lilian Wong from Vancouver to Toronto and their taking on challenging new positions at Tyndale University College in Toronto. We are most grateful to our contributors for their patience and their cooperation to update their chapters.

Many speakers took part in our Meaning Conferences. We want to acknowledge the generous support from the Social Sciences & Humanities Research Council of Canada and the Sir John Templeton Foundation. Several individuals have also consistently supported the Meaning Conferences financially; in particular, we want to recognize Joshua Wong and Donald Jenkins.

The manuscripts published here have gone through at least two rounds of copyediting. We want to thank Holly Klaassen, Belinda Carlaw, and Rebecca Carter-Chand for contributing to the process and Lilian Wong for assuming the responsibility for the final editing.

We also want to say a special "thank you" to the many faithful volunteers, most of them from the Graduate Program of Counselling Psychology of Trinity Western University. Their dedication and enthusiasm have left a deep impression on all the attendees and contributed to the international reputation of our Meaning Conferences.

The Editorial Team

P. T. P. W.
L. C. J. W.
M. J. McD.
D. W. K.

July, 2007

Preface

Some of the most creative minds and most respected academics and clinicians have participated in our Meaning Conferences. These include Erwin Yalom, Howard Gardner, Donald Meichenbaum, Ernesto Spinelli, Kirk Schneider, and Harold Koenig. This volume consists of selected papers from the first three Meaning Conferences, representing theoretical, empirical, and clinical contributions.

Each Meaning Conference focused on a timely and yet timeless theme. The themes for our first three Meaning Conferences were: (1) Searching for Meaning in the New Millennium, (2) Freedom, Responsibility, and Justice, and (3) Transforming Suffering, Loss, and Death through Meaning, Hope, and Faith. Although these are serious and sobering themes, there is an underlying, uplifting message about the human potential for positive change.

In this volume, we have expanded and enriched positive psychology by integrating science with faith, social concerns with the big picture, empirical psychology with phenomenological research, and cognitive-behavioral therapy with existential psychotherapy. We have probed the depths of the human soul and explored the farther reaches of the transcendental reality in order to understand the conditions of human existence.

We hope that you will be informed as well as inspired by the various articles in this volume.

The Editorial Team

P. T. P. W.
L. C. J. W.
M. J. McD.
D. W. K.

July, 2007

About the Editors

Paul T. P. Wong, Ph.D. received his Ph.D. in Psychology at the University of Toronto. At present, he is Professor of Psychology and Chair, Division of Social Sciences and Business Administration, Tyndale University College, Toronto. He has held professorial positions at the University of Texas at Austin, York University, Trent University, and the University of Toronto. He was the founding director of the Graduate Program in Counselling Psychology at Trinity Western University, BC. He is the founding President of the International Network on Personal Meaning (www.meaning.ca), the International Society for Existential Psychology and Psychotherapy (www.existentialpsychology.org) and the Meaning-Centered Counselling Institute. He is a Fellow of the American Psychological Association and Canadian Psychological Association. With more than 120 published articles and book chapters, his current interests cover several areas, from coping with stress to the positive psychology of meaning. Recently he has contributed three chapters to the *Encyclopedia of Positive Psychology*. The second edition of his edited volume, *The Human Quest for Meaning*, was published in 2012.

Lilian C. J. Wong, Ph.D. is Associate Professor of Psychology, Tyndale University College, Toronto. She received her Ph.D. in Counselling Psychology at the University of British Columbia. Her primary research area is multicultural clinical supervision. Her Multicultural Supervision Competencies Questionnaire (developed with Paul Wong) has contributed to the conceptualization and measurement of multicultural supervision competencies. For many years, she has taken an active part in the Round Table Discussions on Hot Topics in Clinical Supervision and Training at APA conventions. Her other research interests include play therapy and grieving in children. She was on the Education Committee of the BC Association for Play Therapy for three years. She is on the Board of the International Network on Personal Meaning (www.meaning.ca) and Vice-President of the Meaning-Centered Counselling Institute. She is co-editor of the *Handbook of Multicultural Perspectives on Stress and Coping* (Springer).

Marvin J. McDonald, Ph.D. is Director of the MA program in Counselling Psychology at Trinity Western University, BC. He is married to Darlys Carlson McDonald and joins her in parenting their two sons, Nathan and Christopher. He publishes in the areas of theoretical psychology, spirituality and health, and professional issues in counselling. He is co-author, with D. W. Klaassen & M. D. Graham, of "Constructivist stances for promoting justice in spirituality research," in J. Raskin & S. Bridges (Eds.), *Studies in Meaning 2: Bridging the Personal and Social in Constructivist Psychology* (pp. 239-263). His more recent publications include "Negotiating justice in psychology: Situating psychology among rival moral orders," in W. Smythe & A. Baydala (Eds.), *Studies of How the Mind Publicly Enfolds into Being*. He is involved with the International Network on Personal Meaning, (www.meaning.ca), and participates in interfaith dialogue activities in his community.

Derrick W. Klaassen, MA, CCC is currently a Ph.D. student in Counselling Psychology at the University of British Columbia. He is a member of the Canadian Counselling Association and the Austrian Society for Logotherapy and Existential Analysis. His clinical and research interests include existential psychology and psychotherapy, cultural psychology, and the role of spirituality and religion in mental health.

About the Contributors

Maureen Angen, Ph.D. is a chartered psychologist and a Canadian Institute of Health Postdoctoral Fellow with the Department of Psychosocial Resources at the Tom Baker Cancer Centre in Calgary, Alberta. She received a Ph.D. in Counselling Psychology from the University of Calgary, Alberta.

Monika Ardelt, Ph.D. is Associate Professor of Sociology and a Founding Faculty Member of the Center for Spirituality and Health at the University of Florida. She received a Ph.D. in Sociology from the University of North Carolina, Chapel Hill. In 1999, Dr. Ardelt was elected as a Brookdale National Fellow to study the similarities and differences between aging and dying well.

Earl D. Bland, Psy.D. is Associate Professor of Psychology, Chair of the Division of Behavioral Sciences and head of the Psychology Department at MidAmerica Nazarene University, also a part-time Director of Counseling & Mentoring at Olathe Bible Church. Dr. Bland received a Psy.D. from the Illinois School of Professional Psychology. He is a licensed psychologist in both Kansas and Missouri.

Adam Blatner, M.D. received his M.D. from the Medical School at the University of California, San Francisco. From 1987-1994, Dr. Blatner was on the faculty of Psychiatry & Behavioral Science, School of Medicine, the University of Louisville, KY. He has also worked in hospitals, clinics, and private practice. He is one of the executive editors of *ReVision: A Journal of Consciousness and Transformation* and co-editor of an anthology on improvisational and interactive drama. He has authored several books, including *Foundation of Psychodrama*, and *Art of Play: Helping Adults Reclaim Imagination and Spontaneity.*

Christine V. Bruun, Ph.D. is Professor of Psychology and Chair of the Department of Psychology at the Rockford College, Rockford, IL. She is interested in developing faith and trust in a college setting.

Marla J. Colvin received her M.A. in Psychology from the University of Illinois. She is on the faculty of the Cuyahoga Community College, teaching courses in Psychology. Her interests include cross-cultural approaches to diagnosis and treatment, development and levels of consciousness, transpersonal psychology, and environmental psychology.

Amy Conlon holds a B.S. in finance from the University of Wisconsin-LaCrosse (WI). She is the Senior Director of Retention Solutions, providing services to campuses through the use of the predictive model for student retention tool *RetentionRT.*

Alvin C. Dueck, Ph.D., a licensed psychologist, is the Evelyn and Frank Freed Professor of the Integration of Psychology and Theology, Department of Clinical Psychology at Fuller Theological Seminary. He received a Ph.D. in Psychology/Education from Stanford University. His scholarly research interests are on the role of religion in therapy, congregational health, and conflict resolution between Christians and Muslims.

Gordon L. Flett, Ph.D. is Professor of Psychology in the Department of Psychology, York University, Toronto, where he holds a Canada Research Chair in Personality and Health. He received a Ph.D. from the University of Toronto. Dr. Flett's research interests include the role of personality factors and depression.

Patricia Frazier, Ph.D. is Associate Professor in Counseling Psychology and Social Psychology in the Department of Psychology at the University of Minnesota, Twin Cities. She received a Ph.D. in Psychology from the University of Minnesota. Dr. Frazier has done extensive research on sexual assault and other traumatic life events. Her research interests include the effects of traumatic events, their potential to create positive life change, and on meaning in life.

Howard Gardner, Ph.D. is the Hobbs Professor of Cognition and Education at the Harvard Graduate School of Education. He received a Ph.D. in Social Psychology/Developmental Psychology from Harvard University. He has authored many books, including, *Frames of Mind*, and *Good Work*. He is best known in educational circles for his theory of multiple intelligences. Most recently, Gardner and his colleagues have launched the GoodWork Project. "GoodWork" is both excellent in quality and exhibits a sense of responsibility with respect to implications and applications.

Marnin J. Heisel, Ph.D. is Senior Instructor in Psychiatry at the University of Rochester Medical School. He received a Ph.D. in Clinical Psychology from York University, and completed a postdoctoral fellowship at St. Michael's Hospital, University of Toronto. With Professor Gordon Flett, Dr. Heisel developed the Geriatric Suicide Ideation Scale (GSIS), an assessment tool for suicidal thoughts among seniors. His research interests include the role of character pathology in suicidality, and end-of-life issues.

Douglas D. Henning, Ph.D. is the Undergraduate Associate Academic Dean and Professor of Psychology at MidAmerica Nazarene University in Olathe, Kansas, and a psychologist at The Rehabilitation Institute of Kansas City. He is a Diplomate in the American Academy of Pain Management. He received a Ph.D. in Counseling & Family Life, Oregon State University. With extensive clinical experience, Dr. Henning has taught in Switzerland, and instructed trainers in marriage and family in Moscow, Russia.

Tara Hyland-Russell, Ph.D. is an Assistant Professor, St. Mary's University College, Calgary, Alberta, and received her doctorate from the University of Calgary. Her research interests include twentieth-century literature, poetry and poetics, women's life writing, critical theory, narrative discourse, children's literature, folk and fairy tales.

Harold G. Koenig, M.D., MHSc. is Associate Professor of Medicine and Psychiatry at Duke University Medical Center. He received a M.D. and M.H.Sc. from the University of California, San Francisco, and completed a fellowship in Geropsychiatry at Duke University Medical Center. He is the director and founder of the Center for the Study of Religion/Spirituality and Health at that institution. He has published extensively in the fields of mental health, geriatrics, and religion. He is editor of the *International Journal of Psychiatry in Medicine*, and founder and editor-in-chief of *Research News & Opportunities in Science and Theology*.

Sameet Kumar, Ph.D. is a Buddhist psychologist trained with Tibetan Buddhist teachers. He received a Ph.D. from the University of Miami. Dr. Kumar works at the Mount Sinai Comprehensive Cancer Center in Miami Beach and Aventura, FL. His areas of expertise are in palliative care, spirituality in psychotherapy, stress management and relaxation, and grief and bereavement. He integrates mindfulness and spirituality in psychotherapy. He is the author of *Grieving Mindfully: A Compassionate and Spiritual Guide to Coping with Loss*.

Ariella N. Lang, RN, Ph.D. is a Canadian Institutes of Health Research postdoctoral fellow in the School of Nursing at the University of Ottawa. Her career has centered around the improvement of care to grieving individuals and their families following the death of a loved one.

Alfried Längle, M.D., Ph.D. is the founder and president (since 1983) of the Society for Logotherapy and Existential Analysis (Vienna). Dr. Längle studied medicine and psychology at the Universities of Innsbruck, Rome, Toulouse and Vienna. After years of hospital work in general medicine and psychiatry, he started a private practice in psychotherapy, general medicine and clinical psychology in Vienna.

Dmitri A. Leontiev, Ph.D., Dr.Sc. is Professor of Psychology at Moscow State University, Russia. He is the Director of the Institute of Existential Psychology and Life Enhancement (EXPLIEN), Moscow, Russia, and Vice-President of Moscow branch of Russian Psychological Society. He is a member of the Board of Directors of ISEPP, editorial board of IJEPP and winner of the Promotional Award of Viktor Frankl Foundation, Vienna (2004).

Joanna Lipari, Psy.D. received her doctorate from Pepperdine University, CA. She has specialized in existential psychotherapy and Geriatric Psychology at the Center for Healthy Aging in Santa Monica, CA. She has held research and clinical positions with the US Veterans at the West Los Angeles Administration. Dr. Lipari also works with adolescents who suffer from severe mental difficulties.

Salvatore R. Maddi, Ph.D. is Professor in the Department of Psychology and Social Behavior at the School of Social Ecology, University of California, Irvine. He received a Ph.D. in Clinical Psychology from Harvard University. Dr. Maddi is a certified clinical psychologist. He specializes in personality, psychopathology, health psychology and creativity, and stress management. He is well known for his research and promotion of hardiness through deepening the attitudes of commitment, control, and challenge to reach individual potentials and cope with stress.

Janette E. McDonald, Ph.D. received her doctorate in Human and Organizational Systems from the Fielding Institute in Santa Barbara, CA. She is an associate professor in the Adult Degree Program /Psychology, Capital University, Columbus, OH. Her scholarly research interests focus on transformative learning experiences for adult learners and end of life issues.

Donald Meichenbaum, Ph.D. is Distinguished Professor Emeritus at the University of Waterloo, and the recipient of the Izaak Killiam Research Fellowship Award. He received a Ph.D. in Clinical Psychology from the University of Illinois, Champaign. Dr. Meichenbaum is one of the founders of cognitive-behavior therapy and the author of numerous books, chapters, and articles, including, *Treatment of Individuals with Anger-Control Problems and Aggressive Behaviors, Treating Post-traumatic Stress Disorder,* and *Coping with Stress.* As reported in the American Psychologist, he was voted "one of the ten most influential psychotherapists of the century," by North American clinicians.

Crystal L. Park, Ph.D. is Associate Professor of Psychology at the University of Connecticut. She received a Ph.D. in Clinical Psychology from the University of Delaware and completed a postdoctoral fellowship at University of California, San Francisco. Dr. Park has published articles on the roles of religious beliefs and religious coping in response to stressful life events, the phenomenon of stress-related growth, and people's attempts to find meaning in or create meaning out of negative life events. She has developed a comprehensive model of meaning as applied to a variety of health-related problems. She is co-editor of the *Handbook of the Psychology of Religion and Spirituality.*

Jordan B. Peterson, Ph.D. is a professor in the Department of Psychology at the University of Toronto and a clinical psychologist. He received a Ph.D. in clinical psychology from McGill University. From 1993 to 1998, he was a professor at Harvard University. Dr. Peterson's current research interests are in self-deception, creativity, achievement, personality, narrative, and motivation. In 1999, he published a book, *Maps of Meaning.*

Alan Pope Ph.D. received his doctorate from the Duquesne University, Pittsburgh, PA. He is an assistant professor for the Department of Psychology at the University of West Georgia and has worked as a bereavement counsellor and psychotherapist. In 2002, he was given a research grant for the Asian Studies Development Program/NEH Summer Institute on Japanese Culture, Honolulu, Hawaii.

Kevin Reimer, Ph.D. is Associate Professor in the Department of Graduate Psychology at the School of Behavioral and Applied Sciences, Azusa Pacific University. He received a Ph.D. from Fuller Theological Seminary and completed postdoctoral fellowships at the University of British Columbia and the University of Oxford. Dr. Reimer's research program includes moral identity in adolescence, altruistic love, and compassionate care in L'Arche and spiritual integration of psychology.

Sarah Sass obtained her B.A from the University of Minnesota, Twin Cities. She is affiliated with the Clinical/Community Division at the University of Illinois. Her research interests are in the cognitive and emotional processing, treatment and prevention of anxiety disorders and depression.

Kirk J. Schneider, Ph.D. is a licensed psychologist and leading spokesperson for contemporary humanistic psychology. He is president of the Existential-Humanistic Institute and an adjunct faculty at Saybrook Graduate School and the California Institute of Integral Studies. Dr. Schneider received a Ph.D. in Psychology at the Saybrook Institute. He has published over 70 articles and chapters and has authored or edited five books, including *The Psychology of Existence: An Integrative, Clinical Perspective* (with Rollo May) and *Rediscovery of Awe.*

William E. Smythe Ph.D. is Associate Professor and head of the Department of Psychology at the University of Regina. He received his doctorate in Psychology from the University of Toronto. His areas of specialization include foundational issues in theoretical psychology, narrative processes in human cognition, the psychology of fiction, metaphor in psychology, personal mythology, folk psychology, and qualitative research ethics. Dr. Smythe is the editor of two books on psychological theory: *Toward a Psychology of Persons* (Lawrence Erlbaum Associates) and (with Angelina Baydala) *Studies of How the Mind Publicly Enfolds into Being* (Edwin Mellen Press).

Ernesto Spinelli, Ph.D. is a Fellow of the British Psychological Society (BPS) and the British Association of Counselling and Psychotherapy (BACP) as well as a UKCP registered existential psychotherapist. After stepping down as Academic Dean of the School of Psychotherapy and Counselling at Regent's College, London U.K., he remains as a Senior Fellow. He has earned a BPS Counselling Psychology Division Award for Outstanding Contributions to the Advancement of the Profession. Dr. Spinelli is the author of numerous articles and several highly respected books on the theory and practise of existential psychotherapy. He is widely recognized as a leading figure in contemporary existential psychotherapy and phenomenological psychology.

Ty Tashiro, Ph.D. is Assistant Professor of Counseling in the Department of Psychology at the University of Maryland, College Park. He received a Ph.D. in Counseling Psychology from the University of Minnesota, Twin Cities. His research interests include interpersonal relationships, affect and social cognition, and stress-related growth.

Bernard Weiner, Ph.D. is Professor of Psychology at the University of California, Los Angeles. He received a Ph.D. from the University of Michigan. In 1965, following two years at the University of Minnesota, he went to UCLA, where he is currently Distinguished Professor of Psychology. Dr. Weiner has published nearly 200 articles, co-authored or edited 15 books, including *An Attributional Theory of Motivation and Emotion*, *Human Motivation: Metaphors, Theories, and Research*, and *Judgments of Responsibility*.

Belinda M. Wholeben, Professor of Psychology, Department of Psychology, Rockford College, Rockford, IL.

Paul T. P. Wong, Ph.D. is Professor of Psychology and Chair of the Division of Social Sciences and Business Administration at Tyndale University College, Toronto. Dr. Wong received his Ph.D. in Psychology at the University of Toronto. He has held professorial positions at the University of Texas at Austin, York University, Trent University, the University of Toronto and Trinity Western University. He is the founding President of the International Network on Personal Meaning (www. meaning.ca), the International Society for Existential Psychology and Psychotherapy (www.existentialpsychology.org), and the Meaning-Centered Counselling Institute.

Jens Zimmermann, Ph.D. is Professor at Trinity Western University, where he teaches English, German, literary theory, and hermeneutics. He received a Ph.D. from the University of British Columbia. Dr. Zimmermann has presented and published numerous articles on the hermeneutics of Calvin, Spinoza, Schleiermacher, Heidegger, Gadamer, and Levinas. He recently published *Recovering Theological Hermeneutics*, a work that unites theological and philosophical traditions.

Introduction: A Quiet Positive Revolution

PAUL T. P. WONG

Positive psychology (PP) means different things to different people, depending on their theoretical perspectives and cultural backgrounds. There is, however, an underlying, unifying theme of PP: Life can be made better for all people, if certain conditions are met. What these conditions are constitutes the subject matter of psychological research. Another characteristic of PP is that it is dynamic, evolving, and ever expanding. As a scientific and social movement, PP cannot be confined to any dogmas carved in stone, because it is always subject to influences by new creative ideas, pressing human needs, and changing circumstances.

The vision of PP articulated in this paper and reflected in this collection of chapters focuses on the big picture of meaning and spirituality. It is a quiet positive revolution without a clarion call to arms, without marching bands, and without an opening salvo of big guns; it does not call for paradigm shift or a drastic change in direction. Raising the somber-colored Banners of Meaning does not have the same currency and power to evoke instant emotions and excite public interest as waving the colorful Flags of Happiness, because meaning is often mistakenly perceived as belonging to the domain of philosophy. In short, it is a positive revolution of: (a) inner awakening, (b) acting out this enlightenment, and (c) working through the practical implications of meaning-based transformation. It is a quiet revolution designed to realize one's potentials and uplift humanity. As such, it is largely under the radar and remains subterranean. It is nevertheless an ongoing grassroots movement, winning the hearts and minds of people, one person at a time. It will continue in the privacy of homes and counseling rooms as well as in public meeting places, such as churches, synagogues, and lecture halls.

THE THREE STAGES OF POSITIVE REVOLUTION

The three stages of this positive revolution are characterized by themes of the first three Meaning Conferences. These are respectively: (a) awakening to the need for meaning, (b) acting out one's responsibility, and (c) working through the power of meaning. This trilogy of positive revolution corresponds to the three basic tenets of Logotherapy: (a) the will to meaning, (b) the freedom of choice, and (c) the meaning of life (Frankl, 1986). I propose that these three stages are involved in both personal and societal transformation.

1

AWAKENING TO THE NEED FOR MEANING

What makes life worth living? What is the good life? There are two approaches to address these fundamental questions, resulting in different research directions and consequences. The first approach is to equate worthiness with happiness. Most of the current PP research focuses on scientific studies of happiness, life satisfaction, and the applications of these empirical findings to facilitate the pursuit of happiness. Unfortunately, the very act of asking: "How can I be happy? How can I pack more happiness into my life?" is seductive—it simultaneously turns the attention to self-interests and dulls one's social responsibility and moral sensitivity. The danger of this happiness orientation is that it often leads to the narcissistic pursuit of personal happiness and success (Schumaker, 2007) and the shallow popularization of PP (Peterson, 2004).

In contrast, an alternative approach is to focus on the quest for meaning. This quest involves a very different motive, process, and destination; it may entail ontological anxiety, risks, setbacks, and self-sacrifices. This vision quest can be likened to navigating a treacherous river or climbing a dangerous mountain. It is not for the faint hearted, who are fearful of confronting the unknown; nor is it suitable for the "softies" who just want to live an easy and pleasant life. The very act of asking, "How can I live a worthwhile life? How can I spend my time in a meaning way?" challenges one to pursue some lofty ideal or higher purpose. One may endure hardships and risk one's life in order to pursue something meaningful and significant, such as climbing Mount Everest or volunteering to defend one's country. Unlike the pursuit of happiness, the human quest for meaning not only reduces one's overall level of positive emotions, but also increases one's likelihood of suffering. However, by embracing the challenge of this vision quest, one experiences the fullness of life and the vitality of feeling intensely alive to a wide range of rich human emotions. Thus the paradox—one finds happiness by losing it, and one finds life by risking it.

This second approach to the good life has several advantages. First, it avoids the pitfalls of the hedonic trap and the rat race. Secondly, it is based on the profound existential insight that authentic happiness will elude us when we intentionally pursue it as if it were our ultimate concern, but will come to us through the back door as a byproduct, when we devote ourselves to live a life that is meaningful and purposeful (Frankl, 1986). Finally, this approach opens up new frontiers of PP research as illustrated by many of the papers in this volume.

Happiness and meaning are closely related: A meaningful life is intrinsically fulfilling and satisfying, and authentic happiness always has a meaning component. But motive matters. If one's primary motive is happiness, it may allure one to a shallow kind of happiness and make one vulnerable to materialism, consumerism, hedonism, and misguided ambitions. If one's primary motive is meaning, it opens up an entirely different vista of heroism and idealism which leads to personal growth and authentic happiness. In short, choosing a slightly different direction can lead to a vastly different journey and destination. How we frame the question of the good life also has important implications for research and applications. Future research needs to compare the impacts of directly pursuing personal happiness and purposefully pursuing a higher purpose.

The International Network on Personal Meaning (INPM; www.meaning.ca) and the International Meaning Conferences focus on a meaning-centered and spiritually oriented positive psychology. In this article, I want to summarize the themes of the first three conferences organized by INPM, just to showcase the rich content and broad parameters of this purpose-driven positive revolution, but only representative papers from these conferences are included in this volume.

The theme for the First Meaning Conference in 2000 was *Searching for Meaning in the New Millennium*. This theme was designed to awaken people's "will to meaning." Frankl (1986) pointed out that this universal primary need for meaning is often blocked by a materialistic culture or misguided egotistic ambitions. One of the main functions of logotherapy is to bring one's existential need for meaning to the conscious level.

Dr. David Myers, keynote speaker at the First Meaning Conference, provided compelling evidence on the decline of personal and social well-being in spite of our continued progress in technology and increase in personal wealth over recent decades. This paradox of success is related to a steady decline in personal philosophy of life or spiritual values. He proposed the need for a social revolution in terms of restoring social capital, such as community, faith, charitable giving, and volunteerism. Dr. Myers' lecture made it very clear that prosperity without purpose leads to disillusionment and emptiness, and progress without social responsibility results in alienation and dehumanization. A winner-take-all economy contributes to conflict, injustice, and an increasing gap between the haves and the have-nots.

Jordan Peterson provided a profound exposition about the different kinds of meaning and the architecture of belief. He proposed that a sense of meaninglessness may lead individuals to identify themselves with some destructive power. Abandonment of meaning exposes one's moral weaknesses and makes one hate life. Therefore, the solution is for human beings to confront the feared unknown and transform it to skills and meaningful representations. We can overcome our fears, hatred, and weaknesses, when we construct and reconstruct stories. Meaning is our basic instinct for survival. In each generation, our conscious capacity to reinterpret religious and mystical narratives enables us to revitalize our essential meaning, which makes human existence possible and peace attainable.

Other keynote speakers included Irvin Yalom, Ernesto Spinelli, and Jeffrey Zeig, who provided profound insights on the important role of meaning, authenticity, and courage in psychotherapy. Sheila McNamee focused on the relational and conversational sources that sustain the process of making meaning. Sheldon Solomon presented his terror management theory as the framework for imbuing the world with meaning and permanence. The positive psychology symposium with C. R. Snyder, E. C. Chang, and C. G. Davis was almost prophetic in framing hope and meaning within the confines of uncertainty and loss—a theme that was later elaborated in the Third Meaning Conference. Muriel James focused on the importance of courage and "the defiant power of the human spirit" in our efforts to discover and create happiness in cruel situations.

Many attendees left the Conference feeling excited about the potential of living a more meaningful and purposeful life in spite of circumstances. Some felt challenged about the need to humanize an increasingly materialistic, competitive, and digital society. The future lies in the discovery and creation of meaning as the basis for survival and resilience. Whenever meaning becomes people's primary concern, their interest in pursuing happiness takes the back seat.

ACTING OUT PERSONAL RESPONSIBILITY

The second stage is to awaken a sense of responsibility in people and empower them to act out their responsibility in every situation. Freedom of choice implies responsibility and accountability. Frankl (1986) has repeatedly stressed that we should not ask what we can get from life, but what life demands of us. Authentic happiness is possible, only when our capacity of freedom is employed to make responsible decisions—decisions that are dictated by our consciences, beliefs, core values, and our best understanding of each situation and life as a whole. We can always retain our attitudinal freedom, even when other freedoms are taken away from us; therefore, we are always responsible and accountable for how we live. The courage to be authentic in every situation and to remain true to our deepest moral convictions endows our lives with singularity and meaning. Therefore, to live meaningfully is to live responsibly.

Just one year after our First Meaning Conference, September 11 exploded into our history and public consciousness. This catastrophe was followed by wars in Afghanistan, Iraq, and other parts of world. Suicide bombings and other forms of terrorist attacks continue to loom ominously on the not-too-distant horizon. As if this was not bad enough, high-profile corporate scandals have rocked the financial world like tidal waves in quick succession: Enron, Arthur Anderson, Adelphia, Tyco, ImClone, and WorldCom. What is next? Are we bracing for the next shoe to drop?

The post-9/11 world reminds us every day that all is not well and it challenges us to conquer whatever evil that threatens human existence, whether it is greed, poverty, abuse of power, or rape against nature. At the same time, it challenges us to be courageous and creative to do what is right and responsible. Positive revolution is about correcting what is wrong as much as creating what is right. We need to ask:

How can we bring out the best in people in spite of their limitations and weaknesses? How can we make the best of the worst situations? How can we live purposefully and responsibly, when so many people have either abused or relinquished their freedoms? Responsibility demands a moral response to the cries of the oppressed, the disfranchised, and the suffering. Responsibility demands empathy and compassion. The spirit of an existential-humanistic positive psychology is captured by the prayer of St. Francis of Assisi:

> Lord, make me an instrument of your peace.
> Where there is hatred, let me sow love;
> Where there is injury, pardon;
> Where there is doubt, faith;
> Where there is despair, hope;
> Where there is darkness, light;
> Where there is sadness, joy.

In view of the above, we chose *Freedom, Responsibility, and Justice* as the theme for our Second Meaning Conference (2002). Responsibility is an antidote to selfishness and egotism. To focus on responsibility is to remind people that the second stage in the quest for meaning is their need for relationship and duty to others. Agency without community, like happiness without purpose, is inherently counterproductive, because no one is an island entirely unto oneself. Our lives become more meaningful and the world can become a better place when we live responsibly. We hoped that the conference and the proceedings could partially achieve this goal.

Howard Gardner's keynote address was on the *Good Work Project* developed by him, Mihaly Csikszentmihalyi and William Damon, and described in a book called *Good Work: When Excellence and Ethics Meet*. His main message was that to be good workers in whatever professions, skills are not good enough; we also need to be moral, ethical, and responsible for the social implications of our decisions and actions. A sense of mission and modeling from good mentors can help counteract the corrupting influences of market forces.

Arun Gandhi's keynote lecture on nonviolence struck a responsive cord among a large audience. Growing up under South Africa's apartheid, Arun was the target of bigoted attacks from other youths. He was full of anger and bitterness because of this painful experience of discrimination. When he was 12 years old, his parents sent him to India to learn how to handle his rage from his grandpa, Mahatma Gandhi. Arun's stay with his grandfather happened to coincide with India's struggle to free itself from British rule. Through modeling and mentoring, Mahatma Gandhi taught Arun precious lessons on how to transform anger and violence to understanding, forgiveness, and love. Therefore, Arun emphasized the importance of educating children and adults that nonviolence is a way of life. Contrary to public beliefs, nonviolence is much more than anti-war demonstrations or passive resistance, because "it's all about life and the meaning of life."

Many other distinguished invited speakers approached meaning and responsibility from different perspectives. Ernesto Spinelli offered an existential view of conflict resolution. Jeffrey Zeig elaborated on the Ericksonian perspective of response-ability and serving the Greater Good. Bernard Weiner gave an attribution analysis of responsibility inference and moral perception. Donald Meichenbaum emphasized the constructive narrative perspective in psychotherapy and highlighted the interventions that nurture hope and foster meaning. John Galvin reflected on existential wisdom of accepting fundamental paradoxes as a way to resolve the dilemma of power and responsibility. The symposium on *A New Measure of Character Strengths for Kids* by K. Dahlsgaard, C. Peterson and M. Seligman focused on the use the Values in Action (VIA) for middle-school children as part of the larger project to discover and cultivate character strengths and virtues in children.

Several speakers were funded by the Sir John Templeton Foundation to focus on the integration of spirituality and health. Harold Koenig gave the Distinguished Public Lecture, which examined the relationship between religious involvement and mental health with a focus on meaning and purpose. He discussed how spiritually inspired meaning and purpose were vital for healing and health. Christina Puchalski spoke on the role of spirituality in health and illness, and emphasized the importance of empathy and compassion. Robert Emmons reminded us that the goodness of one's life lies at least partially outside the self, and he presented research findings on the blessings of cultivating gratitude and personal meaning. Salvatore Maddi highlighted the role of hardiness and existential courage in dealing with anger and depression.

More than one hundred presentations covered different aspects of the conference theme. The overall impact of the Second Meaning Conference was an increase of participants' sense of responsibility to society and humanity and provided a wide range of skills and pathways to act out one's responsibility to the various demands of life. We need different strokes for different folks. After the initial awakening and meaning seeking in Stage 1, people need to do the hard work of fulfilling their responsibilities in Stage 2. Peterson and Seligman's VIA (2004) and Wong's seven pathways to meaning (Wong, 1998) provide various signposts and guidelines for people to discover and develop what they are best at and what matters most so that they can realize their potential and responsibility.

WORKING THROUGH THE POWER OF MEANING

The third stage of positive revolution is working through the transformative power of meaning in difficult situations. The overarching concept of logotherapy (Frankl, 1986) is the optimistic view that meaning can be discovered in the worst of circumstances and that a meaningful future can be built from the rubble of the past. The theme of the third Meaning Conference was: *Transforming Suffering, Loss, and Death through Meaning, Hope, and Faith*. This theme alone makes it clear what an existential positive psychology (Wong, 2009) is all about—it focuses on the human potential for growth and self-transcendence in the midst of existential givens of losses and sufferings. Meaning offers people both an effective protection against the relentless assaults of tragedies and the effective tools to transform sufferings into blessings. In this conference, the focus of positive revolution was shifted from meaning seeking (Stage 1), meaning making, and social responsibility (Stage 2) towards meaning reconstruction and transcendental connections in various boundary situations (Stage 3).

Alfried Längle gave a lecture on the life and work of Viktor Frankl, who embodies the truth that one can realize meaning in the worst circumstances. My presidential address was on *Tragic Optimism in the Midst of Suffering*, which extended Frankl's logotherapy. I provided both a theoretical analysis and empirical evidence on the benefits of a meaning-based and spiritually oriented hope that can survive any kind of adversity. Dan P. McAdams in his keynote address presented both theory and data on the themes of redemption in American life stories, such as religious conversion, spiritual awakening, personal enlightenment, and actualization. These narrative themes reflect the cultural belief in American life that all suffering can indeed be redeemed because of God's special spiritual blessings.

Many other speakers approached the topic of suffering from a variety of cultural lenses. Phil Zylla wrestled with the problem of suffering and articulated the idea of "the God who suffers with us." He presented a Christian theology of suffering that incorporated Dorothee Soelle's concept of lamentation, Henri Nouwen's idea of compassion, and Gutierrez' "spirituality of suffering." Sameet Kumar focused on Buddhist mindful meditation. Koken Otani provided a Buddhist perspective on how to transcend the four inevitable sufferings (birth, aging, illness, and death) through enlightenment and acts of compassion. Chieh-Fang Chi and Heui-min Wu presented the rationale and findings on programs that teach students at all levels of education about the importance of meaning and spirituality; these programs and activities are designed to enhance an appreciation of life and discourage teenage suicide. Nancy Reeves lectured on the spiritual tools for grief therapy.

Two noteworthy keynote addresses funded by the Sir John Templeton Foundation were given by Harold G. Koenig and George F. R. Ellis. Koenig lectured on finding purpose, meaning, and hope in the midst of suffering. He reviewed medical research that examined the well-being, joy, meaning, and purpose among patients with chronic health problems. He also presented a theoretical model to explain how religious faith can positively influence well-being and hope in severe illnesses. George Ellis approached the topic of hope and faith in suffering from an interdisciplinary perspective. Recognizing the inherent limitations of science, and drawing from the South African experience of reconciliation, Dr. Ellis outlined various steps, including forgiveness and kenosis, as the basis of hope for transformation. These steps can generate positive affects in suffering, because they have the capacity to alter the context of action and meaning. There is scope for using suffering towards transformation, even in desperate situations involving military action, provided it is of a highly disciplined kind.

There were also numerous presentations, symposia, and workshops that covered the entire gamut of positive psychology. These included Solomon Katz' scientific studies of spiritual transformation, Richard Tedeschi's posttraumatic growth, Alex Pattakos' meaning of work, William Smythe's mythological perspectives of death and dying, Adrian Tomer's intrinsic religiosity in death attitudes, Alan Pope's research on personal transformation in the loss of parents, and Firestone's approach to creating a life of meaning and compassion.

CONCLUSION

The trilogy of the first three Meaning Conferences presents a good picture of the three stages of positive revolution needed for personal and societal transformation. These stages provide a theoretical framework for positive psychology for research and interventions. Although we can only include a representative sample of the hundreds of presentations during these conferences in this volume, readers can still get some idea of the richness and vitality of a meaning-centered positive psychology.

References

Frankl, V. E. (1986). *The doctor and the soul: From psychotherapy to logotherapy*. New York: Random House, Inc.

Gardner, H., Csikszentmihalyi, M., & Damon, W. (2004). *Good work: When excellence and ethics meet*. Portland, OR: Perseus Books Group.

Peterson, C. (2004). *A primer in positive psychology*. New York: Oxford University Press.

Peterson, C., & Seligman, M. E. P. (2004). *Character Strengths and Virtues: A Handbook and Classification*. New York: Oxford University Press.

Schumaker, J. F. (2007). *In search of happiness: Understanding an endangered state of mind*. Westport, CT: Praeger Publishers.

Wong, P. T. P. (1998). Implicit theories of meaningful life and the development of the Personal Meaning Profile. In P. T. P. Wong & P. S. Fry (Eds.), *The human quest for meaning: A handbook of psychological research and clinical applications*. Mahwah, NJ: Lawrence Erlbaum Associates, Inc.

Wong, P. T. P. (2009). Existential positive psychology: Six fundamental questions about human existence. In S. Lopez (Ed.), *Encyclopedia of positive psychology*. Malden, MA: Blackwell Publishing.

PART ONE

MEANING, SPIRITUALITY, & RELIGIOSITY

The Meaning of Meaning

JORDAN B. PETERSON

Abstract

The world is too complex to manage without radical functional simplification. Meaning appears to exist as the basis for such simplification. The meaning that guides functional simplification may be usefully considered as consisting of three classes. The first class consists of meanings of the determinate world. These are meanings based in motivation, emotion, and personal and social identity. First-class meanings are grounded in instinct and tend, at their most abstract, towards the dogmatic or ideological. The second class consists of meanings of the indeterminate world. These are meanings based on the emergence of anomaly, or ignored complexity. Second-class meanings are also instinctively grounded, but tend towards the revolutionary. The third class consists of meanings of the conjunction between the determinate and indeterminate worlds. These are meanings that emerge first as a consequence of voluntary engagement in exploratory activity and second as a consequence of identifying with the process of voluntary exploration. Third-class meanings find their abstracted representation in ritual and myth, and tend towards the spiritual or religious.

"*Determinate*: Having defined limits; not uncertain or arbitrary; fixed; established; definite" (Merriam-Webster's Collegiate Dictionary, 2003).

The world is too complex to be represented and acted upon without radical functional simplification (Brooks, 1991a, 1991b; Gigerenzer & Goldstein, 1996; Hacking, 1999; Medin & Aguilar, 1999; Simon, 1956). The manner in which human beings manage this complexity is the subject of much debate. It appears that what we experience as meaning allows for such simplification and that meaning

11

ensures that such simplification does not transform itself into inflexible and dangerous stasis. Meaning is a very complex phenomenon, however, even when provisionally defined as an aid to simplification. It therefore appears conceptually useful to consider its manifestation in three broad classes.

The first class of meanings constitutes the mechanism for the establishment of the most basic, universal forms of functional simplifications, commonly regarded as motivations. This class, meanings of the determinate world, includes meanings of emotion, role, and social identity, in addition to motivation. The second class of meanings constitutes the mechanism for the exploration and identification of those aspects of the environment that constantly arise to challenge the integrity of current functional simplifications or determinate worlds. This class, meanings of the indeterminate world, includes the meanings of anomaly or novelty. The third class of meanings constitutes the mechanism for establishing and representing the integrated interaction of the first two classes. This class may be regarded as meanings of the conjunction between determinate and indeterminate worlds. It includes the meanings that arise in the course of exploratory behavior and in the ritualization and subsequent representation of such behavior. Consideration of all three classes provides a portrait of meaning that is simultaneously comprehensive and differentiated.

CLASS 1: MEANINGS OF THE DETERMINATE WORLD
Motivation as the First-Order Solution to the Problems of Self-Maintenance, Self-Propagation, and Complexity

We must survive and propagate in a world whose complexity exceeds our representational and functional capacity. Motivation serves to initially address these problems. A given determinate world is engendered as a consequence of emergent insufficiency, along a basic motivational dimension. The emergence of a particular motivation induces a state of radical world-simplification. Someone deprived of sexual contact, for example, increasingly treats the environment as a place where intimacy might be sought, where lack of sexual gratification constitutes the undesirable beginning state, and physical satiation the desired end state (Gray, 1982; Panksepp, 1999; Rolls, 1999). The motivational significance of beginning-and-end states appears as something primarily given by biology, or secondarily and rapidly derived from biology through learning. We confront the environment, innately, with loneliness, playfulness, hunger, thirst, and sexual yearning (Panksepp, 1999)—even with the desire for a good story. We develop extensive modifications of such concrete beginning and end states through direct learning and abstraction. We will work spontaneously to increase wealth, to take a general example, after coming to understand the polyvalent nature of money.

Motivation does not drive behavior in a deterministic manner. Nor does it simply set goals. A state of motivation is instead an axiom or a predicate of experience; it is something that provides a delimited frame for perception, emotion, cognition, and action (Barsalou, 1983). Motivation provides the current state of being with boundaries and values, which remain unquestioned as long as current action produces its desired ends. These bounded states can be usefully regarded as determinate micro-worlds of experience.

Such determinate worlds are manifold in number, as there are qualitatively different states of motivation, such as hunger, thirst, or lust (Rolls, 1999), and manifest themselves singly and sequentially, as processes of perception, emotion, cognition, and action must be directed towards specified and limited targets (Miller, 1956; Cowan, 2001). Each determinate world contains particularized conceptualizations of the current state of affairs and the desired end, which serve as necessary contrast and target points for the extraction of percepts, the specification of objects of abstract thought, the affect-laden evaluation of ongoing world events, and the selection of motor procedures. Currently functional determinate worlds are productive, predictable, and secure, composed, as they are, of previously encountered, explored, and familiar phenomena.

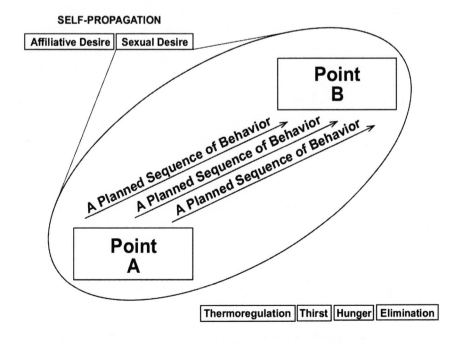

Figure 1. The grounding of a determinate world in motivation

The blueprint of a simple motivation-dependent determinate world is schematically portrayed in Figure 1. This world consists firstly of conceptualizations relevant to the movement from point A, the undesired beginning state, to point B, the desired end state, and secondly of specific motor patterns designed to bring about that movement (Carver & Scheier, 1998). Figure 1 also presents the structural elements of the simplest narrative or story (Peterson, 1999a): I was here, and I went there (by certain means). This simple or normal story (Kuhn, 1970) is akin to the necessary fiction of Vaihinger (1924) and Adler (Ansbacher & Ansbacher, 1956), to the Dasein of the phenomenologists (Binswanger, 1963; Boss, 1963), to the expectancy schema of the behaving animal (Gray, 1982), and to the life space/field of Lewin (1935). Individuals operating within the confines of a given story move from present to future, in a linear track. Two points define such a track. A present position cannot be defined without a point of future contrast. Likewise, a potential future cannot be evaluated (judged affectively as better) except in terms of a present position.

The construction of a simplified determinate world also establishes the functional domain for object perception (Gibson, 1977). The perception of objects is, after all, complicated by the problem of level of resolution: the dividing line between a situation, an object, and the subcomponents that make up that object is far from simply given (Barsalou, 1983; Brooks, 1991a, 1991b). Human beings appear to be low-capacity processors, so to speak, with an apprehension capacity of less than seven objects (Cowan, 2001; Miller, 1956). So it seems that our working memory works in concert with our motivational systems: a good goal requires consideration of no more things than we can track. Perhaps it is in this manner that we determine when to deconstruct a task into subgoals—all goals are motivated; all reasonable goals are cognitively manageable. Figure 1, portraying the frame for emotional response and action, also, therefore, portrays the most basic schema for object and event recognition.

Emotion as a Solution to the Problem of Motivation

Motivations constitute a basic set of solutions to the basic-level problems of human existence. Unfortunately, solutions to problems frequently generate their own problems. The construction of a simplified determinate world helps specify what ends action should pursue, and what phenomena might be considered as objects in that pursuit (Hacking, 1999; Lakoff, 1987; Tranel, Logan, Frank & Damasio, 1997; Wittgenstein, 1968). Action implies trajectory, however, and movement along a trajectory means the action-dependent transformation of experience (as the absolute point of action is to produce desired transformations of experience). Experiential changes produced in consequence of goal-directed maneuvering necessarily have implications for goal attainment—but not only those implications expected or desired. It is the evaluation of implications, including unexpected implications, that constitutes the function of emotion. Emotion might therefore be regarded as a process devoted towards the real-time maintenance of motivation-simplified worlds; it might be regarded as a marker indicating whether the journey to a specified target is proceeding properly or improperly (Oatley & Johnson-Laird, 1987; Oatley, 1999).

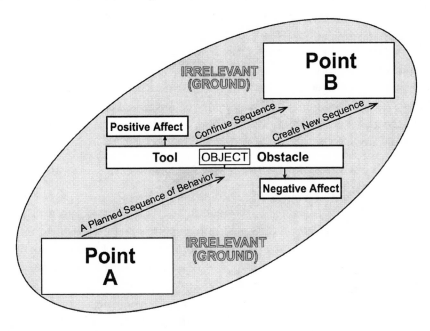

Figure 2. The real-time evaluative role played by emotions

Figure 2 provides a schematic representation of the role played by emotions. Emotional relevance appears as something essentially two-dimensional, in contrast to the multiple domains of motivation. This two-dimensional structure manifests itself because events that occur within determinate worlds have the essential nature of affordances (Gibson, 1977) or obstacles, rather than "objects." Affordances can be utilized to increase the likelihood that a desired end-state might be reached, or to decrease the time-interval until that end-state's manifestation. Obstacles have the reverse nature. Affordances and obstacles can be abstract, as well as concrete. A concrete affordance is a tool. An abstract affordance is a cue that an end-state is likely to manifest itself in the desired manner—a smile, for example, from an attractive individual—while an abstract obstacle is a cue that something has gone wrong.

Affordances are positively valenced—the first dimension of emotion—as they indicate (a) that progress is occurring, and (b) that the structural integrity of the currently operative motivation world may be considered intact. The predictable appearance of affordances is therefore experienced as self-verifying (at least with regards to the delimited aspect of the self currently serving as a motivation-world). Obstacles are, by contrast, negatively valenced (the second emotional dimension), as they indicate that progress has been halted or is in danger. More importantly, they suggest that the current determinate world may not be functional. It is less disruptive to encounter an obstacle that merely requires the switching of means than it is to encounter an obstacle that invalidates a motivation-world, as such. This means that emotional significance may be usefully considered in its within- and between-world variant forms (Peterson, 1999a). This is an observation with important implications for the meanings of identity.

Identity as a Solution to the Problems of Motivation and Emotion

I am capable of second-order representation, so I know that I will desire companionship, and shelter, and sustenance, and exploratory engagement, so I conjure up a determinate world where I can work to obtain tokens that may be exchanged for such things. The pursuit of those tokens then becomes something meaningful. And I conjure up such an abstracted, delimited space to keep my basic motivational states regulated, and act cautiously so that I do not accidentally fall under the domination of negative emotion. And so one might say that a third form of determinate-world meaning can be identified—one that is much closer to abstract conceptualization and to social being than to basic motivation or emotion. I have a stake in the maintenance of my determinate worlds, regardless of their particular content. They take time, energy, and courage to construct, and are therefore valuable. They simplify the world and hold its complexity in check. They suit my needs and regulate my emotions. I am emotionally attached to them. I identify with them. So personal identity is, in its simplest form, the acceptance of a given motivation world as a valid aspect of the self.

More complexly, however, identity constitutes a solution to the problem of organization posed by the diverse motivational aspects of lower-order meaning. First is the issue of sequencing: in what order should particular motivation-worlds be allowed to manifest themselves, in the course of a given day, or week, or year? Second is the closely related issue of hierarchical import: what motivational worlds should be granted priority of value? When I am faced with a conflict between affiliation and productivity, for example, which do I choose? This problem is, of course, rendered far more complex by the fact of social being. The others who surround me are also rank ordering their values hierarchically and implementing their motivational worlds, while constantly exchanging motivational and emotional information with one another. The structure of my identity is therefore determined not only by my own motivations and emotions (and my decisions with regards to their relative rank) but by the fact that all others are making analogous decisions. That means that personal identity shades into the social; it means that personal and social identity is the emergent and even "unconscious" (i.e., automatic and unplanned) consequence of the cooperative/competitive establishment, sequencing and rank ordering of determinate worlds. So, the third form of meaning tends towards identity in the personal guise and ideology in the social, as specific modes of being are integrated under the rubric of general ritual and abstract conception, at levels of order that transcend the individual (Peterson, 1999a).

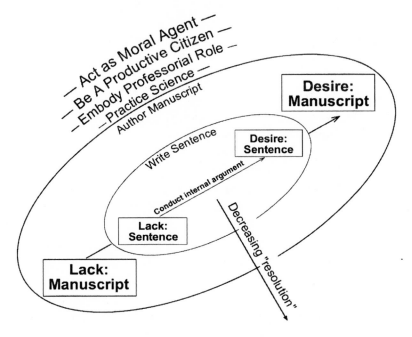

Figure 3. Identity as the sequencing and rank ordering of determinate worlds.

Figure 3 schematically portrays a representation of identity, which constitutes the organization of motivational and emotional states. At the highest level of resolution, identity consists of the motor patterns that constitute a given behavior ("write sentence," in the current example) and the perceptions, cognitions and emotions that are relevant to that behavior. At lower levels of resolution (or higher levels of abstraction), behaviors are organized into functional and theoretically homogeneous groupings, which may reasonably be considered classes. High-resolution levels of behavioral operation constitute sub-elements of low-resolution conceptualizations (Carver & Scheier, 1998; Powers, 1973) and are governed (i.e., sequenced, hierarchically rank-ordered, and evaluated) in consequence of their relevance as affordances, obstacles or irrelevances, construed in relation to those lower-resolution conceptualizations. So I write a sentence, and attend to the specific topic of that sentence while doing so. Then I decide where that sentence should be placed, calculate its comparative importance, and evaluate it for quality—but I do this by switching to the lower-resolution determinate world "author manuscript" and use that world as the frame for my decisions. In turn, I consider "authoring manuscripts" as a subelement of the determinate world "practice science," and so on, up the hierarchy of abstraction from the purely personal to the shared social (Peterson, 1999a).

CLASS 2: MEANINGS OF THE INDETERMINATE WORLD
Anomaly as a Consequence of the Insufficiency of Determinate Motivation Worlds

Personal identities and social roles, unfortunately, also are characterized by emergent insufficiencies. The most serious of these might be regarded as the problem of the dead past. The environment is entropic, while tradition is static (hence "the state"). The sequenced and hierarchically arranged determinate worlds generated by those who inhabited the past may, therefore, become inadequate because of the dynamic transformations that constitute the present. This is the problem of constraint by the world—it is the problem not of matter, but of what matters, the problem not of the object, but of what objects (see Norretranders, 1998). The environment is complex beyond comprehension, yet I must act on it. So I simplify it, in a functional manner (relying on motivation and tradition) but its complexity still emerges when I least expect it. Such emergent complexity manifests itself uncontrollably in numerous ways: as flood, war, illness, new technology, new belief, or ideology (Peterson, 1999a). This means that world delimitation may solve a particular problem, but can never provide a solution to the more general "problem of problems"—the ineradicable emergent complexity of the world. This implies, as well, that tradition can never satisfy, in any final sense. Too much human vulnerability necessarily remains present. This is true regardless of the content of tradition (lawyer versus doctor or Muslim versus Jew) or its existence as personal role or social identity (Peterson, 1999b).

This all means that meaning is the significance of our determinate worlds, the implication of the events that occur during the enaction of those worlds, and the sequenced and hierarchical structures that we use to organize motivation and emotion psychologically and socially. This explication is relatively comprehensive but still fails to deal with a whole complex class of meaningful phenomena. Determinate positive and negative events occur as the world unfolds in the course of goal-directed activity. Irrelevant things occur, too, of course, but they are in some important sense never realized (as you cannot pay attention to all activity, but only to all relevant activity). But what does one make of anomalous events? Some occurrences are neither good nor bad—nor immediately eradicable as meaningless. These are generally occurrences that are not understood, not explored, and cannot be placed into the context of the current motivational world. What can be done in such cases? What is not comprehended but is still undeniably extant must logically be experienced as paradoxical (Jung, 1967, 1968; Gray, 1982; Peterson, 1999a): negative, in potential, and positive, in potential, and irrelevant, in potential (and self and world in potential, as well).

There is something even deeper and more mysterious about the anomalous event. At some point in the process of psychological development, however hypothetically localized that point must be, all events are anomalous. That implies that the construction of forms of reference that allow for the determinate classification and utilization of objects, situations, and abstractions is something dependent on the extraction of information from the overarching and ever-emerging domain of the anomalous. It is for all these reasons that the anomalous must be regarded as meaningful, a priori, and that the meaningful anomaly might well be regarded as the ground of determinate being itself.

Figure 4a and 4b schematically portray class 2 meaning, associated with the emergence of world complexity or anomaly, of the "within" and "between" determinate-world types. Figure 4a portrays the consequences of emergent anomaly, rapidly adjudicated as nonrevolutionary (i.e., the encounter with something unexpected, in the course of goal-directed activity, within the context of a given determinate world). An anomalous occurrence is not initially an object (an affordance or obstacle). It is, instead, the re-emergence of ignored ground. As such, it first produces an undifferentiated state of affect, weighted in most cases towards the negative—as caution is an intelligent default response to evidence of error (Dollard & Miller, 1950; Gray, 1982). A within-determinate-world anomaly is something that can be merely circumvented, however, without eradicating the protective and simplifying structure of that world. If you are accustomed to walking down a hallway to an elevator, a carelessly placed chair in the middle of that hallway would constitute such an anomaly. You can still get to the elevator, but you have to step around the chair. Such a situation will produce a brief flurry of indiscriminate affect, immediately quelled by classification ("misplaced chair") and appropriate action. This is process within normal limits.

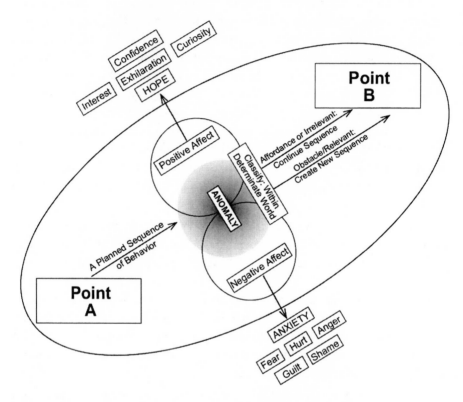

Figure 4a. Emergence of within-determinate-world complexity

Insofar as the goals of current behavior remain unchallenged, the means may switch repetitively without undue alarm. If a dozen plans fail to reach a given goal, however, the functional integrity of the determinate world itself becomes questionable. This questioning process may occur because of the emergence of "anxiety," "frustration," "disappointment," or "anger" as a consequence of repeated failure. Under such conditions, it becomes reasonable to rethink the whole story—the current determinate world. Perhaps where you are is not as bad as you think; alternatively, another somewhere else might be better. This process of more dramatic error-driven reconsideration and categorical reconstruction is portrayed in Figure 4b.

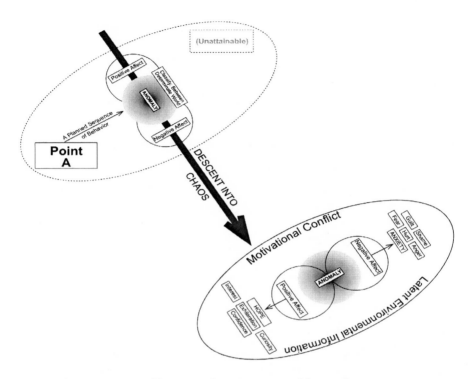

Figure 4b. Emergence of between-determinate-world complexity

Figure 4b portrays the consequences of anomaly resistant to categorization within the confines of the current determinate world. This situation arises when a problem that cannot be easily solved makes itself manifest. You have a career, for example, as a typesetter. But new technology makes your skills obsolete. Experience can no longer be properly constrained by your habitual role. This means that you must construct a new determinate world—even a different hierarchy—to deal with the new situation. Such construction does not occur, however, without energy (Roland, Erikson, Stone-Elander & Widen, 1987) and without cost (the cost is signaled by the emergence of negative affect). Reconstrual of the environment is substantively difficult. What should be done, when one's livelihood disappears? What should be felt? What should be perceived? In the interim, before such things are specified, experience consists of a descent into chaos—the no-man's land between decisions. This frequently hellish place is ruled by conflicting motivations. Basic regulatory systems strive to obtain dominance over and bring order to the currently dysregulated world. Emotions compete to guide behavior: anger, fear, guilt, hurt, or even exhilaration, if the disrupted world was ambivalent in value (e.g., perhaps you did not like your job). More complexly, new information reveals itself as a consequence of the eradication of the limits placed on perception by the now-disrupted determinate world. Perhaps you are hurt beyond tolerance by your invalidation. Perhaps you learn a valuable lesson. The information that makes such learning possible is in the same "between-decision" domain as the emotional and motivational chaos attendant upon failure (Jung, 1952, 1967, 1968; Peterson, 1999a).

Orienting and Exploration as a Solution to the Problem of Anomaly

We know that whatever exists is more complicated than whatever is specified by our current determinate world. We know that we must perform radical simplifications of the world, in order to operate in it. This means that whatever exists might be regarded as the sum of all we assume, plus all that is left over. This implies that "all that is left over" may constantly present itself as something with the capacity to "correct" the insufficiencies of our current simplified but situationally functional stance. Then the question immediately arises: What is the consequence of the emergence of such corrective information? Here might be proposed a radical answer: It is the direct revelation of meaning (Binswanger, 1963; Boss, 1963). This implies that the world, as it truly exists, reveals itself as paradoxical meaning, long before it reveals itself as determinate significance, as irrelevance, or even as object or fact (because something is novel long before it becomes a recognizable object and the construction of fact requires the active participation of other people).

It is something fascinating to note that the facts themselves appear in concordance with this pragmatic inversion of materialist reality. Let us take, for example, the processes underlying a diverse range of animated activities—animal as well as human. It is an accepted axiom of neo-psychoanalytic (Adler, in Ansbacher & Ansbacher, 1956; Jung, 1952), cybernetic (Weiner, 1948), behavioral (Gray, 1982), cognitive (Miller, Galanter & Pribram, 1960), psychobiological (Panksepp, 1999), narrative (Bruner, 1986) and social-psychological (Carver & Scheier, 1998) theories that human behavior is goal-directed, rather than simply driven. Let us start with an attempt to integrate the well-defined animal-experimental/behavioral formulations of Jeffrey Gray (1982), Jaak Panksepp (1999), and Edmund Rolls (1999).

These modern behaviorists speak the operational, empirical language of stimulus and reinforcement. When such a researcher refers to broadly positive emotional states, for example, he/she says "consummatory" or "incentive reward." In general, the experience of such states will produce an increase in the future likelihood of immediately preceding behaviors. Consummatory reward, specifically, means occurrences that will bring the current determinate world to a satisfied end. Incentive reward means occurrences. Incentive reward, specifically, signals or cues consummatory reward. When a modern behaviorist refers to negative emotional states, by contrast, he says "punishment" or "threat." In general, the experience of such states will produce a reduction in the future likelihood of immediately preceding behaviors. Punishment, specifically, means occurrences that will produce angry, depressive, or flight-oriented responses. Threat, specifically, signals or cues punishment.

Why is all this relevant? Well, consummatory and incentive rewards have meaning—"repeat preceding behavior" or "continue on the same (potentially) productive path"—experienced as affect. That affect is somnolent pleasure and the momentary lessening of general motivation, in the case of consummatory reward, and hope, curiosity, excitement, and interest, in the case of incentive reward. Punishment and threat have opposite meaning—"do not repeat preceding behavior" or "discontinue movement on this counterproductive trajectory"—also experienced as affect. That affect is hurt (disappointment, frustration, anger, pain), in the case of punishment; anxiety (fear, worry, concern), in the case of threat. And it should be stressed that such meaning is not only relevant for behavior, but for entire determinate worlds. Such worlds are supported (reinforced) by their success and eradicated, or at least threatened, by their failure, even when that success or failure is something only imagined.

Once again, what does one make of anomaly? A meaningful goal-directed schema is established, serving to specify the objects of apprehension and the motor-programs matched to those objects. A goal-relevant world of comprehensible simplicity emerges, accompanied by procedures known to be effective in that world. Everything irrelevant to that domain of concern is ignored (i.e., virtually everything). When the plan is a good plan the desired end is obtained—but nothing novel is learned. It is because things are learned only when desired ends are not obtained that error, signaling anomaly, serves as the mother of all things.

The appearance of the informative anomalous produces its own determinate world, manifested as the orienting complex (Gray, 1982; Halgren, 1992; Halgren, Squires, Wilson, Rohrbaugh, Babb & Crandell, 1980; Ohman, 1979, 1987; Sokolov, 1969; Vinogradova, 1961, 1975). The beginning point of that world constitutes the insufficiency of present knowledge, and the desired end point the functional classification of the presently anomalous emergent phenomenon. Anomaly draws attention inexorably to itself, so that increased intensity of sensory processing and increased exploratory activity may be brought to bear upon it. Such processing and exploration means examination of the anomalous from the perspective of various alternative determinate worlds (Is it relevant to another motivational state?) and from various emotional perspectives (Can it serve as an affordance or obstacle? Can it be classified into the same domain as other irrelevant "objects," and regarded as ground?). This process of effortful classification constitutes (a) the elimination of possibility from the infinite, indeterminate domain of the anomalous to the finite domain of a determinate world; (b) the reworking of identity, which is the sum total of all such determinate worlds; and (c) the process by which identity originally comes to be, in the course of spontaneous exploratory activity (Peterson, 1999a). The determinate world that guides anomaly exploration has as its end-point the promise or potential of the unknown, which has more the nature of an incentive (Gray, 1982), than a consummatory reward (as promise is a cue for consummation, rather than its object). So it might be said that the exploratory spirit is something under the control of incentive, serving a consummatory function. This is in keeping with the more abstract "need" of curiosity.

CLASS 3: MEANINGS OF THE CONJUNCTION BETWEEN THE DETERMINATE AND INDETERMINATE WORLDS
Metaidentity as a Solution to the Problem of Identity

Now, just as the meaning that creates the determinate world guiding exploration is more abstract than the meaning that constitutes primary motivation, so the identity that incorporates the exploratory spirit is more abstract than the primary identity organizing basic-level motivation. Meanings of primary identity are solutions to the problems that emerge as a consequence of operation within the determinate worlds of motivation and emotion. Individual roles and beliefs, merged through ritual or ideological means into social identities, regulate the intrinsic meanings of life, bringing intrapsychic and social order to the conflict-laden chaos of need and want. Members of identifiable groups become predictable to themselves and others by sharing a hierarchy of determinate motivation-worlds. This predictability, this cooperative reduction to ground, is a great cognitive and emotional relief. It remains, however, eminently vulnerable. All roles and ideologies, no matter their level of sophistication, can be undermined by emergent complexity. We, therefore, gerrymander specific solutions in the manner of engineers and strive to maintain our identities—but these are not, and never can be, complete. This means that a third class of meaning must emerge, to address the metaproblem of emergent complexity. This third class manifests itself directly in two situations and indirectly as a form of metanarrative when its situation-specific processes attain symbolic embodiment and representation.

Class 3 meanings arise first when a determinate world has been rendered invalid, as a consequence of the emergence of some troublesome anomaly. The anomaly initially manifests itself experientially, in the guise of a war of motivations and emotions—emotions that are primarily negative (for defensive reasons) in the immediate aftermath of task failure (Dollard & Miller, 1950). But anomaly does not only signify failure. Equally, it signifies possibility, as the manifestation of the previously unrevealed complexity of the world. This complexity may be transformed, may be utilized as an affordance or as a means of reconstructing failed determinate worlds. The very act of harnessing emergent possibility is meaningful.

Class 3 meanings arise, as well, in the case of full satiation, where all basic-level states of motivation have met their consummatory destiny and, therefore, have temporarily ceased to dominate the determinate world of experience. This second situation arises because the metaproblem of the possible problem still lurks ineradicably when full satiation has been reached and because exploration constitutes the only possible solution to that metaproblem. Immersion in exploration, undertaken for playful, curious and fantasy-driven reasons, also constitutes a higher-order encounter with meaning.

Simple determinate worlds find their communicable expression in the simplest story: "I was here and that was insufficient, so I went there." Description of the vicissitudes encountered in the course of such a journey adds interest to the basic plot (Oatley & Johnson-Laird, 1987; Oatley, 1999). Complex characters, pursuing many simple stories, represent hierarchically structured identities. But the most complex and fascinating story is a metanarrative: a story that describes the process that transforms stories (Jung, 1952; Neumann, 1954; Peterson, 1999a). It is identification with this process of story transformation that constitutes metaidentity, predicated upon recognition that the human spirit constructs, destroys, and rejuvenates its worlds, as well as merely inhabiting them. Such identification constitutes the most fully developed revelation of class 3 meaning.

Figure 5 portrays the process of voluntary determinate world eradication and exploration-predicated reconstruction. This transformational process is both perilous and enriching. It is perilous because descent into the motivational and emotional chaos extant between determinate worlds is stressful, in the truest sense of the word. It is enriching because unexplored anomaly contains information whose incorporation may increase the functional utility or the very nature of one or more determinate worlds. This makes involvement in the process of transformation a "metasolution" (a solution to the problem of problems). It appears, at least in principle, that this metasolution constitutes a capstone of emergent meaning—a true capstone, beyond which no further emergence of solution is necessary. The complex structure of this solution has remained, to this day, essentially implicit in mythology as abstracted and compelling drama and may be acted out usefully and productively in the absence of explicit understanding. Its implicit existence is the consequence of the imitation and dramatic abstraction of the ideal, i.e., the consequence of admiring, distilling the reasons for admiration, and portraying those reasons in ever-more potent ritual and literary forms, in a process of highly functional fantasy spanning generations (Peterson, 1999a).

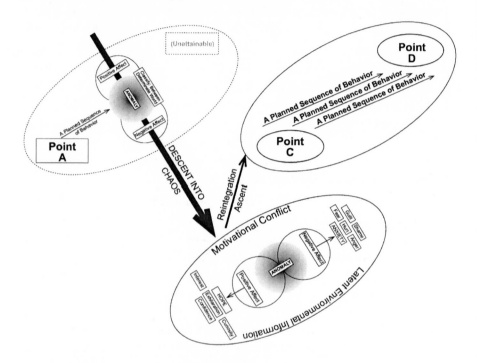

Figure 5. Metaidentity, or the transformation of determinate worlds.

Figure 5 has the structure classically identified as central to complex narrative: steady state, breach, crisis, and redress (Bruner, 1986; Jung, 1952; Eliade, 1965), or, metaphorically, paradise, encounter with chaos, fall, and redemption (Peterson, 1999a). This third complex class of meaning is dramatic in its means of representation, and religious in its phenomenology. Direct religious experience appears equivalent to immersion in the meanings driving exploratory activity, as has been described by Rudolf Otto (1958) as a paradoxical combination of *mysterium fascinans* and *mysterium tremendum* (awe and terror in the face of the absolute unknown). Dramatic representation of this transformative process, presented "unconsciously" as an aid to mimicry, takes the form of hero mythology. Such mythology is the abstracted portrayal of courageous approach to anomaly, investigation of its properties, functional categorization, and recategorization as a consequence of that investigation, and subsequent communication of the results to the social world.

Although such dramatic representation is abstract, and is communicated symbolically, it is not entirely explicit, and remains embedded in the patterns of myth and literature. We are motivated, and know we are motivated, so we can represent and understand the state of motivation. Likewise, we are emotional, and can represent the state of emotion. We are novelty processors, no less universally, but do not completely understand this ability, nor explicitly appreciate its absolutely central place in our adaptive striving. It is a remarkable and telling fact that such appreciation has emerged, nonetheless, in an implicit fashion, and is headed up the hierarchy of abstract representation (Peterson, 1999a). Here we will take a detour into grounds that are richly meaningful in the third-class sense and provide a psychological interpretation for phenomena that have as of yet remained opaque to the searching eye of science.

If a phenomenon is truly universal, it should pick up abstracted representation over time, just as the constituent elements of personality have become encapsulated in the languages of the world (Goldberg, 1992). But the processes that make up class 3 meaning are complex and dynamic—more like "procedures," "contexts," or "situations," than things—and cannot easily be named. So they have not precisely garnered lexical representation. Instead, they have been represented dramatically, as characters immersed in plots (Peterson, 1999a). The basic character is the hero; the basic plot is confrontation with the unknown, and the subsequent creation or reconstitution of the ever-threatened determinate world of experience. The creator of culture (i.e., the creator of the personal and social identity that regulates object perception, abstract thinking, motivation, and emotion) is the individual who voluntarily faces the unknown and carves it into useful categories.

The ancient Sumerian arch-deity Marduk, for example, voluntarily faces Tiamat, the abysmal monster of chaos and mother of all being. This voluntary encounter enables Marduk to create "ingenious things" in consequence (Heidel, 1965; p. 58, 7:112-115), and to serve as the creator of the habitable world of man. Mircea Eliade states, with regards to such stories:

> It is by the slaying of an ophidian monster—symbol of the virtual,
> of "chaos," but also of the autochthonous—that a new cosmic or
> institutional "situation" comes into existence. A characteristic feature,
> and one common to all these myths, is the fright or a first defeat of
> the champion.... (1978a, p. 205)

The courageous capacity embodied by Marduk was also the process upon which functional reconstruction of traditional categories and habits rested (Peterson, 1999a; 1999b), according to the Sumerians. As *Namtillaku*, Marduk was the god who restored all "ruined gods, as though they were his own creation; [t]he lord who by holy incantation restore[d] the dead gods to life" (Heidel, 1965; p. 53, 6:152-6:153). Whatever Marduk represented also served as the ritual model of emulation for the Sumerian emperor and as the very basis for his sovereignty. This all means that the Sumerians implicitly recognized, at the dawn of history, that particular beneficial modes of being (determinate worlds) were dependent for their existence on the general pattern of action incarnated by Marduk (Peterson, 1999a).

In the great Egyptian dynasties similar ideas prevailed. The Egyptian Pharaoh was simultaneously regarded as the force that created truth, justice, and order (*ma'at*) from chaos, and as the immortal embodiment of Horus, who brought his once-great father, founder of Egyptian tradition, back from the dead (Eliade, 1978a). Similar patterns of narrative ideation necessarily underlie religious traditions of diverse origins, as the social regulation of determinate worlds drives individuals to universally embody and then to dramatize adaptive forms. A few examples include: the collapse of Buddha's protected childhood existence, attendant on his discovery of mortality, and his rebirth, illumination, and return to the community; Moses' exodus from tyranny, his descent through the water into the desert, and his subsequent journey to the promised land; Adam and Eve's tempted fall, the profane subsequent existence of mankind, and humanity's eventual redemption by Christ, the second Adam (Jung, 1968; Peterson, 1999a). Figure 5, which describes the archetypal processes of the transformation of category and habit, also schematically portrays the death of the childhood personality, its descent to the underworld, and its reconstruction as an adult, dramatized and facilitated by initiatory ritual (Eliade, 1965; 1985), as well as the hero's voluntary journey into and return from the lair of the treasure-hoarding dragon (Jung, 1952; 1968). Figure 5 also presents a cognitive stage transition (Piaget, 1977), an epiphany, an awakening, and a paradigmatic revolution, in a somewhat broader sense than that originally meant by Kuhn (1970) (Peterson, 1999a).

CONCLUSION

The determinate world of experience, simultaneously internal presupposition and external social construction, constitutes order, security, tyranny, yang, set up against chaos, indeterminacy, unpredictability, danger, possibility, yin. Order is inherently unstable, as the chaos or complexity encapsulated by previous effort continually conspires to re-emerge. New threats and anomalies continually arise, as the natural world ceaselessly changes. These threats may be ignored, in which case they propagate, accumulate, and threaten the integrity of the current mode of being. Alternatively, the unknown may be forthrightly faced, assimilated, and transformed into a beneficial attribute of the renewed world. Upon this

grammatical edifice is erected every narrative, every theory of personality transformation—perhaps every system of truly religious thought (Peterson, 1999a).
Error must be recognized and then eliminated, as a consequence of voluntary
exploration, generation of information, and update or reconstruction of skill and
representation. Things that are bitter, feared, and avoided must be approached and
conquered, or life finds itself increasingly restricted, miserable, and hateful. Our
greatest stories therefore portray the admirable individual, engaged in voluntary,
creative, communicative endeavor; they portray that individual generating a
personality capable of withstanding the fragility of being from such endeavor. We
are thus prepared to find sufficient sustenance in stories portraying the eternal
confrontation with the terrible unknown, and its transformation into the tools
and skills we need to survive. If we act out such stories, within the confines of
our own lives, then the significance of our being may come to overshadow our
weakness. It is in the hope that such a statement might be true that we find the
most profound of the many meanings of meaning.

References

Ansbacher, H. L., & Ansbacher, R. R. (1956). *The individual psychology of Alfred Adler: Selections from his writings.* New York: Harper Torchbooks.

Barsalou, L. W. (1983). Ad hoc categories. *Memory & Cognition, 11*, 211-227.

Binswanger, L. (1963). *Being in the world.* New York: Basic Books.

Boss, M. (1963). *Psychoanalysis and daseinsanalysis.* New York: Basic Books.

Brooks, A. (1991a). Intelligence without reason. *MIT Artificial Intelligence Laboratory: Artificial Intelligence Memo 1293.*

Brooks, A. (1991b). Intelligence without representation. *Artificial Intelligence, 47*, 139-159.

Bruner, J. (1986). *Actual minds, possible worlds.* Cambridge, MA: Harvard University Press.

Carver, C. S., & Scheier, M. F. (1998). *On the self-regulation of behavior.* New York: Cambridge University Press.

Cowan, N. (2001). The magical number 4 in short-term memory: a reconsideration of mental storage capacity. *Brain and Behavioral Sciences, 24*, 87-114.

Dollard, J., & Miller, N. (1950). *Personality and psychotherapy: An analysis in terms of learning, thinking, and culture.* New York: McGraw-Hill.

Eliade, M. (1965). *Rites and symbols of initiation: The mysteries of birth and rebirth* (W. R. Trask, Trans.). New York: Harper and Row.

Eliade, M. (1978a). *A history of religious ideas: Vol. 1. From the stone age to the Eleusinian mysteries.* Chicago: University of Chicago Press.

Eliade, M. (1978b). *The forge and the crucible* (2nd ed., S. Corrin, Trans.). Chicago: University of Chicago Press.

Eliade, M. (1985). *A history of religious ideas: From Mohammed to the age of reforms.* Chicago: University of Chicago Press.

Gibson, J. J. (1977). The theory of affordances. In R. Shaw & J. Bransford (Eds.), *Perceiving, acting and knowing* (pp. 67-82). New York: Wiley.

Gigerenzer, G. & Goldstein, D. G. (1996). Reasoning the fast and frugal way: Models of bounded rationality. *Psychological Review, 103*, 650-669.

Goldberg, L. R. (1992). The development of markers for the big-five factor structure. *Psychological Assessment, 4*, 26-42.

Gray, J. A. (1982). *The neuropsychology of anxiety: An enquiry into the functions of the septo-hippocampal system.* Oxford, U.K.: Oxford University Press.

Hacking, I. (1999). *The social construction of what?* Cambridge, MA: Harvard University Press.

Halgren, E. (1992). Emotional neurophysiology of the amygdala within the context of human cognition. In J. P. Aggleton (Ed.), *The amygdala: Neurobiological aspects of emotion, memory and mental dysfunction* (pp. 191-228). New York: Wiley-Liss.

Halgren, E., Squires, N. K., Wilson, C. L., Rohrbaugh, J. W., Babb, T. L., & Crandell, P. H. (1980). Endogenous potentials generated in the human hippocampal formation and amygdala by infrequent events. *Science, 210*, 803-805.

Heidel, A. (1965). *The Babylonian genesis.* Chicago: University of Chicago Press (Phoenix Books).

Jung, C. G. (1952). Symbols of transformation: An analysis of the prelude to a case of schizophrenia (R. F. C. Hull, Trans.). *The collected works of C. G. Jung: Vol. 5. Bollingen Series XX.* Princeton, NJ: Princeton University Press.

Jung, C. G. (1967). Alchemical Studies (R. F. C. Hull, Trans.). *The collected works of C. G. Jung: Vol. 13. Bollingen Series XX.* Princeton, NJ: Princeton University Press.

Jung, C. G. (1968). Psychology and alchemy (R. F. C. Hull, Trans.). *The collected works of C. G. Jung: Vol. 12. Bollingen Series XX.* Princeton, NJ: Princeton University Press.

Kuhn, T. S. (1970). *The structure of scientific revolutions* (2nd ed.). Chicago: University of Chicago Press.

Lakoff, G. (1987). *Women, fire, and dangerous things: What categories reveal about the mind.* Chicago: University of Chicago Press.

Lewin, K. (1935). *A dynamic theory of personality.* New York: McGraw-Hill.

Medin, D. L., & Aguilar, C. M. (1999). Categorization. In R. A. Wilson & F. Keil (Eds.), *MIT Encyclopedia of cognitive sciences.* Cambridge, MA: MIT Press.

Merriam-Webster's collegiate dictionary (11th ed.). (2003). Springfield, MA: Merriam-Webster.

Miller, G. A. (1956). The magical number seven, plus or minus two: Some limits on our capacity for processing information. *Psychological Review, 63*, 81-97.

Miller, G. A., Galanter, E., & Pribram, K. (1960). *Plans and the structure of behavior.* New York: Holt, Rinehart and Winston.

Neumann, E. (1954). *The origins and history of consciousness* (R. F. C. Hull, Trans.). New York: Pantheon Books.

Norretranders, T. (1998). *The user illusion* (J. Sydenham, Trans.). New York: Penguin.

Oatley, K., & Johnson-Laird, P. N. (1987). Towards a cognitive theory of emotion. *Cognition and Emotion, 1*, 29-50.

Oatley, K. (1999). Why fiction may be twice as true as fact: Fiction as cognitive and emotional simulation. *Review of General Psychology, 3*, 101-117.

Ohman, A. (1979). The orienting response, attention and learning: An information-processing perspective. In H. D. Kimmel, E. H. Van Olst, & J. F. Orlebeke (Eds.), *The Orienting Reflex in Humans* (pp. 443-467). Hillsdale, NJ: Erlbaum.

Ohman, A. (1987). The psychophysiology of emotion: An evolutionary-cognitive perspective. In P. K. Ackles, J. R. Jennings, & M. G. H. Coles (Eds.), *Advances in Psychophysiology: A Research Annual* (Vol. 2, pp. 79-127). Greenwich, CT: JAI Press.

Otto, R. (1958). *The idea of the holy.* Oxford, U.K.: Oxford University Press.

Panksepp, J. (1999). *Affective neuroscience.* Oxford, U.K.: Oxford University Press.

Peterson, J. B. (1999a). *Maps of meaning: The architecture of belief.* New York: Routledge.

Peterson, J. B. (1999b). Individual motivation for group aggression: Psychological, mythological and neuropsychological perspectives. In L. Kurtz (Ed.), *Encyclopedia of Violence, Peace and Conflict* (pp. 529-545). San Diego, CA: Academic Press.

Piaget, J. (1977). *The development of thought: Equilibration of cognitive structures* (A. Rosin, Trans.). New York: Viking.

Powers, W. T. (1973). *Behavior: the control of perception.* Chicago: Aldine.

Roland, P. E., Erikson, L., Stone-Elander, S., & Widen, L. (1987). Does mental activity change the oxidative metabolism of the brain? *Journal of Neuroscience, 7*, 2372-2389.

Rolls, E. (1999). *The brain and emotion.* New York: Oxford University Press.

Simon, H. A. (1956). Rational choice and the structure of the environment. *Psychological Review, 63*, 129-138.

Sokolov, E. N. (1969). The modeling properties of the nervous system. In I. Maltzman & K. Coles, (Eds.), *Handbook of Contemporary Soviet Psychology* (pp. 670-704). New York: Basic Books.

Tranel, D., Logan, C. G., Frank, R. J., & Damasio, A. R. (1997). Explaining category-related effects in the retrieval of conceptual and lexical knowledge for concrete entities: Operationalization and analysis of factors. *Neuropsychologia, 35*, 1329-1139.

Vaihinger, H. (1924). *The philosophy of "as if:" A system of the theoretical, practical, and religious fictions of mankind* (C. K. Ogden, Trans.). New York: Harcourt, Brace, and Company.

Vinogradova, O. (1961). *The orientation reaction and its neuropsychological mechanisms.* Moscow: Academic Pedagogical Sciences.

Vinogradova, O. (1975). Functional organization of the limbic system in the process of registration of information: Facts and hypotheses. In R. Isaacson & K. Pribram (Eds.), *The hippocampus, neurophysiology, and behavior* (Vol. 2, pp. 3-69). New York: Plenum Press.

Wiener, N. (1948). *Cybernetics: Or, control and communication in the animal and the machine.* Cambridge, MA: Technology Press.

Wittgenstein, L. (1968). *Philosophical investigations* (3rd ed., G. E. M. Anscombe, Trans.) New York: Macmillan.

Author Note

This work was supported by the Social Sciences and Humanities Research Council of Canada.

The Phenomenon of Meaning:
How Psychology Can Make Sense of It

DMITRY A. LEONTIEV

For it's not the things that feed his spirit, but rather the links between the things.
Not the diamond, but some relations between people and the diamond may feed him.
Not the sand, but some relations established between the sand and the tribes. Not the
words in a book, but some relations existing in the book between and beyond words,
relations that are love, poem, and Lord's wisdom.

A. de Saint-Exupery

MEANING AS PROBLEM

Misunderstanding is almost always warranted when one speaks of meaning. During the second half of the twentieth century, one could hardly find another psychological concept used as eagerly and widely, on the one hand, and as vaguely and loosely, on the other hand. One constantly feels something very important and promising in this word, but when using it, a protean or versatile nature is thus revealed, avoiding any strict definition (except for logical and linguistic definitions that are far too narrow from a psychological point of view). As a result, meaning provides a common (or neutral) territory for dialogue between academic science and the practical industry of psychotherapy and psychological help that function without exact definitions.

While working on my Ph.D. during the mid-1980s, I found over 25 distinct, originally theoretical views of personal meaning in psychological sources, not to speak of the linguistic and semantic conceptions of meaning as an impersonal reality (Leontiev, 1996). It certainly proves that there is a persistent need for a clearer understanding of meaning in psychology. The concept of meaning is at home in both everyday speech and in academic discourse; it is also at home in fundamental and applied research, in "depth" (Freudian) and "height" (Vygotskian) approaches, and in the traditional and humanistic paradigm. And the postmodern situation in present-day psychology requires that we get in touch with the reality

33

we study, rather than observe it distantly (Shotter, 1990). Today, it is more favorable than ever for the concept of meaning, which helps to transcend, as well as to link different contexts together. Meaning corresponds to objective, subjective, and intersubjective or "conversational" reality; and, it relates to consciousness, the unconscious, behavior, personality, as well as interpersonal processes. Whatever one studies, one cannot miss the importance of meanings.

Freud (1917/1953) discovered that whatever we do, it always means something. Adler (1932/1980) brought us to the realization that "human beings live in the realm of meanings" (p. 1). Frankl (1967) persuaded us that meaning is what our life actually is directed at, and guided by. The main problem is to discover what meaning is, and correspondingly, what one should seek in one's search for meaning. Until now, meaning remains an insightful metaphor rather than a scientific concept.

An obstacle is the English language, where the single word *meaning* denotes a striking multitude of phenomena while other languages use different words for different things. For instance, in German there is a clear conceptual opposition of *sinn* (sense) versus *bedeutung* (meaning), and this opposition plays a central role in all the humanities. The first pole of this opposition most often denotes subjective personalized meaning rooted in an individual's life, or a deep value-laden, cultural meaning. The second pole represents a culturally invariant elementary meaning (such as word meaning), which can be shared by a common community of language speakers. The same opposition exists in Russian with *smysl* (sense) versus *znachenie* (meaning). In English, however, the word *meaning* covers both poles (private, individual, personal, existential, idiosyncratic, and subjective, on the one hand, and public, collective, cultural, verbal, shared, and objective, on the other hand), and it is used for notions having almost nothing in common: for example, Freudian or Adlerian *sinn* (rooted in an unconscious dynamic), and Vygotskian *znachenie* (understood as a unit of condensed sociocultural, pragmatic experience). Two key dichotomies—*private versus public* and *individual versus collective* (Harre, 1983)—which are fairly well conceptualized both in German and in Russian, dissolve in the English word *meaning*. It is no wonder that the pioneers who first introduced the concept of meaning (beyond a purely linguistic context) in the humanities, were German-speaking (E. Husserl, W. Dilthey, E. Spranger, M. Weber, S. Freud, C. Jung, A. Adler), and Russian-speaking (G. Shpet, M. Bakhtin, L. Vygotsky) authors.

It is not only the problem of translating foreign texts into English that makes these difficulties evident. Some authors, using the concept of meaning, have to describe meaning on different levels in different ways (Kreitler & Kreitler, 1972; Carlsen, 1988). In fact, at these different levels we discover somewhat different realities, but language still fails to catch some of the important distinctions. One possible way would be to use the English word *sense* in a conceptual opposition *sense* versus *meaning*, especially considering its etymological closeness to the German *sinn*. "The word 'sense' (*sinn*) stems from the Old High German verb *sinnan*. In the old days *sinnan* meant: to be on the way towards a goal" (Boss, 1988, p. 115). Unfortunately, the word *sense* is rarely used in this context (rare examples: Bugental, 1976; Gendlin, 1981), and it usually evokes associations with sensory processes rather than with the dynamics of the individual personality.

A systematic analysis of different definitions and other ways of using the concept of meaning in psychology and in the humanities (beyond a purely linguistic context) reveals only two basic properties that may serve as a commonly accepted point of departure: (a) a meaning of an object, event or action exists only within a definite context; in different contexts the same object has different meanings, and (b) meaning always points to some intention, goal, reason, necessity, including desired or supposed consequences, or instrumental utility. In short, defining the meaning of anything presupposes placing it into some intentional context. This is not, however, a purely cognitive operation, resulting only in a new level of understanding. Making sense of our actions, as well as making sense of outside events, gives our activity a totally new quality.

MEANING AS A REGULATING PRINCIPLE

The existing approaches to meaning can be classified through the understanding of the ontological nature of meaning; for example, it may be interpreted as objective reality, subjective reality, or conversational reality. Another dimension of classification is the view of the functional levels of meaning. Meaning can be understood as *the meaning*, the single ultimately integrative reference point inside the person, or as *a meaning* representing an element of ever-present mechanisms connected with the ongoing regulation of behavior and cognition (see Leontiev, 1996, for details). The second dimension seems to me to be even more important than the first. Paradoxically, the more weight is ascribed to this concept, the less important it becomes in the explanation of human life. I suppose we may take for granted that human life is a self-regulated or self-controlled process. Any explanation in terms of regulation presupposes an idea of: (a) the criteria of regulation, that is, the desired state or ideal to which the system is supposed to strive, and (b) the psychological mechanisms that are supposed to make the system move toward this criteria. The second point is far more important, because we may change the criteria, with the mechanisms being maintained, and the system would then keep functioning in the same way, just in another direction; however, if we change the regulating mechanisms, we then change the principles of the entire process of functioning. The least important aspect in the Adlerian revolution against Freud was his change of libido for the striving for power and superiority as the ultimate criteria of regulation; the most important aspect was the shift from past causes to anticipated goals as the motives of actions. It may also be that the transformation of the regulating mechanisms will also change the criteria. For example, in Maddi's (1971) theory the predominance of psychological needs over biological and social ones results in different mechanisms of behavioral regulation that change the whole direction of personality development.

Meaning, as a psychological concept, is a very important explanatory principle for human behavior and life inasmuch as it differs from animal behavior and life. However, today it would be too simplified to understand human behavior simply as meaning-seeking behavior based on responses to stimuli, operant conditioning, social learning, and defense mechanisms. Meaning is much more than the ultimate level or integral criterion: it is a principle of the regulation of behavior functioning at all levels.

Psychology recognizes other regulating principles, and in reality there is no one regulating principle of human behavior. In what I call the *Multiregulation Personality Model* (Leontiev, 1999), six competing regulative principles are described for human behavior, and the list may not be complete. Phenomenologically, this model describes the varieties of logic of behavior, specified by the answer to the question: "Why do you (and people in general) behave the way you (they) do?" Although these principles are described as pure cases, in actual behavior they seem to merge into more or less complicated systems, where actual behavior is usually multicontrolled, except in some cases of pathology.

1. *The logic of drive gratification* underscores the response: "Because I want (need, strive to do) something."

2. *The logic of responding to stimuli* underscores the response: "Because something or someone provoked or teased me."

3. *The logic of learned habits and dispositions* underscores the response: "Because I always (use to) behave this way."

4. *The logic of social norms and expectations.* The relevant answer: "Because this is the way one should behave and most people behave this way in this situation."

5. *The logic of a life-world, or the logic of meaning.* The relevant answer: "Because this is important for me, this matters."

6. *The logic of free choice.* The relevant answer: "Why not?"

Logic 1, 2, and 3 are common for humans and animals. The manifestations of logic 4, the logic of social norms and expectations, though distinctively human, characterize an impersonal, hypersocialized individual, a "social animal," which corresponds to the conformist path of personality development, as understood by Maddi (1971).

Logic 5 is only inherent in humans, due to the fundamental difference between humans and animals, which is explained by several thinkers in very similar terms: For animals there is nothing but the environment; however, for humans, there is the world (Vygotsky, 1934/82, p. 280; Frankl, 1982, p. 116). All animal behavior (i.e., logic 1, 2, and 3) is tied to the immediate environment and to internal impulses, in other words to the situation of the "here and now"; and, all of the sources of its determination lie within the (external + internal) situation. We find no factors influencing animals besides the actual external stimuli and the actual internal urges (drives and programs). Unlike animals, humans are able to relate their activity to their entire *life-world* rather than to an actual situation; their activity is determined by the world at large, as opposed to the environment. This means that by following this logic in human action, reasons and incentives that are located far beyond the situation, including distant consequences and complicated connections, are then taken into account together with immediate incentives. It is not a purely rational logic, or a purely cognitive capacity, though cognitive schemes play an important role in the regulation processes based on this logic. Personality, as a psychological category, appears as an organ or a system of mechanisms, providing regulation of human activity throughout the entire structure of an individual's relations to the world, behaving according to the logic of meaning. A life-world, however, not only includes the world in which one lives and to which one relates, but it also includes one's inner world. The inner world is not a picture or reflection or image of the outer world; the main function of the inner world is to *make sense* of the objects and events of the outer world in the context of an individual's life.

The six principles of logic may be treated as six dimensions of human behavior. Every action can be split into six vectors, with each of the vectors representing a projection of the whole action related to the dimension of this or that logic. Keeping the proposed model in mind, we will first notice *considerable individual differences* in the use of all six principles. The most important understanding at this point is that different people transcend immediate personal urges and needs into the realm of meanings to different degrees. Second, it is evident that there are *developmental trends and successions* with respect to all of the logical principles mentioned. Third, clinical psychology provides enough evidence for separate types of *distortions* of these regulatory systems; in particular, psychopathy presents the distortion of meaning-based regulation that result in behavior according to momentary urges. The ability of self-control, characteristic of a psychologically sound person, presupposes the balanced development of all six (or, at least, the first five) regulatory systems; the dominant role should belong to the highest, distinctively human, ones.

The relationship between these higher laws of the regulation of behavior and the lower ones has been brilliantly expressed by Hegel (1927): "Circumstances or urges dominate a person only to the extent to which he allows them to do so" (p. 45). A person is thus able to both allow the lower principles of logic to guide the definite action, and not to allow certain things to happen. In a similar context, Rollo May (1967) described a distinctively human capacity as being able to deliberately take either the position of an active subject, or that of a passive object.

It follows from the considerations listed above that human beings act in accordance with different regulating principles, or logic, some of which are inherited from the animal world, and some of which relate to being distinctly human. Relations between animal and human potentialities of behavior within an individual are ones of competition, rather than of fighting or even submission. Both possibilities are open for us in many diverging points of bifurcation: the ability of acting as any other animal would do, or to act as only humans are able to. It is beyond the scope of this paper to dwell on the human drama of choosing between these options. However, what is the most important point in this context is the *meaning-based regulation* that gives one the possibility of transcending behavior determination both by internal impulses and learned programs, and by actual external stimulation. In other words, meaning offers a person a high degree of freedom from what is determined. A personal life-world ultimately maintains the capacity of creating a new intentional context for human activity. This is best exemplified by the following story: A number of active members of nobility were in the opposition movement in Russia, the so-called Decembrists, who had openly revolted against Czar Nikolaus I in December, 1825. Ultimately they lost, and were arrested and finally banished to a penal colony in Siberia. A colony officer strongly disliked them, and, wishing to destroy the young men morally, made them carry heavy stones from one place to another, then back, again and again. They were about to lose their minds and their spirit with this meaningless labor, but then the solution appeared. They found the meaning to their predicament: They started carrying the stones quickly, with accurate precision, in order to infuriate the officer and to make *him* lose his spirit. In the end they were most successful.

An animal responds to a stimulus representing the actual environment. Human action is guided by a meaning representing one's personal life-world. A meaningful action is a mediated action—mediated by a life-world. You act meaningfully, or are regulated in a meaningful or human way, if your action (however local it may be) takes into account the whole life-world of yourself, spreading far beyond the actual situation. Behaving according to the logic of a personal life-world, or according to the principle of meaning, is taking into account the entire multitude of personal contexts that matter, rather than only the "here and now" urges and demands. However, to have your behavior controlled by meaning, by your own personal life-world, you should have your life-world developed enough to provide meanings that differ from those stemming from the immediate situation.

THE ONTOLOGY OF MEANING

We find meaning first of all through our mind—we perceive, imagine, or recollect things not as exact projections, but as having some personal meaning for us, a meaning that manifests itself through image transformations (see Leontiev, 1990). But it would be too hasty to call meaning a subjective reality, although this *phenomenological dimension of meaning*—its direct representation in consciousness—is quite important.

We find meaning, then, in various effects on behavior and on performance at large. If we ask young boys to hold their breath for as long as possible, then ask them to beat their previous record, and then ask them to imagine a partner to compete with, the results will normally increase (Aidman, 1988). What we accomplish with this method is to help find additional meaning through enlarging the context of one's own actions, resulting in improved performance. I call these effects the *behavioral dimension of meaning*.

The most important aspect, however, is that both phenomenological and behavioral manifestations of meaning are derivatives of the third aspect that I call the *ontological dimension of meaning*. What we see in traditional psychological research are emotional responses and evaluations, psychodynamics, changes in perceptual images or other cognitive representations, changes in performance, direction, and results of activity. We see no meaning. Any attempts to distinguish between personal meaning and emotion, personal meaning and connotation, personal meaning and attitude, *inter alia*, remain futile until we leave behind the psychological processes and events by transcending them into the realm of personal-world relationships. In order to discover the meaning of an action, an object, or an event for any person (including ourselves), we must investigate the person's life-world, disclosing the links between the given action, object, or event, and everything that is important for him/her in the world. The concept of the world does not belong within the scope of psychology, and a person's underlying ontological links to the world cannot be empirically assessed or measured. Nevertheless, many questions belonging to different branches of general psychology cannot be answered in the fashion of an empirical science only, without postulating some basic ontological structure and considering this structure within a theoretical explanation. The ontological links are theoretical constructions that are not noticeable or detectable; however, they serve as a necessary element of psychological explanation, as an independent variable that does not contain a psychological nature. The sum total of these links defines the *life meaning* of the given action, object, or event, that is its place and role in the person's life. To define the meaning of some object, event, or action for anyone is to put it into the context of the person's life as a whole.

The meaningful links that embody the living fibers of a life-world can also explain why something unimportant may become important. These links can be expressed in colloquial words: for the sake of, to prevent, to escape, to provide, to facilitate; it is a sign of, it warns, it helps, it brings something closer, it is important, etc. The links and interrelations define the whole structure. This point is illustrated precisely by the example offered by J. Nuttin (1984, p. 71): A student may try hard to study well in order to win his parents' approval, or, he may try hard to win his parents' approval in order to obtain the possibility to study in the first place. What we encounter here are not just two different motives, but two different *means-end* structures or links of *meaning*.

Conditioning is simply a very special case of establishing links of meaning. More often these links have another nature than conditioning; it is a matter of the dynamics of life, the flow (Csikszentmihalyi, 1990), rather than training. Generally, the structure of meaning includes three elements: a *carrier of meaning* (the meaning of what we are discussing); the *source of meaning* (an element or a structure of the context that gives meaning to the carrier); and the *meaning-link* (i.e., the psycho-logical aspect of the connection between the carrier and the source). Meaning flows along the trajectories of meaningful links from sources to carriers that become sources for new carriers, etc. Some aspects of this dynamic structure have been conceptualized by different theorists in different ways: for example, as psychodynamics (Freud, 1917/1953), valence (Lewin, 1935), expectancy x value model (Tolman, 1951), goal instrumentality (Vroom, 1964), personal construct systems (Kelly, 1955), psycho-logics (Smedslund, 1984), valuation (Hermans, 1998), etc.; however, each of these approaches only includes certain types of links of meaning.

The links of meaning represent the core of the phenomenon of meaning because they can be found in the ontological dimension alone. All of the knots along the trajectories of meaning, within the living tissues of the network of the life-world that complete the web of meaning, belong to this dimension. This dimension is the key to the triadic, three-dimensional structure of meaning: only within the ontological dimension can one find the links between the elements of the personal life-world, the links that can explain certain psychological effects. I call this the principle of ontological mediation: behavioral and phenomenological effects of meaning reflect ontological dynamics (what is going on between you and the world). A person can study meaning with any kind of research tools inasmuch as one can take into account the ontological dynamics as the primary reality explaining all of the psychological effects (though psychological instruments don't capture this reality directly). Otherwise, one will study emotions, connotations, or whatever, but not meaning. This is why the problem of personal meaning escapes any positivistic approach (in the traditional sense of this word).

MEANING-BASED REGULATION AS THE MEASURE OF HUMANITY

A psychologist sees meaning phenomena as manifested in the phenomenological dimension (i.e., selecting, transforming, or emotionally coloring of the images), or in the behavioral dimension (i.e., energizing, blocking, or directing the activity). The relationship between these manifestations and the ontological links of meaning represents a "converted form" (Mamardashvili, 1970). This concept presumes that some content being transposed onto another substratum is being transformed according to the functional properties of the new substratum, like the narrative of a novel being transformed into a movie script: both are quite different texts, but, in a sense, they are one.

There is a long tradition of theoretical and experimental studies of phenomenological and behavioral manifestations of meaning-based activity regulation (usually called sense regulation) in Soviet/Russian psychology (Leontiev, 1991, 1998). The most integral concept dealing with sense regulation is the concept of the *sphere of sense* related to the personality (Bratus, 1990), that I would define as the system of *refracted personal meanings* incorporated into the mechanisms of human cognition and practical activity that control this activity, according to the logic of the personal life-world.

The most comprehensive account of this tradition is given in my recent works (Leontiev, 1999), where I propose a highly complex, theoretical model of structure and functioning of meaning-based regulation in human cognition and practical activity. What I consider to be most important is that individuals evidently differ in their capacities of meaning regulation. Six individual variables relevant to this sphere have been proposed:

- The most important is general teleological versus causal orientation, doing things for the sake of something rather than because of something.

- The quantitative measure of meaning as a factual presence in life, e.g., as measured by Purpose-in-Life test (Crumbaugh & Maholick, 1964).
- Value/need ratio in meaning sources. This point deserves a much more detailed description, for which I have no place here (see Leontiev, 1998).
- Structural coherence of personal meanings within personality structure (e.g., Leontiev, in press).
- The capacity of reflexive awareness of one's relations to the world.
- Sound integration of past, present, and future orientations.

Numerous studies of sense regulation in different forms of mental pathology have revealed that: (a) although in most cases the sphere of sense is usually damaged, the changes are nonspecific with respect to the classification of diseases, (b) most of the pathological or maladaptive changes concern structural mechanisms of regulation rather than meanings themselves, and (c) with mental pathology, the more mature the person is when the disease begins, the less are the changes within sense regulation, as a rule, and the prognosis of recovery will be better.

However, studies of delinquents as subjects, without a manifested mental pathology, have provided a much clearer picture of specific distortions of meaning-based regulation, as well as the sense sphere of personality. In particular, juvenile delinquents, as compared to non-delinquents, (a) tend to be reactive rather than proactive, (b) have lower scores on the Purpose-in-Life test, (c) have a weak and distorted role of values, (d) have poorly constructed personal meanings, (e) show poor reflexive awareness, and (f) are centered in the present, having a distorted orientation of the future (Leontiev, 1999). In other words, this sample exemplifies the underdevelopment of the capacity of meaning regulation that can be labeled as a special metapathology (Maslow, 1976) of meaning-based regulation of behavior. Considering that meaning-based regulation represents a specifically human way of relating to the world, what we meet in delinquents is some deficit of humanity, or "human diminution" (Maslow, 1976), rather than a pathology in the exact meaning of the word. Interestingly enough, in our studies with juvenile delinquents, we have also discovered a "delinquent" personality pattern in a number of participants from the control sample as well. Being psychologically disposed as delinquents, the subjects seem to have been lucky enough not to get into conflict with the law.

CONCLUSION

During the entire last century, mainstream psychology tried to study human behavior in its subhuman manifestations only. By adding the dimensions of meaning, and meaning regulation, the mechanisms of activity obtained a completely new quality—a specifically human one. This does not imply, however, that we must totally break with mainstream psychology. Maslow (1976) stated that a completely new theory of motivation must be written for self-actualizing persons. I would state that we must somewhat rewrite the old theory rather than throw it away. The challenge is whether we can describe and investigate human activity as qualitatively different from animal behavior, while incorporating all of the subhuman mechanisms as well, and to demonstrate how and why a human being may choose to behave either in a human or in a subhuman way. This is the challenge for the next millennium, carried over from the twentieth century, the century that experienced both the godlike heights of the human spirit, and the complete betrayal of humanity.

References

Adler, A. (1980). *What life should mean to you*. London: George Allen & Unwin. (Original work published 1931)

Aidman, E. V. (1988). Development of means of activity control: Today's vision of Lev Vygotsky's ideas. In F. Eros & G. Kiss, *Seventh European CHEIRON Conference* (pp. 150-153). Budapest, Hungary: Hungarian Psychological Association.

Boss, M. (1988). Is psychotherapy rational or rationalistic? *Review of Existential Psychology and Psychiatry, 19*, 115-127.

Bratus, B. S. (1990). *Anomalies of personality*. Orlando, FL: Paul Deutsch.

Bugental, J. F. T. (1976). *The search for existential identity*. San Francisco: Jossey-Bass.

Carlsen, M. B. (1988). *Meaning-making: Therapeutic process in adult development*. New York: W. W. Norton & Co.

Crumbaugh J. S., & Maholick L. T. (1964). An experimental study in existentialism: The psychometric approach to Frankl's concept of noogenic neurosis. *Journal of Clinical Psychology, 20*(2), 200-207.

Csikszentmihalyi, M. (1990). *Flow: The psychology of optimal experience*. New York: Harper Perennial.

Frankl, V. E. (1967). *Psychotherapy and existentialism*. New York: Simon & Schuster.

Frankl, V. E. (1982). *Der Wille zum Sinn* [The Will to Sense] (expanded ed.). Bern, Switzerland: Huber.

Freud, S. (1953). Introductory lectures on psychoanalysis. In J. Strachey & A. Freud (Eds.), *The standard edition of the complete psychological works of Sigmund Freud (Vols. XV, XVI)*. London: Hogarth.

Gendlin, E. T. (1981). *Focusing* (2nd ed.). Toronto, ON: Bantam Books.

Harre, R. (1983). *Personal being: A theory for individual psychology*. Oxford, U.K.: Basil Blackwell.

Hegel, G. W. F. (1927). *Philosophische Propadeutik* [Philosophical prevention]. In Samtliche Werke [Collected works] (Vol. 3). Stuttgart, Germany: Frommann.

Hermans H. J. M. (1998). Meaning as an organized process of valuation: A self-confrontational approach. In P. T. P. Wong & P. S. Fry (Eds.), *The human quest for meaning* (pp. 317-334). Mahwah, NJ: Lawrence Erlbaum Associates.

Kelly, G. A. (1955). *The psychology of personal constructs.* New York: Norton.

Kreitler, H., & Kreitler, S. (1972). *Psychology of the arts.* Durham, NC: Duke University Press.

Leontiev, D. A. (1990). Personal meaning and the transformation of a mental image. *Soviet Psychology, 1990, 28*(2), 5-24.

Leontiev, D.A. (1991). The concept of personal sense through the decades. *Studi di Psicologia dell'Educazione, 3,* 32-40.

Leontiev, D. A. (1996). Dimensions of the meaning/sense concept in the psychological context. In C. Tolman, F. Cherry, R. van Hezewijk, & I. Lubek (Eds.), *Problems of theoretical psychology,* (pp. 130-142). New York: Captus University Publications.

Leontiev, D. A. (1998). Motivation through personal sense: Activity theory perspective. In P. Nenniger, R. Jaeger, A. Frey, & M. Wosnitza (Eds.), *Advances in motivation* (pp. 7-22). Landau, Germany: Verlag Empirische Paedagogik.

Leontiev, D. A. (1999). Psikhologiya smysla [The psychology of personal meaning]. Moscow: Smysl.

Leontiev, D. A. (in press). Approaching world view structure with ultimate meanings technique. *Journal of Humanistic Psychology.*

Lewin, K. (1935). *A dynamic theory of personality: Selected papers.* New York: McGraw-Hill.

Maddi, S. (1971). The search for meaning. In W. J. Arnold & M. M. Page (Eds.), *Nebraska symposium on motivation* (pp. 137-186). Lincoln, NE: University of Nebraska Press.

Mamardashvili, M. K. (1970). Forma prevraschennaya [Converted form]. *Filisofskaya entsiklopediya* [Philosophical encyclopedia] (Vol. 5, pp. 386-389). Moscow: Sovetskaya entsiklopediya.

Maslow, A. H. (1976). *The farther reaches of human nature.* Harmondsworth, U.K.: Penguin.

May, R. (1967). *Psychology and the human dilemma.* Princeton, NJ: Van Nostrand.

Nuttin, J. (1984). *Motivation, Planning, and Action: A Relational Theory of Behavior Dynamics.* Leuven: Leuven University Press; Hillsdale, NJ: Lawrence Erlbaum Associates.

Shotter, J. (1990). Getting in touch: The metamethodology of a postmodern science of mental life. *The humanistic psychologist, 18*(1), 7-22.

Smedslund, J. (1984). What is necessarily true in psychology. In J. R. Royce & L. P. Mos (Eds.), *Annales of Theoretical Psychology* (pp. 241-272). New York: Plenum.

Tolman, E. C. (1951). A psychological model. In T. Parsons & E. Shils (Eds.), *Toward a general theory of action* (pp. 277-361). Cambridge, MA: Harvard University.

Vroom, V. H. (1964). *Work and motivation.* New York: Wiley.

Vygotsky, L. S. (1982). Problema razvitiya v strukturnoi psikhologii [The problem of development in the structural psychology]. In *Sobranie Sochineniy* [Collected Works] (pp. 238-290). Moscow: Pedagogika.

The Search for Meaning in Life
and the
Existential Fundamental Motivations

ALFRIED LÄNGLE

Abstract

Personal meaning is a complex achievement of the human spirit and is found in the individual's confrontation with the challenges of the world and one's own being. How can people find orientation in the midst of the innumerable possibilities that characterize our present day and how can this orientation be realised? Phenomenological and empirical research have shown that there are three existential motivations that precede a fourth motivation concerned with finding meaning. The first motivation is framed by the question, "How can one relate to the fact of being in the world?" The second turns the question around and asks, "How can one relate to the fact of having a life?" The third, "How can one relate to the fact of one's own individual identity (self)?" Individuals are fundamentally looking for a greater context and values for which they want to live. Personal existential meaning (Frankl's Logotherapy) derives from this. This paper describes the four fundamental aspects of existence that form a matrix for the psychopathological understanding of psychic disorders and provide a background for clinical interventions. They represent the structure and model of modern existential analytical psychotherapy.

AN INTRODUCTION TO MEANING

Viktor Frankl once came along and showed me a little drawing that he had come across in a newspaper. His bright spirit, with which Frankl was always combining casual happenings with deeper insights, was the source of his humour and wit. The drawing Frankl found that day was of an arrow shot at a plain wall where it was stuck. A man with a bow in his left hand was standing next to the wall painting the sign of a target around the arrow.

Frankl, commenting on this drawing, said: "Look at that, this picture shows exactly what is not meant by meaning! This man is constructing a meaning about an arbitrary action. He tries in retrospect to make a senseless action meaningful by giving it a meaning, to give the appearance of a meaning. But existential meaning is never arbitrary nor is it a construction, if it is supposed to give structure and support to one's life. Such a meaning must be based on given facts, must be hewn out of reality and cannot be changed deliberately!"

Frankl described the concept of meaning as follows: "We do not just attach and attribute meanings to things, but rather find them; we do not invent them, we detect them" (Frankl, 1985, p. 31). Meaning, from an existential analytic and logotherapeutic context, is understood as a correlation of two given facts: the *demand of the situation,* and *one's understanding of oneself,* (i.e., what a person thinks and feels in terms of who they are or should be).

As I write this paper, the demand of the situation for me, as I understand it, is to find out what the reader might be interested in while reading such a paper and to correlate this with my experience, my view, and investigation. The importance of this is my meaning. For those reading this paper, the meaning may be following the text or correlating it with personal experience or current thinking and considering what is of higher importance right now: to continue the reading or to continue one's own thought. Thus, meaning is a Gestalt emerging from the midst of both inner and outer reality. What I wish to outline here is the idea that personal meaning is a complex achievement of the human spirit (or noëtic potential, as Frankl preferred to call it so as to make a clear distinction from a religious understanding of that term). Personal meaning is a nonphysical power underlying our conscience, our mind, our capacity to feel and to sense, and even our body. The nature of the spirit is dialogical. As a dialogical force it brings us into continuous confrontation with other people, other things, and with ourselves. This dialogical interaction lays the ground for a basic prerequisite of existence: for detecting what is possible in the midst of the given facts. All of that which is not yet fixed represents the existential field waiting to be realized. Through our spirit, we are directed towards dialogue and relationship, where we realize possibility, where we realize what is waiting for us, what might challenge us, reach out to us or invite us. This is our existential actuality and as an existential reality, it is at the same time our future. It is through our spirit that we are capable of separating the factual, what is given, from what is possible thereby creating the specifically human dimension of existence (Frankl, 1985, p. 19, 79, 134).

The possibilities within this world implicate our human potential; we shape our existence through these possibilities. "Existence" means having a chance to change things for the better, to experience what is of value and to avoid or to eliminate what could be damaging or harmful. Possibilities provide us with directions to which we can orient ourselves. This is an essential orientation of human beings, not a superficial one. Being directed towards what is possible, what is yet to be fulfilled, what is waiting for us in each and every situation corresponds perfectly to the essence of our spirit—a spirit that is looking out for participation, dialogue, creativity, and possibility. We see the essential task of existence to be one of finding this correspondence between our potential for participation (for creativity, action and encounter) and what is possible, what is needed, what is undone, what we see and feel and understand to be waiting for us, despite the possibility of risk and error.

A PRACTICAL GUIDE TO MEANING

Viktor Frankl (1973) gave a general guide for finding meaning. Finding meaning requires an attitude towards the world. Frankl wrote:

> We must perform a kind of Copernican Revolution, and give the question of the meaning of life an entirely new twist. To wit: It is life itself that asks questions of man.... It is not up to man to question; rather, he should recognize that he is questioned, questioned by life; he has to respond by being responsible; and he can answer to life only by answering for his life. (p. 62)

This attitude is in fact a phenomenological attitude, an openness of the mind free from personal interest, an attitude directed towards the essence of the situation, an attitude that allows one to be reached or even to be captured by the situation.

If the essence of a situation is valuable in itself, if it cannot be made better for example, if it is seemingly perfect, then we are left to enjoy, to admire and to simply experience. A marvelous sunset, a beautiful face, music by Mozart, and a painting by Picasso qualify as examples of what Frankl termed experiential values and one avenue to meaning.

If under different circumstances this openness leads us to an imperfect situation, a situation that requires some intervention for improvement, we may perceive the circumstance as both valuable but requiring something for its improvement. Such a situation requires either a suitable activity in the world, such as speaking to a person, writing a letter, cooking a meal, etc. or mental or spiritual activity in one's inner world, which means a change of attitude towards the world, life, oneself, or the future. Frankl included creative and attitudinal values as the two other avenues to meaning.

All phenomenological perceptions reveal possibilities for action. This action can take the form of subjective experiencing, of working, of reflection, or one's own attitude. These possibilities, because of their inherent "demand quality" (*Aufforderungscharakter*) create a field of tension, which Frankl (1985) called "existential dynamics" (p. 35). Frankl's key to meaning is a more philosophical approach, elaborating the appropriate attitude and subsequently providing the necessary substance or "grain" for a fulfilling existence.

From a more psychological point of view, existential analysis describes the key for a fulfilling existence in finding a way of living with inner consent. This inner consent relates to what we do, to what we commit ourselves, or to what we choose to omit. In other words, inner consent is a continuous activity that underlies any fulfilled existence and the finding of meaning.

This activity consists of a two-sided dialogue. One is directed towards the outside with such questions as: What appeals to me? What attracts or challenges me? Where am I needed, and what do I want to do in this situation? For example, is what I am reading at this moment interesting to me, does it challenge me, does it speak to me in some way so that I might see what I can do with it?

The other dialogue runs inwardly. Whatever I decide to do, I cannot leave myself aside to experience meaning. We, therefore, always live with the question of whether we agree with our decisions. To put it more concretely, this inner agreement is a process of contacting the deepest feelings that arise in any situation. We have to take them seriously. I am not speaking about anxiety, mood, delight, or the like, for they too have their meaning. When our deepest and purest emotions correspond with our intentions and plans, then we live with inner consent, our inwardly felt or spoken "yes." Inner consent enables us to stand on our own, stand as a unique individual and realize ourselves by meeting the demands of the situation. Meaning, in our definition, creates a harmony between inner experience and outer action.

The process I have described provides an encapsulated definition of existential analysis and possibly of existential psychotherapy in general: to help a person find a way of life wherein they can give their inner consent to their own actions.

A scientific definition of existential analysis describes it as phenomenological-personal psychotherapy with the aim of enabling a person to experience his or her life freely at the spiritual and emotional levels, to arrive at authentic decisions and to come to a responsible way of dealing with himself or herself and the world around him or her (Längle, 1993; 1995; 1999a). This reflects Frankl's teaching, in which he stated that a person's existence is characterized by freedom, by the capacity for decision and by responsibility (Frankl, 1959; 1973, xxiv). Each of these three steps contains the most important asset of existential analysis: a person's own inner consent.

THE FOUR FUNDAMENTAL CONDITIONS FOR A FULFILLED EXISTENCE

If we scrutinize the themes that concern us throughout our lives, they are related to four fundamental realities. These four fundamental realities have been supported by empirical and phenomenological work in psychotherapy over the last 20 years. As spiritual beings we are essentially confronted with:

- The world in its factuality and potentiality.
- Life with its network of relationships and its feelings.
- "Being oneself": existing as a unique, autonomous person.
- The future which we shape equals our development through our activities.

Human existence is based on these fundamental realities. They are the four cornerstones of existence according to modern existential analytical theory. Yalom (1980) has described quite similar fundamental existential realities. Yalom's categories highlight the common existential emphasis on the tragic dimensions of human existence:

- Freedom in the sense of groundlessness.
- Death.
- Isolation in the sense of loneliness.
- Meaninglessness/absurdity.

Although Yalom's categories correspond largely to our four existential realities, existential analysis, in the tradition of Frankl, emphasizes the elements of possibility and potential that mark human existence. As a comparison therefore:

- Groundlessness implies the world with its supporting structure.
- Death means having a life with growth and temporality.
- Loneliness arises from the uniqueness of each person.
- Meaning relates to a contextual understanding of one's own existence and of one's activities which are directed towards a worthwhile future.

Our categories can nevertheless be called "existential" for one central reason: They claim our own inner position towards them. Each of the four existential realities leads us into a process that demands an exchange or even a dialogue. This exchange or dialogue helps to form our own notions about the quality and content of our subjective reality. Dialogue and encounter require us to decide how we want to relate. This challenges us; it challenges our activities and our response to alter and work on our reality until we can give our inner consent—a consent not merely for what we do but for how we live. There is, of course, always the possibility of failing, experiencing loneliness or feelings akin to an emotional death. We might experience feelings of futility or "absurdity" as Camus and Sartre have described. But the four cornerstones of existence offer a chance to entrust ourselves to external structures and contents (Längle, 2001). As structures of human existence, these realities are basically involved in every motivation and can therefore also be called the "fundamental existential motivations" (Längle, 1992; 1993; 1994a; 1997; 1998a,b,c; 1999a,b; 2002, June). These fundamental existential motivations (i.e., cognition, feelings and values, and decision and meaning) result in arriving at an inner consent. As basics of human existence, these motivations are relevant in all areas where an individual stands in the center, such as education, pastoral counseling, prevention of diseases, coaching, management training, and organizational structures.

The First Fundamental Condition for a Fulfilled Existence

The first condition arises from the simple fact that I am here at all, and that I am in the world. Where do I go from here? Can I cope with my being there? Do I understand that I exist? As an old German saying from the 12th century goes, loosely translated: "I don't know where I am from, I don't know where to, I wonder why I am so glad." I am here, this is me—how is that even possible? This seemingly self-evident fact can lead to questioning of great depth. If I really think about this, I realize that I cannot truly comprehend it. My existence appears like an island in an ocean of ignorance and alludes to connections that surpass me. The most adequate attitude towards this incomprehensible fact is one of astonishment. Basically, I can only be astonished that I am here at all.

But I am here, which puts the fundamental question of existence before me: I am—can I be? To bring these questions to a practical and manageable level, I might apply them to my own situation. I then ask myself: Can I claim my place in this world under the conditions I live within *and* the possibilities I have before me? This demands three things, namely, protection, space, and support. Do I enjoy protection, acceptance, and do I feel at home somewhere? Where do I find support in my life? If the answer to the above is negative, it will result in restlessness, insecurity, and fear. But if I do have these three things, I will be able to feel trust in the world and confidence in myself, maybe even faith in God. The sum of these experiences of trust is a fundamental trust; a trust that I have a profound and enduring support in my life.

It is not enough to find protection, space, and support, however. I also have to seize these conditions, to make a decision in their favor, to accept them. My active part in this fundamental condition of being here is to accept the positive aspects and to endure the negative ones. To accept means to be ready to occupy the space I am in, to rely on the support given and to trust the protection bestowed on me; in short "to be here" and not to flee. To endure requires the fortitude to accept whatever is difficult, menacing, or unalterable, and to tolerate what cannot be changed. Life imposes certain conditions on me; the world has its laws to which I must adapt. This idea is expressed in the word "subject" in the sense of "not independent," of being subject to something or someone. On the other hand, these same conditions of the world are reliable, solid, and steady despite the boundaries they may impose. I can allow them to be and accept them if I can be at the same time. To accept means letting the other be, whether a person, a thing, or a situation. It means that I can be and the other can be equally because there is still enough space for me and the circumstances do not threaten my being here. Individuals procure themselves the space they need for being with their ability to endure and to accept the conditions of their lives. If this is not the case, psychodynamics take over the guidance of a person's life in the form of coping reactions in order to secure "being here" (Dasein) (Längle, 1998a). Each fundamental motivation has four types of reactions:

- The basic reaction type.
- The paradoxical reaction type or "activism," which is a displacement activity, a hyperactivity.
- The third type of coping reaction is a specific aggression (Längle, 1998b).
- The final type of coping reaction is akin to a feigned death, a semi-paralysis. A person's activity level is greatly reduced and feelings are deadened.

When the first existential motivation is in danger or not sufficiently realized, the basic coping reaction is avoidance or flight; the displaced reaction is over-activity or compulsive behavior (i.e., fighting bacteria by compulsive washing). The aggressive reaction takes the form of destruction such as hate; and "feigned death reaction" is denial or pretending to be nonexistent. If any of these coping reactions are insufficient to stem the psychodynamics that have emerged, they get fixed and psychopathology arises. In cases where a lack of protection, space, and support is present, fear and anxiety arise.

The Second Fundamental Condition for a Fulfilled Existence

Once individuals have their space in the world, they can fill it with life. Simply being there is not enough. We want our existence to be good, since it is more than a mere fact. It has a "pathic dimension," which means that life does not simply happen but rather we experience, suffer, or enjoy it (from the Greek *pathos*, suffering, used, e.g., in "psycho-pathology"). Being alive means to cry and to laugh, to experience joy and suffering, to go through pleasant and unpleasant things, to be lucky or unlucky, and to experience what is worthwhile and what is worthless. As happy as we can be, we can also suffer deeply. The amplitude of emotionality is equal in both directions, whether this suits us or not.

I am, therefore, confronted with the fundamental question of life: I am alive—do I like this fact? Is it good to be here? It is not only strain and suffering that can take away the joy of life. It may also be the shallowness of daily life or the neglecting areas of one's life that make life stale. Do I truly live? In order to seize my life and to love it, I need three things: relationship, time, and closeness. We can verify the "presence of life" by asking: Do I have relationships in which I feel closeness, for which I spend and give my time, and in which I experience community? What do I take time for? Do I take time for valuable things, worthy of spending my time on? To take time for something means to give away a part of one's life and spend it with someone or something. Can I feel close by maintaining closeness to things, plants, animals, and people? Do I allow the closeness of someone else? If relationships, closeness, and time are lacking, longing will arise, followed by distancing—a coldness—and finally depression. If these three conditions are fulfilled, however, I experience myself as being in harmony with the world and with myself and I can sense the depth of life. These experiences form the fundamental value, the most profound feeling, for the value of life. Whenever we experience something of value, this fundamental value is touched upon. It colors our emotions and represents a yardstick for anything we might feel to be of worth. Our theory of emotion and theory of values correlate with this (Längle, 2003).

And yet, it is not enough to have relationships, time, and closeness. My active participation and my consent are also required. I must seize life by engaging in life. When I turn to other people, to things, animals, intellectual work, or to myself, I turn towards life. When I move towards something or someone, allow myself to get close, allow myself to be touched, I experience life as vibrant. By fully acknowledging what is before me, I not only experience life as vibrant, I equally experience such things as loss and grief. If I am to move freely in life, my consent to being touched by life is necessary. The basic coping reaction at this level is regression; over-protection or a striving for achievement are "activistic" reaction types. The aggressive behavior is fury or rage which does not lead to destruction but leads towards the agitation of other persons with the impulse towards obtaining or improving a relationship. Resignation and apathy are reactions that mimic a "feigned death." If these reactions cannot neutralize the problem or the loss, depression arises.

The Third Fundamental Condition for a Fulfilled Existence

The first two fundamental conditions are, however, not sufficient in themselves for a fulfilling existence. In spite of my being related to life and to people, I am aware of my being separate and different. There is a singularity that makes me an "I" and distinguishes me from everybody else. I realize that I am on my own, that I have to master my existence myself, and that I am essentially alone and perhaps even solitary. But, there is so much more that is equally singular. The diversity, beauty, and uniqueness that exist in all dimensions of life, produce feelings of awe and respect in me.

In the midst of this world, I discover myself unmistakably, I am with myself, and I am given to myself. This puts before me the fundamental question of being a person: I am myself—may I be like this? Do I feel free to be like this? Do I have the right to be what I am and to behave as I do? This is the plane of identity, of knowing oneself, and of ethics. In order to succeed here, it is necessary to have experienced three things: attention, justice, and appreciation. Again, we can verify this third cornerstone of existence in our own life by asking: Who sees me? Who considers my uniqueness and respects my boundaries? Do people do justice to me? What am I appreciated for? How do I appreciate myself? If these experiences are missing, solitude, hysteria, and a need to hide behind shame will result. If, on the contrary, I have experienced attention, justice, and appreciation, I will find myself, find my authenticity, and find my self-respect. The sum of these experiences builds my self-esteem, who I am at my core.

In order to be oneself, it is not enough to simply experience attention, justice, and appreciation. I also have to say "yes to myself." This requires my active participation. I have to look at other people, to encounter them. At the same time I have to delineate myself, stand on my own, and refuse whatever does not correspond to my sense of self. Encounter and regret are the two means by which we can live authentically without ending up in solitude. Encounter represents the necessary bridge to the other. It makes me experience another person's essence as well as my own; discovering the "I" in "you." My participation with and appreciation of others create an equal appreciation for who I am. When these elements are missing, I may react by distancing myself or leading a life of hyperactivity. The typical aggressive reaction consists of annoyance, anger, and reproach. A paralysis or resignation at this level leads to dissociation of bodily integrity, dividing and splitting of emotion and cognition. If these reactions do not suffice to neutralize the hurt, they get fixed and histrionic symptoms and/or personality disorders arise.

The Fourth Fundamental Condition for a Fulfilled Existence

If I can be here, love life, and find myself within these, the conditions are fulfilled for the fourth fundamental condition of existence; I recognize my life and what it is all about. It does not suffice to simply be here and to have found oneself. In a sense, we have to transcend ourselves if we want to find fulfillment and to be fruitful. Otherwise we would live as if in a house where nobody ever visits.

Life's transitory nature puts the question of the meaning of our existence before us: I am here for what purpose? Three things are needed: a field of activity, a structural context, and a value to be realized in the future. We can ask ourselves practical questions, such as: Is there a place where I feel needed, where I can be productive? Do I see and experience myself in a larger context that provides structure and orientation to my life; where I want integration? Is there anything that should still be realized in my life? If this is not the case, the result will be a feeling of emptiness, frustration, despair, and frequently addiction. If, on the contrary, these conditions are met, I will be capable of dedication and action and finally, my own form of religious belief. The sum of these experiences adds up to the meaning of life and leads to a sense of fulfillment.

If a person fails systematically to reach meaning, their coping reactions will be a provisional attitude towards life as a basic reaction together with a "disorganized day-to-day attitude toward life" and "collective thinking" (Frankl, 1973, p. xvi). Idealization and fanaticism are main forms of hyperactivity along with indignation, aggressive games, and cynicism. Fatalism (Frankl, 1973, p. xvi), loss of interest, apathy, and nihilistic attitudes, can be seen as forms of internal paralysis. Nihilistic attitudes in particular are, from all evidence, a form of spiritual deadening. Disorders at this level lead frequently to addictions.

It does not suffice to simply have a field of activity, to have our place within a context and to know values to be realized in the future. A phenomenological attitude is needed. As each situation places a question before me, an attitude of openness represents the existential access to meaning in life. "What does this hour want from me, how shall I respond?" (Frankl, 1973, p. xv; p. 62). The meaningful thing is not only what I can expect from life, but, in accordance with the dialogical structure of existence, it is equally important what life wants from me, and what the moment expects from me, and what I could and should do now for others as well as for myself. My active part in this attitude of openness is to bring myself into agreement with the situation, to examine whether what I am doing is really a good thing: for others, for myself, for the future, for my environment. If I act and if I respond to these questions, my existence will be fulfilling. Viktor Frankl (1982) once defined meaning as "a possibility against the background of reality"

(p. 255). In another context (Frankl 1985) he referred to the potentialities under-lying the meaning: "The potentialities of life are not indifferent possibilities; they must be seen in the light of meaning and values. At any given time only one of the possible choices of the individual fulfills the necessity of his life task" (p. 57).

The notion of valuable possibilities is further endorsed by the theory of fundamental existential motivations and brings the concept of meaning into an even more concrete definition as, "The most worthwhile (the one of greatest value) and realistic possibility present in a given situation and one for which I feel I should decide." Existential meaning is therefore what is possible here and now, on the basis of facts and reality. What is possible for me may be what I need now, or what is the most pressing, valuable, or interesting alternative. To define and redefine this continually is an extremely complex task for which we possess an inner organ of perception capable of reducing this complexity to livable propor-tions: our sensitivity as well as our moral conscience.

Besides existential meaning there is an ontological meaning. This is the overall meaning in which I find myself and which does not depend on me. It is a philo-sophical and religious meaning; the meaning the creator of the world must have had in mind. I can perceive it through divination and in faith (cf. Längle, 1994b).

The importance of the ontological meaning for understanding life (cf. Längle, 2002, p. 60ff.) is illustrated simply by the following story Frankl once told. When the cathedral at Chartres was being built, a traveler came along and saw a man sitting at the roadside, cutting a stone. The traveller asked the man what he was doing there. "Don't you see," the man replied, "I am cutting stones!" Nonplussed the traveler continued on his way. Around the next bend, he saw another man, also cutting stones. Again he stopped and asked the same question. "I am cutting cornerstones," was the reply. Shaking his head, the traveler continued on once again. After a while he met a third man who was sitting in the dust and cutting stones just as the others had been. Resolutely the traveler walked up to him and asked: "Are you also cutting cornerstones?" The man looked up at him, wiped the sweat from his brow and said: "I am working at a cathedral."

References

Frankl, V. E. (1959). Grundriß der Existenzanalyse und Logotherapie. In V. E. Frankl, V. V. Gebsattel, & J. H. Schultz, *Handbuch der Neurosenlehre und Psychotherapie* (pp. 663-736). Munich, Germany: Urban & Schwarzenberg.

Frankl V. E. (1973). *The doctor and the soul: From psychotherapy to logotherapy.* New York: Random House.

Frankl V. E. (1982). *Ärztliche Seelsorge.* Vienna, Austria: Deuticke.

Frankl V. E. (1985). *Psychotherapy and existentialism: Selected papers on Logotherapy.* New York: Washington Square Press.

Längle A. (1992). Was bewegt den Menschen? Die existentielle Motivation der Person. *Existenzanalyse, 16*(3), 18-29.

Längle A. (1993). *Antrag auf Anerkennung der Existenzanalyse als psychotherapeutisches Fachspezifikum durch das Österreichische Bundesministerium für Gesundheit.* Unpublished manuscript, Vienna.

Längle A. (1994a). Lebenskultur-Kulturerleben. Die Kunst, Bewegendem zu begegnen. *Bulletin, 11*(1), 3-8.

Längle A. (1994b). Sinn-Glaube oder Sinn-Gespür? Zur Differenzierung von ontologischem und existentiellem Sinn in der Logotherapie. *Bulletin der GLE, 11*(2), 15-20.

Längle A. (1995). Logotherapie und Existenzanalyse - eine Standortbestimmung. *Existenzanalyse, 12*(1), 5-15.

Längle A. (1997). *Modell einer existenzanalytischen Gruppentherapie für die Suchtbehandlung.* Vienna, Austria: Facultas.

Längle A. (1998a). Verständnis und Therapie der Psychodynamik in der Existenzanalyse. *Existenzanalyse, 15*(1), 16-27.

Längle A. (1998b). Ursachen und Ausbildungsformen von Aggression im Lichte der Existenzanalyse. *Existenzanalyse, 15*(2), 4-12.

Längle A. (1998c). Lebenssinn und Psychofrust - zur existentiellen Indikation von Psychotherapie. In L. Riedel (Ed.), *Sinn und Unsinn der Psychotherapie* (pp. 105-124). Basel, Switzerland: Mandala.

Längle A. (1999a). Existenzanalyse—Die Zustimmung zum Leben finden. *Fundamenta Psychiatrica, 12*, 139-146.

Längle A. (1999b). Die existentielle Motivation der Person. *Existenzanalyse 16*(3), 18-29.

Längle A. (2001). Psychotherapie—Methode oder Spiritualität? Zum Verhältnis von Immanenz und Transzendenz am Beispiel der Existenzanalyse. In H. Schmidinger (Ed.), *Geist–Erfahrung–Leben. Spiritualität heute* (pp. 177-206). Innsbruck, Austria: Tyrolia.

Längle A. (2002). *Sinnvoll leben. Logotherapie als Lebenshilfe.* Freiburg, Germany: Herder.

Längle A. (2002, June). *Existential Fundamental Motivation.* Paper presented at the International Conference on Motivation WATM – 8th Workshop on Achievement and Task Motivation, Moscow.

Längle A. (2003). Wertberührung–Bedeutung und Wirkung des Fühlens in der existenzanalytischen Therapie. In A. Längle (Ed.), *Emotion und Existenz* (pp. 49-76). Vienna, Austria: Vienna University Press WUV-Facultas.

Yalom I. D. (1980). *Existential psychotherapy.* New York: Basic Books.

Editors' Note

Translation by Godela v. Kirchbach, English language consultation provided by Britt-Mari Sykes, University of Ottawa, and Christopher Wurm, Adelaide.

Meaning, Hermeneutics, and Ethics: Post-Postmodern Subjectivity

JENS ZIMMERMANN

Abstract

Starting from the assumption that theories of meaning and concepts of selfhood are inseparably interwoven, this paper takes the current philosophical turn toward ethics as a revival of humanistic concerns in order to argue for a formulation of selfhood as hermeneutical, ethical, and social that goes beyond both modernist and postmodernist views of the self. Drawing on the works of Michael Polanyi, Emmanuel Levinas, and John Macmurray, I argue that being human entails the creating of meaning, requires a personal-relational framework, and needs an irreducible ethical boundary. These essential elements of the self, however, require the readmittance of the religious into our discussion about what it means to be human.

After the linguistic turn, philosophical reflection has entered a new phase, the so-called ethical turn. After years of deconstructing both the human subject and its arrogant aspirations to divinity or absolute knowledge through metaphysics, postmodern philosophy has begun to realize that deconstructing the human self can become as dehumanizing as the god-like self of its metaphysical predecessors. Postmodernism has succeeded in replacing the Cartesian or scientific epistemology of absolute certainty, objective detached knowledge and its concomitant atomized self (cognito) with the equally dogmatic position that all knowledge is interpretation and that all interpretation is determined by economics of desire, power, and capital. The self becomes a mere construct, even if a required one for the sake of identity, an identity tenuously held together by the constantly shifting interpretation of the determinant forces of culture, economics, and power. A determinist self and the godlike self share the same problem: They are inhuman. We can neither live up to godhood ("I can know things with absolute certainty") nor does a determinist self truly allow for ethical accountability among ourselves ("Ideology made me do it"). Hence the renewed interest in reconstructing the human subject is driven by the need to secure a fixed aspect of the human self which may serve as an anchor for ethics; it is in effect a return to the ancient humanistic question: "What does it mean to be human?" Yet this return occurs after the deconstruction of modernist (and sometimes caricatures of) Cartesian subjectivity and thus offers real possibilities for a more holistic articulation of the human subject which no longer views the human self as a disembodied mind or soul but includes such constitutive factors of selfhood as emotions, agency, linguistic-cultural embeddedness, and sociality.

There are, to be sure, still unresolved issues that obstruct a truly open, inter-disciplinary dialogue on subjectivity. These concerns are voiced mainly in the natural sciences and philosophy. The scientist is afraid that introducing the role of emotions and cultural influences to our interpretation of reality will vanquish the achievements of objective knowledge and open the door for rampant subjectivism and relativism. Since the scientist knows that radical relativism does not work in the empirical world of research, he/she soon loses interest in discussions of subjectivity.

The philosopher, on the other hand, fears that a renewed discussion of subjectivity will permit metaphysical and, worst of all, theological presuppositions to be smuggled into the discussion and regress from the postmodern achievement of the closure of metaphysics and the consequent rejection of metanarratives. I want to address both of these concerns by drawing on the thought of three important thinkers of the twentieth century: Michael Polanyi, John Macmurray, and Emmanuel Levinas. All three of them point out the limit of scientific epistemology which presupposes a limited view of the self. Furthermore, all three figures indicate that the possible consequence of the return to ethics is a renewed discussion of religion: The question is not so much whether one chooses to be religious or secular but rather that both outlooks go wrong when relying on either an atomized or constructivist self. The way forward lies in the conception of the self as social, ethical, and rational, a conception of the human, which, on philosophical grounds, is inseparable from either the metaphysical or the religious.

MICHAEL POLANYI: TO BE HUMAN IS TO INTERPRET

Usually the German philosopher Martin Heidegger is given credit for dismantling Cartesian epistemology and overcoming its concomitant subject-object division through his existential hermeneutics. In his early lectures on the hermeneutics of facticity, Heidegger states that hermeneutics is not a method, nor a doctrine about understanding, but our very mode of existence:

> Hermeneutics is not an artificially devised mode of analysis which is
> imposed on Dasein and pursued out of curiosity.... The relationship
> between hermeneutics and facticity is not a relationship between the
> grasping of an object and the object grasped.... Rather, interpreting
> is itself a possible and distinctive of the character of the being of
> facticity. Interpreting is a being which belongs to the being of factical
> life itself. (p. 13)

Heidegger's insight is quite limited, for the reduction of understanding to self-understanding, as the "wakefulness of Dasein for itself" is problematical in its egocentrism. Heidegger's main point is, however, that we are homo interpretans, a hermeneutical being with the essential characteristic of meaning making. One who has expressed this idea much more clearly than Heidegger and who provides a corrective to Heidegger's definition of hermeneutics as self-understanding is the scientist and philosopher Michael Polanyi. In his last publication entitled *Meaning* (1975), Polanyi argues that the making of meaning is what makes us human, and that interpretation is not just self-understanding or the wakefulness of self, but is the only way of coming to terms with reality.

Polanyi's (1975) accomplishment is to refute science's monopoly of real, factual knowledge by showing how the same interpretive approach underlies both the human and the natural sciences. According to Polanyi, the Cartesian culture on whose soil the modern sciences matured, is obsessed with a desire for impersonal knowledge and absolute certainty. Modern scientific culture has inadvertently declared the human subject as split between knowledge (impersonal, objective facts) and belief (subjective, unverifiable faith). Polanyi argues, however, that all knowledge is personal, and that even the most rigorous scientific procedure requires personal commitment, imagination, and intuition. These human qualities are required for the production of meaning in any field, and together they form what Polanyi calls "tacit integration."

According to Polanyi (1975), knowledge consists in the ordering of facts or events (subsidiaries) within a greater framework (focus). In this act of integration, the subsidiary facts have meaning insofar as they contribute to the construction of the greater framework or goal.

Polanyi (1975) illustrates this "tacit integration" by describing a blind man probing an object with his stick. The man's coordinated bodily movements and even the stick are mere subsidiaries to the focus of determining the nature of the object under investigation. Polanyi makes two important points. First, the blind man "indwells" his stick. He cannot be critically aware of the stick while it serves him as a probe. If he does, his focal point is lost. For the duration of his investigation, he trusts and relies critically on the stick.

Secondly, the man's determinations of the possible nature of the object's nature move in a hermeneutical circle. His imagination and intuition, based on past experiences, project a hypothesis which is subsequently verified or corrected by his probing. Such, Polanyi (1975) argues, is the nature of all knowing, both in the sciences and in the humanities. Contrary to scientist's popular self-image, this act of integration and the validity of a cast of hypotheses depend not on a formal, empirically verifiable procedure but on an educated hunch: "It is only the imagination that can direct our attention to a target that is as yet unsupported by subsidiaries" (p. 57). Polanyi calls these educated hunches "perceptive anticipations," and believes that this anticipatory integration occurs not only in our interpretation of linguistic utterances but is "actually found at work in every deliberate human action" (p. 59). Moreover, intuition fueled by the imagination is informed by hope and passionate commitment. Even the scientist is always personally involved and never detached from his project. Polanyi thus confirms the philosophical insight of Hans-Georg Gadamer that personal involvement and prejudgments are not to be avoided but form the very canvas on which we create meaning. We should now be able to see that all our knowledge is inescapably indeterminate (Polanyi, 1975, p. 61).

In sum, all processes of knowing (including those of science) in no way resemble an impersonal achievement of detached objectivity. They are rooted throughout (from our selection of a problem to the verification of a discovery) in personal acts of tacit integration and not in explicit operations of logic. Scientific inquiry is accordingly a dynamic exercise of the imagination and is rooted in commitments and beliefs about the nature of things. According to Polanyi (1975), the very structure of knowing demands personal involvement: We dwell in the subsidiaries (in our theories, beliefs, commitments, etc.) and bring them to bear focally on an interpretation. In fact, the projection of an interpretation (a coherence) requires that the subsidiaries remain subordinate to the greater goal. When we bring the subsidiaries into focal awareness, the greater paradigm is lost and integration becomes impossible. Thus, the scientific ideal of detached knowledge, where each single fact is not only verified by empirical evidence but also held in critical abeyance while formulating a hypothesis, is not only illusory but actually undesirable because of its opposition to how perception and scientific discovery actually work. As Polanyi (1975) puts it,

> Scientific inquiry is accordingly a dynamic exercise of the imagination
> and is rooted in commitments and beliefs about the nature of things.

It is a fiduciary act. It is far from skepticism itself. It depends upon
firm beliefs. Nor should it ever give rise to skepticism. Its ideal is the
discovery of coherence and meaning in that which we believe exists;
it is not the reduction of everything to a meaningless jumble of atoms
or accidentally achieved equilibrium of forces. (p. 63)

Thus science itself is merely another expression of our basic hermeneutical
desire to make sense of the world around us. To be human means to create meaning,
to unite the fragmentary elements of our existence into a coherent story; whether
this story is expressed in scientific, religious or artistic terms, all these forms of
human self-expression are an attempt to interpret human existence within an
objective reality.

Polanyi's work shows that the creation of meaning requires a meta-narrative.
Interpretive metanarratives are moral ideals because through them we try to understand how and to what end reality works. Hence the interpretation of facts and
experiences do not require an amoral point of view but involvement of personal
moral ideals and beliefs. Polanyi (1975) points out the great danger in the otherwise well-meant desire for scientific detachment and amorality. Man is a moral
animal and needs to fill and act on his inclination for moral ideals. The scientific
requirement of moral detachment has led to the suspicion of all moral ideals and
sentiments (nihilism). In fact, however, moral ideals were simply replaced with
material purposes. When nihilists become political activists for whatever cause,
their homeless moral passions are poured into a purely materialistic framework
of purposes: "The moral needs of man, denied expression in terms of ideals, are
injected into a system of naked power to which they impart the force of a blind
moral passion" (p. 17). For example, the scientific enterprise is only possible
under the assumed ideal of a cosmological, universal tendency toward unfolding
meaning.[1] Thus, when scientists insist on the impersonal and value-free knowledge
which supposedly sets their discipline apart from the human sciences, they not
only deny the very structure of their own research but they also pave the way for
the destruction of humanity because the scientific myth of impersonal knowledge
leaves no room for ethics. Polanyi (1975) wrote: "As long as science remains the
ideal of knowledge, and detachment the ideal of science, ethics cannot be secured
from complete destruction by skeptical doubt" (p. 29). A scientistic—and hence
naturalistic—worldview collaborates with nihilism in suspecting all moral ideals
as illusory. Polanyi argues that the most disastrous ideologies in the scientific age,
Nazism, Stalinism, and Communism, have thrived on this naturalistic naiveté. In
the absence of a natural moral order, homeless moral passions were poured into

the purely immanent, materialistic framework of purposes provided by Hitler, Stalin, and Lenin.

Polanyi's (1975) indictment of scientism as dehumanizing applies with equal force to the postmodern denial of metanarratives. In Polanyi's terms, the dogmatic dismissal of frameworks of coherence with universal intent is inhuman, for such dismissal effectively prevents tacit integration. Both postmodernism and scientism alike focus on the subsidiaries, with the only difference that these subsidiaries are facts in the sciences and personal, or at best communally valid, stories in the post-modern context. The effect, however, is the same. Even though in postmodernism we are allowed to create meaning, the universal intent of our interpretation of reality is denied. Thus, what makes meaning meaningful, namely, its claim as an interpretation of a universally valid truth claim is thus condemned to opinion. If Polanyi is correct, the very virtue of postmodernism, the denial of metanarratives in order to avoid totalization and oppression, turns out to be a dehumanizing vice. So we need metanarratives, but what kind of ethical restraints can prevent them from forcing the particular individual into a totalizing metanarrative? Are not ethical norms themselves oppressive? The Jewish thinker Emmanuel Levinas has given a great deal of thought to this problem.

EMMANUEL LEVINAS: TO BE HUMAN IS TO BE ETHICAL

The validity of Levinas' (1998) claim that the human self is primarily ethical in nature depends on his interpretation of Western philosophy. In its obsession with self-understanding and the concomitant movement towards self-consciousness, Western philosophical thought equates the conscious self with activity. The "I" is always the initiating agent, aiming at control and systematization and thus denying the primacy of the subject (p. 59). Levinas (1969/1998) believes that all of Western philosophy from its beginnings to the present age is premised on an "imperialism of the same" because it defines knowledge as dependent on totality and egology (p. 39). Things can only be known to the backdrop of a neutral, totalizing matrix, whether this be Spinoza's substance or Heidegger's Being, and are recognized only as representations to the respective meaning-giving framework of a knowing ego. In this economy of the same, the self represents things to itself; it com-prehends (French: prendre—to grasp), that is, it tries to grasp and represent to itself other beings in their totality. Western philosophy is thus obsessed with control: The positing of the non-I depends on economy of the same over the other and denies the transcendent element required for our mutual responsibility and the recognition of difference.

Much like Martin Heidegger, Levinas thus advances another panoramic view of Western philosophy: Against Heidegger's portrayal of Western thought as the forgetfulness of Being, Levinas characterizes philosophical history from its inception to the present as "egology," or, more trenchantly, as atheism. Both terms describe our equation of the knowing subject with mind or consciousness, insisting that all knowledge and understanding proceeds from the self and its attempt to grasp things and thereby excludes genuine input of knowledge from the outside. While Levinas is not interested in revelatory religion in the commonly understood sense either, he wants to preserve the radical otherness or alterity that it conveys. For Levinas the human other (l'Autrui), like God, is irreducible to an interpretive theme and encounters me as exterior, radical otherness, a master who teaches me in a personal face-to-face relation.

Western philosophy, by contrast, tends to dehumanize the Other by objectifying him. In rather colonial fashion, we like to conquer things by knowing them, rather than attending to their self-disclosure, letting the other thing or person really speak to us by "caressing it" as a lover would the object of her love rather than interrogating it (Levinas, 1969/1998, p. 258). Such megalomania leaves no room for revelation in either the biblical or the philosophical sense. In light of this development, Levinas's goal is to recover the idea of infinity inherent in every human being. He believes that already in Plato, but particularly in Descartes, we find the notion that each self contains the idea of infinity whose very existence indicates transcendence and breaks the egocentric mode that stands in the way of the ethical relation.

This infinity, argues Levinas (1969/1998), is the presence of the Other in me, his ethical demand on me. Only in such a way can we achieve the necessary balance of a unique self that is at the same time open and accountable to others. The irreducible individuality of the I, rather than its subsumption into a totality of objective morality, also calls for "a privileged place with regard to responsibilities for which no one can replace me and from which no one can release me. To be unable to shirk: this is the I" (p. 245).

Levinas reminds us that philosophy is eminently practical: How we conceive of selfhood determines how we act. His primary illustration for this truth is the fundamental ontology of Martin Heidegger who is often credited with dismantling the modernist subject and whose thought has greatly shaped postmodern thought. Levinas, too, had drunk deeply at the well of Heidegger's criticism of Western metaphysics and upheld its claim to have uncovered our original rationality and thereby achieved a turn away from the objectifying explanatory approach of positivist philosophy toward a concrete philosophy of existence (Altwegg, 1988).

Heidegger's commitment to Nazi movement, however, shocked Levinas into a more critical appraisal of Heidegger's thought. Levinas writes: "I was shaken in my conviction that an unbridgeable gap eternally separates the insane and criminal hatred, which evil proclaimed on the pages of *Mein Kampf*, from the intellectual acuity and extreme analytical virtuosity of *Being and Time*" (Altwegg, 1998, p. 110). Levinas has come to see what he considers the most profound philosophical effort of the twentieth century not merely as compatible with evil but as part of the dehumanizing legacy of the twentieth century.[2]

Levinas sees the principal connection between Heidegger's philosophy and Hitler's totalitarian regime in shared view of the self as object. In Heidegger's fundamental ontology, the subject still remains an object of thought that is to be understood. Other human beings are reduced to objects of understanding that are situated within the horizon of being and thus placed beyond the particular. In other words, while Heidegger attempts to deconstruct Cartesian metaphysics, his thought still follows the Western philosophical tradition obsessed with self-understanding and a movement toward self-consciousness.

Still unable to break free from Western thought, Heidegger cannot handle real difference in others. Heidegger's very decentering of the modern Cartesian subject subordinates the relations between beings to the totalizing structures of being, "metaphysics to ontology, the existentiell to the existential." Levinas (1998) argues that the notion of understanding as disclosure in Heidegger, as a letting be, collapses the differences between a human being and any other object (p. 5). Against Heidegger, Levinas insists that the human subject is not something disclosed by Being, but is its own individual being who reveals himself only through the address of discourse. Consequently, not the impassive contemplation of Being, but the active discourse motivated by sympathy and love should characterize our interhuman relations.[3] Even Heidegger's sociality, his Miteinandersein, rests on an ontological relation in which mutual understanding is predicated upon the disclosing horizon of Being. For Levinas (1998), such a relation does not recognize individuality; it is just one more system which assimilates the individual to the reflexive consciousness. In the proper face-to-face relation, by contrast, the Other circumscribes a unique and passive subjectivity which can only disclose itself to me through careful and respectful address (p. 7).

Levinas (1998) concludes his critique of Heidegger with his famous call to ground human relations not in ontology but in ethics:

> The relation to the other is therefore not ontology. This bond with
> the other is not reducible to the representation of the other, but to his
> invocation, and [this bond] in which invocation is not preceded by an
> understanding I call religion. The essence of discourse is prayer. (p. 7)

Against any totalizing discourses, Levinas wants to affirm the human by setting it apart as holy and sacred. Ethics exists prior to reflection, and ethics requires transcendent grounding from which it can break open totalities (p. 57). The iron cage of abstract, and thus inhuman, terminology resulting from philosophy's reduction of the self to consciousness requires Levinas' use of religious conceptuality in expressing his idea of ethics as first philosophy. Already in his early work, *Totality and Infinity*, Levinas (1969/1998) implies a religious dimension of ethics by anchoring the transcendent self in God as the ultimate Other. For Levinas, the face of the other person bears the trace of God and as such grounds his otherness as an ethical demand.[4] True humanism, according to Levinas, requires a Messianic, eschatological transcendent dimension that has been neglected by Western philosophical and scientific thought. The philosopher Simon Critchley (1999) gives the best summary of Levinas' humanism:

> Levinas' point is that the humanity of the human signifies
> precisely through this inability to be autarchic, where the subject is
> overwhelmed by an alterity that it is unable to master. The subject is
> no longer the self-positing origin of the world; it is a hostage to the
> other. Humanism should not begin from the datum of the human
> being as an end-in-itself and the foundation for all knowledge,
> certainty, and value; rather, the humanity of the human is defined by
> its service to the other. Levinasian ethics is a humanism, but it is a
> humanism of the other human being. (p. 67)

Levinas' demand for an ethical self strikes at the root of both modern cultural and philosophical individualism: Intellectual, social, and economic egoism is untenable in light of an ethically constituted self. Before we think or act we are already subject to an ethical demand from our fellow human beings.

Levinas appears on the philosophical scene like an Old Testament prophet, pronouncing the ethical demand with a gravity and urgency reminiscent of Isaiah's demands for justice. His insistence of the self's passivity as hostage to the Other's demand gives rise to equal concerns regarding my own freedom. Moreover, Levinas' account seems to bypass human reason with its unequivocal, prereflective demand of the other in me. The ethical relation takes place at the level of sensibility, not at the level of consciousness; "the ethical subject is a sensible subject, not a conscious subject" (Critchley, 1999, p. 65). A more nuanced account of the Other is offered by the British philosopher John Macmurray and his concept of the self as person in relation.

JOHN MACMURRAY: TO BE HUMAN IS TO BE IN RELATION

In his Gifford Lectures, John Macmurray (1961) argues that being human is to be a person in relation and that viewing the self as an isolated, mental construct is wrong both biologically and philosophically. On the level of biology, Macmurray argues against the still popular view of Homo sapiens as rational animal. He contends that for too long have we let Greek thought govern our ideas of the human. Aristotle defined the human in analogy to his observation of plant and animal life as an organic entity which unfolds in its adaptation to the environment from an instinctual to a rational mode of existence. Macmurray objects that this view inverts the nature of the self as person. We are, of course, organisms, but our organic nature is not what makes us human. Being a person in relation does. The organic aspect is a negative which is subservient to the personal and to which we can descend from the category of the personal. There is, however,

> no way for thought to ascend from the organic to the personal. The organic perception of man excludes, by its very nature, all the characteristics of human beings. To include them, we must change our categories and start afresh from the beginning. (Macmurray, 1961, p. 47)

According to Macmurray (1961), we are genetically motivated from infancy by the desire for personal communication rather than by the mechanics of environmental adaptation. A baby does not ascend to rationality but requires it from the beginning because its life depends upon rational activity (p. 47). Macmurray concludes: "We are not organisms, but persons. The nexus of relations which unites us in a human society is not organic but personal. Human behavior cannot be understood but only caricatured if it is presented as adaptation to the environment" (p. 46).

Instead, humans are first and foremost made to be cared for; we are designed for communication. Communication sets the human apart from the plant and animal life and is fundamental in all personal experience and determines its form. From the need to communicate derive our personal motivations to action: love, fear, and hatred. We require love, we fear to be isolated from community, and we respond with hatred to those who deny us communication. Human rationality is thus motivated by emotions, which presuppose a human Other so that our actions motivated by these emotions are incomplete without reference to a personal Other. Likewise, knowledge is from the very first knowledge of the personal Other with whom I am in communication, who responds to my cry and who cares for me. According to Macmurray, this emotional reason "is the very starting point of all knowledge and is presupposed at every stage of its subsequent development" (1961, p. 76).

Besides the dehumanizing organic analogy bequeathed on us by science, philosophy has handed down to us an equally distorting image of the self as mind. Macmurray (1991) believes that just as science mistook a negative aspect of humanness, the organic, for our actual positive human nature, so philosophy erred when it considered the thinking self as the starting point of apperception. Macmurray objects that the self is not a mind but primordially an agent: "The Self has its being only in its agency, and its reflective activities are but negative aspects of this agency. The Self as "the Mind," which is the Self as non-agent, is a non-entity" (p. 15).

The wrong starting point of the solipsistic thinker, unimplicated in the dynamic relatedness of our existence, soon transforms itself unwittingly into an existential solipsism: "We are imprisoned in an 'egocentric predicament,' and there is no way out. We are committed to explaining knowledge without reference to action" (Macmurray, 1961, p. 21). This disembodied view of the self leads to all kinds of unnecessary philosophical problems and inventions. It creates, for example, the infamous philosophical problem of other minds, a non-issue if the "I do" precedes the "I think." It also engendered the "faculty psychology" of mind and will, a dualism which Enlightenment thinkers tried to overcome by positing a common rationality: "If we think logically, we think the same thing in the same connection; if we act rationally, we all do the same thing in the same circumstances" (p. 19). This philosophical sleight of hand, however, conceals any real substantive differences by forcing every person into the same pattern of logic and reason. These differences are then relegated into the realm of the irrational and psychological so that we may escape into "a logical heaven, where error and evil cease to trouble us, where the clash of our mutual contradictions is stilled and the struggle of our antagonistic purposes resolved" (p. 20). Once the self has been split, philosophy has to invent a universal rational mind in order to find common rational ground. Objective truth thus becomes pure access to substantive universal reason which demands in turn an isolated, reflective existence through the negation of personal prejudices, emotions, and the particular historical existence of other selves.

What, however, does objective truth actually mean? It certainly does not mean impersonal knowledge nor does it mean scientific knowledge. We have come to think of science as objective and equate impersonal knowledge with truth. Yet, the term "objective" does not mean true, for objective statements are often false. Nor is the term "scientific" synonymous with correct for "the tracks of science are littered with scientific theories which have been abandoned as incorrect. If our generation tends to associate truth with science and objectivity, the association rests upon no logical implication, but only upon an emotional prejudice in favour of science" (Macmurray, 1961, p. 31). We can, and indeed we must, for reasons of analysis and reflection, look at people impersonally.[5] The person as object is, however, merely an abstraction from our true human nature as persons in relation. Our misunderstanding of what constitutes objectivity is influenced by another commonly accepted dualism, a dualism stemming from the Stoics' distinction between reason and the passions which tries to purge the emotional involvement of our actions. Here, reason is commonly associated with the mind and passion with human agency and the will. We thus contrast two forms of behavior: "The one rational and objective, the other subjective or emotional. The first has an intention, but no motive; the second a motive but no intention, since the motive fully accounts for the behavior which flows from it as a cause determines its effect" (p. 32). Objective knowledge is deemed free while subjective knowledge is deemed determinate and explicable through cause and effect.

Macmurray (1961) believes that exorcising "the ghost of the old faculty psychology which still haunts our philosophies" with its metaphysical fictions of mind and will allows for a more holistic conception of reason: "We can insist that all our activities, whether practical or theoretical, have their motives as well as their intentions, and are sustained by an emotional attitude" (p. 33). Hence human reason becomes, "the capacity to act and only in a secondary and derivative sense the capacity to think, that is to say, to pursue a merely theoretical intention" (p. 26). In this way rationality encompasses the entire scope of our emotions, motivations, and historical-cultural situatedness; the dualism of a rational and an empirical self disappears (p. 27).

Macmurray's (1961) relational self thus defines objectivity as relational knowledge. His concept of emotional reason is nothing less than a hermeneutic stance which defines us as human by replacing an erroneous instrumental view of reality with apperception motivated by love. Genuine love is never introspective and selfish. Hence emotional reason simply means being open to reality, "maintaining and increasing our sensitiveness to the world outside irrespective of whether it gives us pleasure or pain" (p. 51).

CONCLUSION

Clearly, meaning is bound up with our conceptions of selfhood. When the self disappears, meaning also vanishes. We enter the new millennium after passing through the modernist view of the self as autonomous and the postmodern dismantling of these very aspirations to epistemological divinity. Both views, however, are detrimental in their dehumanization of meaning: by making meaning an impersonal affair of scientific and universal reason, the one empties meaning of its humanness and makes it effectually meaningless. By denying metanarratives and universal aspects of humanness, the other deprives us of our human need for communication and meaning making in its very advocacy of tolerance, plurality, and difference. Ironically, while modern and postmodern conceptions of selfhood were motivated by their noble quest for human freedom from oppression, they both end up by denying our humanity.

It is their failure, however, which allows us to conceive of the self and meaning in a more human way. In light of our examination, the self emerges as neither an individual consciousness nor as a mere construct but as a socially constituted, relational entity whose effort to make sense of the world is grounded in its primary need of communication. To be human not only entails meaning making, for which metanarratives are required (Polanyi's argument) but meaning can only exist within a social context and its inherent ethical demand of the other person (Levinas' point). For human knowledge to be objective, and objective should mean knowledge that is true to its object, it must correspond to who we are as persons. To be objective and rational hence means to include all that makes us persons (Macmurray's conclusion).

Such a view of rationality as openness necessarily includes the religious as the primary source for interpretive frameworks of ethical and social quality.[6] Macmurray, for example, believes that the whole nature of religion is bound up in the assertion that all men are equal and that fellowship is the only relation between persons (p. 205). Religion is the highest form of such fellowship. Similarly, Levinas' ethical demand is essentially a religious demand. Thus as we set the tone for discussions of our selfhood and meaning—in short, of our humanity—this desire for a new humanism should not neglect the religious, an essential element of our subjectivity.

References

Altwegg, J. (Ed.). (1988). *Die Heidegger-Kontroverse*. Frankfurt am Main, Germany: Athenäum.

Critchley, S. (1999). *Ethics, politics, subjectivity*. London: Verso.

Heidegger, M. (1999). *Ontology – The hermeneutics of facticity* (John Van Buren, Trans.). Bloomington, IN: Indiana University Press.

Levinas, E. (1969/1998). *Totality and infinity*. Pittsburgh, PA: Duquesne University Press.

Levinas, E. (1998). *Entre nous*. New York: Columbia University Press.

Macmurray, J. (1992). *Reason and emotion*. London: Faber and Faber.

Macmurray, J. (1961). *Persons in relation*. London: Faber and Faber.

Polanyi, M. (1975). *Meaning*. Chicago: University of Chicago Press.

Polanyi, M., & Prosch, H. (1977). *Meaning*. Chicago: University of Chicago Press.

Endnotes

1. "We are thus able to think that real discovery in science is possible for us because we are guided by an intuition of a more meaningful organization of our knowledge of nature provided by the slope of deepening meaning in the whole field of potential meanings surrounding us" (Polanyi, 1975, p. 178).

2. Levinas is convinced of Heidegger's ongoing agreement with Nazi politics, or at least of his nonrepentance concerning his Nazi involvement by three evidences. First, even after his separation from the movement did he continue to wear the swastika. Second, in his last Spiegel interview, Heidegger remains inexplicably silent about the Holocaust and its implications for his philosophy. Levinas judges this silence to be "evidence of the soul's complete closedness [Verschlossenheit] toward sensitivity and like a condoning of the horrible" (Altwegg, 1988, p. 104). Third, this insensitivity is confirmed by an analogy Heidegger made between technology and the cremation of Jews in his unpublished Bremen lectures of 1949 (*Das Gestell*): "Farming is now a motorised industry of nourishment [Ernahrungsindustrie], in principle the same as the fabrication of corpses in Gas chambers and death camps [Vernichtungslagern], the same as the blockade and starvation of countries, the same as the manufacturing of nuclear bombs [Wasserstoffbomben]."

3. Levinas writes: "Is our relation with the other a letting be? Is not the independence of the other achieved through his or her role as one who is addressed? Is the person to whom we speak understood beforehand in his being? Not at all. The other is not first an object of understanding and then an interlocutor. The two relations are merged. In other words, addressing the other is inseparable from understanding the other" (Levinas, 1998, p. 6).

4. In fact, one way of understanding Levinasian ethics is to see them as the Jewish version of the later Christian concept of human dignity as grounded in the imago dei.

5. Here Macmurray offers a needed qualification to Levinas, who seems to regard any objectification of the other human being as dehumanizing.

6. Of the three basic expressions of human rationality, science, art, and religion, Macmurray believes religion to be the highest form. Scientific reason remains abstract, and artistic expression remains too individualistic. Religion describes our interpersonal relations. According to Macmurray (1992), reason is revealed most strongly in the religious because here reason "reveals itself in the capacity to go beyond individual prejudice, bias and self interest, and to think and act in terms of a reality that is beyond ourselves and bigger than ourselves" (p. 202).

The Role of Hardiness and Religiosity in Depression and Anger

SALVATORE R. MADDI

As personal stances out of which interaction with the world is conducted, hardiness and religiosity have certain similarities and differences. The major similarity is that both personal stances are spiritual, rather than material. The spiritual nature of religiosity is obvious, as it leads the person to think in terms of a higher order of meaning that emphasizes honesty, justice, courage, and other values that transcend mere materialism. Although perhaps less obvious, hardiness is also spiritual rather than material; it provides the courage and motivation to find positive meaning, stay involved, keep trying, and grow in wisdom regardless of whether one's life is easy or difficult (cf. Maddi, 1986, 2001, 2002, June).

The major difference between hardiness and religiosity is in the source of spirituality and direction. In religiosity, the source and direction for spirituality is some supernatural order, typically a view of god or gods who have responsibility for the universe. In contrast, the source and direction of spirituality in hardiness is the person's subjective struggle to interpret, order, and influence experiences so as to provide meaning in an otherwise indifferent universe.

Despite the difference just specified, both hardiness and religiosity are considered resources in maintaining and enhancing performance and health in whatever circumstances come your way (e.g., Atchley, 1997; Bergin, 1983; Bartone, 1999; Clark, Maddi, 2002; Maddi & Kobasa, 1984; Maddi & Hess, 1992). In particular, these spiritual resources are most protective as stressful circumstances mount. The process whereby performance and health are maintained and enhanced under stress is similar for both hardiness and religiosity. Specifically, both constitute a set of beliefs that provide the courage and motivation to cope effectively and participate in socially supportive interactions.

There are now rapidly growing bodies of research evidence showing that hardiness and religiosity each does indeed maintain and enhance performance and health under stress (e.g., Atchley, 1997; Bartone, 1999; Bergin, 1999; Clark, Friedman, & Martin, 1999; Fitchett, Rybarczyk, DeMarco, & Nicholas, 1999; Fry, 2000; Genia, 1998; Idler & Kasl, 1997; King, King, Fairbank, Keane, & Adams, 1998; Kobasa, Maddi, Puccetti, & Zola, 1986; Koenig, Cohen, Blazer, Pieper, Meador, Shelp et al., 1998; Maddi & Hess, 1992; Maddi & Khoshaba, 1994; Maddi & Kobasa, 1984; Maddi, Wadhwa, & Haier, 1996; Maddi, 2001, 2002, 2002, June; Matthews, McCullough, Larson, Koenig, Swyers, & Milano, 1998; McCullough, Hoyt, Larson, Koenig, & Thoresen, 2000; McIntosh, Silver, & Wortman, 1993; Wallace & Forman, 1998; Westman, 1990; Weibe & McCallum, 1986). Interestingly though, there does not appear to have been much effort thus far to compare the effects of hardiness and religiosity. So, several colleagues and I (Maddi, Brow, Khoshaba, & Vaitkus, 2003) decided to study the roles of hardiness and religiosity in depression and anger. It seemed clear to us that both hardiness and religiosity should provide people with the courage and motivation to cope and interact effectively, so as to avoid depression and anger. In this, we were conceptualizing depression and anger as signs of negative meaning, or meaninglessness resulting from ineffective coping and nonsupportive interactions. More exploratory in our minds was the question of what the combination, or interaction, of hardiness and religiosity would show.

RELATIONSHIP OF HARDINESS AND RELIGIOSITY

We were able to collect relevant data on 53 senior U.S. Army officers attending a one-year supplementary educational program at an appropriate training facility. They completed relevant questionnaires. Needless to say, among the variables assessed were religiosity and hardiness.

Religiosity was assessed by the Duke Religion Index (DRI), which comprises five rating-scale items concerning organizational, nonorganizational, and intrinsic religiosity (Sherman, Plante, Simonton, Adams, Harbison, & Burris, 2000). Organizational religiosity involves the public practice of your religion, e.g., attending congregational ceremonies. Nonorganizational religiosity involves the private observance of your religion, e.g., saying prayers at night. Intrinsic religiosity involves incorporating your religion into all aspects of your life. At least one study (Sherman et al., 2000) has reported adequate internal-consistency reliability for this test. Numerous studies have shown this test's validity (cf. Sherman et al., 2000). In our study, the DRI items showed intercorrelations ranging from .39 to .85, and correlations with total religiosity ranging from .71 to .86. For our study, the

DRI was supplemented by two additional rating-scale items addressing intrinsic religiosity. That these additional items are compatible with the Duke test is shown by intercorrelations of items ranging from .46 to .85, and by correlations with the total DRI score of .88 and .93.

Hardiness was assessed by the Personal Views Survey III (PVS III), comprised of 30 rating-scale items concerning the attitudes of commitment, control, and challenge (Maddi & Khoshaba, 1998). Those strong in commitment believe that staying involved with the events and people in their world is the best way to find meaning and satisfaction. Those strong in control believe that continuing to struggle to influence the outcomes that are going on increases the likelihood of having an effect on them. Those strong in challenge believe that it is most fulfilling to continue to learn and to grow in wisdom from one's experiences, whether they are positive or negative. As to test reliability, several studies (e.g., Maddi & Khoshaba, 1998) have shown the PVS III to have adequate internal consistency and stability. There are by now numerous studies attesting to this test's validity (cf, Maddi & Khoshaba, 1998). In our study, commitment, control, and challenge showed the expected intercorrelations with each other, and high correlations with total hardiness.

In our study, there was a moderate, positive correlation between hardiness and religiosity. This statistically significant correlation indicates that the two measures share some variance, but are hardly the same thing. Going further, the total religiosity score showed significant positive correlations with the commitment and control components of hardiness, but no correlation with the challenge component. This suggests that while remaining involved with and attempting to influence the world around you is consistent with religiosity, continuing to grow in personal wisdom through interpretations of one's experiences may be too individualistic for religious convictions.

RELATIONSHIPS WITH DEPRESSION AND ANGER

The participants in our study also completed the Center for Epidemiological Studies Depression Scale (CESD), a 20-item questionnaire designed by Radloff (1977) to measure depressive symptomatology in the general population. Although there is no currently agreement on subscales for this test, research shows that it assesses depressed mood, feelings of guilt and worthlessness, helplessness and hopelessness, psychomotor retardation, loss of appetite, and sleep disturbance (Hann, Winter, & Jacobsen, 1999). Internal consistency and stability estimates for the CESD have been adequate, and there is also evidence of its convergent and divergent validity (Radloff, 1977; Hann et al., 1999).

Also administered was the State-Trait Anger Expression Inventory (STAXI), a 44-item, multidimensional measure developed by Spielberger (Impara & Plake, 1998). This test assesses state anger (reactions to specific events), trait anger (general disposition), angry temperament (expressing anger with little or no provocation), angry reaction (reaction to criticism), anger-in (withholding expressions of anger), anger-out (directing anger toward others), anger control (how frequently one attempts to control anger), and anger expression (how frequently one expresses anger). Bishop and Quah (1998) have reported adequate internal consistency and stability reliability for this test, along with better validity than another measure of anger.

In our study, we found that both hardiness and religiosity were negatively correlated with depression at about the same moderate, though significant, level. Further, hardiness was negatively related at a statistically significant level to anger-in, trait anger, anger expression, angry reaction, and total anger. In contrast, religiosity showed only one significant finding, and that was a negative relationship with anger-in. This suggests that hardiness is a better protection against anger in general than is religiosity.

Next, to determine the unique contribution of hardiness and religiosity to depression and the anger variables that yielded significant correlations, multiple regression analyses were run. Data were controlled for gender, age, and race. Hardiness and religiosity were centered for purposes of evaluating their possible interaction.

The regression analysis examined both the main and interaction effects of hardiness and religiosity on depression and the relevant anger variables. When hardiness and religiosity are purified of the effects of each other, only hardiness shows a significant main effect of negatively predicting depression. This suggests that the previously mentioned negative correlation between religiosity and depression is due to the degree to which the DRI measures hardiness.

Further, in the regression analysis, the interaction of hardiness and religiosity is also a significant negative predictor of depression. In an attempt to understand this finding, we graphed the relationship between religiosity and depression for subgroups high, medium, and low in hardiness. For participants low in hardiness, a negative relationship exists between religion and depression. Participants medium in hardiness showed a similar, but less strong pattern. But, for participants high in hardiness, the relationship between religiosity and depression appears to have diminished. Their level of depression remains relatively unchanged over all levels of religiosity and, interestingly, they score highest in depression among the three hardiness subgroups when religiosity is high. Overall, the findings suggest that hardiness is a better negative predictor of depression than is religiosity, and that the latter may even have a paradoxical effect when hardiness is high.

Regression analyses also point to the greater role played by hardiness than religiosity in anger. Significant main effects for hardiness, but not for religiosity, are shown for the negative prediction of anger-in, trait anger, anger expression, angry reaction, and total anger. This suggests the greater role of hardiness than religiosity in the avoidance and control of anger. Significant interaction effects appear only for anger-in, and angry reaction. As was done for depression, we graphed the relationship between religiosity and these anger variables for subsamples low, medium, and high in hardiness. The outcome was similar to that of depression; namely, there appeared to be a negative relationship between religiosity and anger variables for participants low in hardiness, but this trend disappears, and even reverses, as hardiness increases. Overall, hardiness emerges as more important than religiosity in keeping anger from developing, and under control if it develops.

MECHANISMS WHEREBY HARDINESS AND RELIGIOSITY HAVE THEIR EFFECTS

The findings mentioned thus far indicate that hardiness may be more effective than religiosity in helping people to avoid depression and anger. This highlights the importance of scrutinizing the relative power of hardiness and religiosity in leading people toward effectiveness in coping with stressful circumstances, and deriving social support from interactions.

Relevant to investigating this, our sample of officers completed questionnaires concerning their coping and social interaction efforts, and their experiences of stress and strain. As to coping, the participants completed all the items of the COPE test (Carver, Scheier & Weintraub, 1989), except those referring to one's religious beliefs. The utilized items of this test were organized into two scales, one of transformational (or problem-solving) coping, and the other of regressive (or denial and avoidance) coping (Maddi & Hightower, 1999). These two scales have been shown, in one study (Maddi & Hightower, 1999), to have adequate internal consistency reliability and construct validity. Transformational coping should be more effective than regressive coping in helping people avoid depression and anger. As to patterns of social interaction, the participants were administered items based on Moos' (1979) questionnaire charting the social support experienced at work and in private life. Used in numerous studies, this questionnaire appears to have adequate reliability and validity.

As to the stressfulness of ongoing circumstances, items were included that tap the subjective experience of both acute stresses (i.e., disruptive changes) and chronic stresses (i.e., continuing mismatches between what you want and what you get). Used in several previous studies (c.f., Maddi, 2002; Maddi & Kobasa, 1984), this stress measure has shown adequate construct validity. Strain is the organism's arousal response to stresses, and was measured using the total score from the Symptom Check List – 90 (Derogatis, Lipman, Rickels, Uhlenhuth & Covi, 1974). This approach has shown adequate reliability and validity in previous studies.

The bivariate correlations of hardiness and religiosity with these variables showing possible mechanisms indicate that hardiness is, as expected, negatively related to stress and strain, and positively related to transformational coping, work support, and private life support. In contrast, while religiosity is negatively related to stress, strain, and regressive coping, it is unrelated to transformation coping, work support, and private life support.

To clarify these relationships further, multiple regression analyses were conducted in order to purify hardiness and religiosity of their effects on each other, and to study the interaction of these two predictors. These analyses show that there are main effects for hardiness, but not for religiosity, on stress, strain, transformational coping, work support, and private life support. The only significant interaction effect is for strain, and there are no significant effects for regressive coping. Graphing the significant interaction effect for strain leads to results similar to what was found for depression and anger. Specifically, when hardiness is low, religiosity protects against strain. But when hardiness is high, religiosity appears positively related to strain. Overall, it is hardiness, and not religiosity, that demonstrates the expected mechanisms that would lead to protection against such performance and health problems as depression and anger.

THE RELATIVE POWER OF HARDINESS AND RELIGIOSITY

The results of our study show rather clearly that it is hardiness and not religiosity that encourages effective coping and social support interactions such that stress, strain, depression, and anger are minimized. In the regression analyses, it is hardiness and not religiosity that produces main effects on the dependent variables.

Further, the significant interaction effect of hardiness and religiosity on depression, anger-in, angry reactions, and strain deserves further attention here. The graphing of the relationship between religiosity and the dependent variable for participants low, medium, or high in hardiness produces an invariant pattern. When hardiness is low, there is a negative relationship between religiosity and the dependent variables. This suggests that religiosity can be helpful in the absence of hardiness. But when hardiness is high, the relationship becomes paradoxically positive between religiosity and the dependent variables! Perhaps there is a conflict between hardiness and religiosity such that, when both are strong, strain, depression, and anger follow. After all, hardiness emphasizes an individual struggle to find meaning and fulfillment, whereas religiosity emphasizes more passively adopting a credo for life that is predetermined and relatively unchangeable. When one's past life results in both hardiness and religiosity being simultaneously strong, personal conflict may result that could spur emotional difficulties.

Needless to say, one limitation of our study is its use of the DRI, which is only one of the various measures of religiosity that is available. Further, our sample was relatively homogeneous—senior military officers—and that may limit the generalizability of the results. Clearly, more studies comparing hardiness and religiosity need to be done.

Nonetheless, our results encourage us to reflect on the possibility that something more secular—such as the existential courage constituted by hardiness—may be more powerful in the process of maintaining and enhancing performance, development, and health than is the typically supernatural belief systems of religiosity. Both hardiness and religiosity are spiritual in nature, but the former emphasizes individual resources, whereas the latter emphasizes universal givens, in the effort to find meaning and direction in life.

FURTHER REFLECTIONS ON RELIGIOSITY

Let us speculate further on religiosity from the secular standpoint of hardiness. It is typical of religions to postulate a god or gods, who have created our world, ourselves, and the rules whereby we must navigate that world. Once a god-figure has been postulated, it is only natural to speculate on its appearance and manner of functioning. In this, humans tend to take an anthropomorphic approach, because it is difficult to conceptualize much else. So, the god-figure is often attributed a sex (in recent centuries, typically male), a humanoid appearance (typically the look that is most admired), a manner of operating (typically rewarding good, and punishing bad behavior), helpers (e.g., lesser gods, angels, disciples), and even an alter ego (which is the embodiment of evil).

Once formulated, a religion has many effects on people. It imparts the meaning of feelings and events, organizing them into what are good and what is bad. In this, you have a basis for moral evaluation of not only your own behavior, but that of others as well. As to coping, you have an unchanging moral basis for struggling to achieve certain ends, for desisting from other ends, and for stoical survival or retaliation when you are victimized. As to social interaction, you define your community by those who share your religious beliefs, and react to others either benevolently (e.g., by proselytizing) or by rejection or hostility. Although there is some room in all this for individual decisions, the emphasis is on a formulated moral system of meaning and action that applies to all, and does not change, regardless of ongoing events.

The ubiquitous tendency to anthropomorphize god-figures without realizing that this has been done is a major danger in religious belief systems. Anthropomorphizing opens the way for projecting our unresolved conflicts onto religious systems, as Freud recognized. Speculate with me for a moment. Imagine a large group of people whose family life involves an authoritarian, even despotic father, a powerless mother distrusted for her sexual appeal, and children who are treated like burdens, and required to toe the line, having little enjoyment or rights. What religious credo is such a group of people likely to develop and endorse?

The answer is a religion of fire and brimstone. The god-figure will likely be a male, imbued with absolute power, and given to unforgiving brutality in keeping his flock in line. Flock members will be seen as weak, given to selfish, immoral behavior, and requiring the punishment their god is quick to give out. Flock members will work hard to overcome their seemingly inherent immorality, and be quick to see outsiders as heathen, dangerous enemies reveling in the very inherent immorality that is such a threat.

In this, a likely reaction to heathens would be to express the tendency toward punitive retaliation for bad behavior that is built into religions of fire and brimstone through violence ranging from holy wars (if the flock feels organized and powerful enough) to terrorism (if desperation and hopelessness abounds in the flock). Those involved in such aggression do not see it as incompatible at all with their god-figure and credo, and feel no guilt for, but rather pride in what they do, as it seems like god's work.

Of course, it is also possible for the anthropomorphic projection process to produce a religion emphasizing love and encouragement, rather than fire and brimstone. Presumably, the development of such a religion builds on a group of people whose family life emphasizes a relatively egalitarian atmosphere, in which both parents love and respect each other and their children, and see their role as guiding and supporting their children in the journey toward expression of ethical values and principles. The resulting religious credo is likely to emphasize a view of humans as essentially good, though distractible, naïve, and in need of guidance, and a god-figure who is forgiving, supportive, and appreciative of human efforts to improve. In all this, flock members are likely to love and support each other, react to transgressions with forgiveness and corrective assistance, and see the people outside the flock as potential members to be proselytized, rather than as enemies to be fought. In religions of love, there is much less threat of wars and terrorism, but still an established, unchanging sense of the good life and how it must be led that can limit individual development. Interestingly, examples of religions of love are rare, with Unitarian Universalism being the clearest contemporary example.

FURTHER REFLECTIONS ON HARDINESS

Although religions of love come as close as a religion can to hardiness, there is still an insurmountable difference. Because hardiness does not postulate a god-figure and an unchangeable credo of acceptable behavior, it provides less basis for immortalizing family conflicts through a projective process. Consequently, hardiness can legitimately advocate a personal developmental process in finding meaning through immersing oneself in interaction with others and events (commitment), struggling to have an influence on outcomes (control), and continually learning from one's resulting experiences (challenge). That the resulting life will be admirable, rather than reprehensible, is rendered likely by the fact that, because this life is not led in isolation, commitment involves cooperation, control involves credibility, and challenge involves creativity (Maddi, Khoshaba, & Pammenter, 1999).

Needless to say, hardiness as an approach to life derives from existentialism (e.g., Maddi, 1986, 2001, 2002, 2002, June). Interestingly, the first glimmers of existentialism surfaced in the context of religiosity. At the beginning of Christianity, for example, there was the Gospel of Thomas (Meyer, 1986), in which Christ was quoted as dissuading his followers from worshiping him, and encouraging them instead to look within themselves to find God. This is a clear admonition to finding one's own way through individualistic pursuit of meaning. Perhaps this downplaying of an unchangeable credo for all, administered by an all-powerful god-figure, is why Thomas' Gospel was never included in the Bible.

Another existential foray from within religiosity was initiated by Søren Kierkegaard, the nineteenth century Christian minister and theologian from Denmark. The first fulsome existentialist, Kierkegaard (1954) emphasized that everything we do in life constitutes a decision. Each of these decisions can be made in a way that pushes us toward the future, or holds us back into the past. Choosing the future is best, because it stimulates development by bringing new information and meaning, whereas choosing the past leads to stagnation. Developmentally valuable though it is, choosing the future brings with it ontological anxiety, or the fear of uncertainty. But choosing the past is even worse, as it brings with it ontological guilt, or the sense of missed opportunity and stagnation. With repeated choices of the past, ontological guilt accumulates, in a process that starts with boredom, transitions into a sense that one is wasting time, and ends with what Kierkegaard (1954) called "the sickness unto death," or the conviction that life is meaningless.

To lead a vibrant and meaningful life, one must regularly choose the future despite the ongoing ontological anxiety and doubt that it will bring (Kierkegaard, 1954). As aid in tolerating ontological anxiety, Kierkegaard (1954) feels that one needs the religious faith that, in choosing the future, one brings oneself closer to God. After all, he proposes that God is the prototypical decision maker for the future, having created the world and continuing its evolution. It is those who regularly choose the future who will achieve paradise after death.

In advocating that people choose the future, Kierkegaard is not in any way insisting that they toe the line of some preconceived, unchangeable credo of right and wrong. They will find their own way, as did God. With such an individualistic message, it is not surprising that Kierkegaard's fellow ministers came to regard him as a heretic, and that he was generally considered dangerous and rejected by Danish society. Living in isolation, he wrote book after book under a pseudonym, for fear of more retaliation.

Also in the nineteenth century, the American theologian and minister, Ralph Waldo Emerson (1940) evolved from a more traditional religiosity into the view he called transcendentalism. This view emphasizes that although there is indeed a universal force influencing all our lives, it is not lodged in a god-figure, but rather in the universal human capability for finding essential meaning through observing and interpreting every day experience. As he went further and further in this existential direction, Emerson finally had to tell his congregation, during his service one Sunday, that he could not continue to be their minister, as he no longer believed in a god-figure. Shock and horror followed, and Harvard University stopped him from teaching in their Divinity School.

In the twentieth century, Paul Tillich (1952), also a theologian, continued this line of thinking. He agreed with Kierkegaard that everything we do constitutes a decision made for the future or the past, and that choosing the future brings ontological anxiety. He also agreed that choosing the future is the way of development and wisdom, insisting that "the god above God is doubt," or ontological anxiety (Tillich, 1952). That Tillich was not summarily rejected by the religious community is a sign of how much things had changed by then. In his time, it was not unusual to encounter so-called "God is dead" theologies.

Considering Tillich's rejection of a god-figure, it is not surprising that he did not emphasize faith in God as that which helps you tolerate the anxiety of uncertainty, but rather the more individualistic, secular "courage to be." To my mind, hardiness is an operationalization of the existential courage Tillich was talking about (Maddi, 1986, 2001, 2002, June). As such, it makes sense that hardiness facilitates maintenance and enhancement of performance, conduct, morale, stamina, and health under stress (cf. Maddi, 2002).

ARE EXISTENTIALISM AND HARDINESS MORAL STANCES?

It should be recognized that all of the philosopher-theologians mentioned thus far would have regarded existentialism as moral, in the sense that it aids people in avoiding the superficial semblance of moral behavior that can result from organizational religiosity, with its vulnerability to social desirability. Kierkegaard (1962) even went so far as to assume an inborn need for loving. Further, if they were alive now, these existentialists would point to the immorality of terrorism as an even deeper moral critique of conventional religiosity from the standpoint of existentialism.

Indeed, the twentieth century nontheologian who also championed the existential position, the Frenchman Jean Paul Sartre (1956), insisted that it necessarily fell outside of the religious context. Nonetheless, he devoted considerable effort to exploring how the individualistic search for meaning could be as moral as any religious conviction. First and foremost in this was his admonition, shared with other existentialists, that because we formulate our own lives through the decisions we make, we are therefore responsible for what we think, feel, and do. If we do not like our lives, we cannot blame others, feel victimized, and either strike out at them or justify any sort of fiendish behavior on our part. Because we have formulated our lives, it is up to us to make them acceptable to us and to those around us whom we love and admire. That there is no freedom without responsibility is a strong basis for recognizing that existentialism is hardly immorality.

Further, Sartre (1956) argued that as our lives are inextricably led in interaction with others, their evaluations of our behavior make a deep impression on us to be the best human beings we can be. In this, he had no patience for superficialities, such as physical beauty, and material wealth. After all, it was Sartre who declined the Nobel Prize when it was offered to him, on the grounds that he did not wish to fall into superficiality by being tempted to define himself as "a great man." He thought it safer to continue to choose the future, and learn along the way.

Still further, Sartre (1956) insisted, along with other existentialists, that not everything is possible, just because we are inveterate decision makers. There are givens that simply cannot be altered. For example, with my anatomy and physiology, I am unable to give birth to a child. Less unchangeable, but still givens while present, are laws of the land, and even the social norms that people have come to regard as important. Why, for example, did no one come to this meeting nude? Laws and norms are especially relevant, because to violate them by our decisions means that we have to pay the consequences. Therefore, they ride hard on selfish, irresponsible decision making, as paying the consequences usually means radically limiting our freedom. This shows that it is in our own self-interest to work within existing laws and norms as we try to formulate our lives.

The emphasis of all this is that the existential life stance is not a celebration of immorality. Rather, it assumes that human beings are essentially good, ready to live responsibly, be close to others, and respect what is regarded as important to us all. This is in contrast to the common religious belief that humans are given to immorality, and must be controlled by an imposed moral credo.

Hardiness fits into the existential frame of reference. The attitude of commitment leads you to want to be inextricably involved with the people and events in your world. The control attitude leads you to the conviction that you deeply influence what is going on in your life. And the challenge attitude encourages you to keep learning from the resulting experiences, so that you can find meaning and wisdom. In all this, hardiness assumes that humans have both social and psychological needs (Maddi, 2002, June). The social need leads you to want continuing contact, communication, and solidarity with the others around you. And the psychological need, based on the continual information requirements of the big-brain humans that have evolved, leads you to search continually for the stimulation provided by new experience. Put the two needs together, and that is the human basis for the value of deepening social relationships in the direction of intimacy and caring, rather than mere contractuality.

Given this, I submit that hardiness is not likely to lead in the direction of immorality, as this would jeopardize the increasing intimacy of ongoing and new social relationships. Thus far, the research evidence showing that hardiness leads to enhanced performance, leadership, morale, stamina, and health under stress (Maddi, 2002), while consistent with morality, does not test it directly. The closest bit of evidence we have is that, among adolescents, there is a negative relationship between hardiness and drug or alcohol use (Maddi, Wadhwa, & Haier, 1996). In this study, substance use was measured not only by self-report, but by urine screens as well. Although further studies are needed for full empirical validation, what we know thus far indicates that hardiness enhances conduct. This is certainly consistent with the view that hardiness is a morale stance, despite its individualistic stance on finding meaning through one's own decisions.

References

Atchley, R. C. (1997). The subjective importance of being religious and its effect on health and morale 14 years later. *Journal of Aging Studies, 11*, 131-141.

Bartone, P. T. (1999). Hardiness protects against war-related stress in Army reserve forces. *Consulting Psychology Journal, 51*, 72-82.

Bergin, A. E. (1983). Religiosity and mental health: A critical reevaluation and meta-analysis. *Professional Psychology, 14*, 170-184.

Bishop, G. D., & Quah, S. H. (1998). Reliability and validity of measures of anger/hostility in Singapore: Cook & Medley Ho Scale, STAXI and Buss-Durkee Hostility Inventory. *Personality and Individual Differences, 24*, 867-878.

Carver, C. S., Scheier, M. F., & Weintraub, J. K. (1989). Assessing coping strategies: A theoretically based approach. *Journal of Personality and Social Psychology, 56*, 267-283.

Clark, K. M., Friedman, H. S., & Martin, L. R. (1999). A longitudinal study of religiosity and mortality risk. *Journal of Health Psychology, 4*, 381-391.

Derogatis, L. R., Lipman, R. S., Rickels, K., Uhlenhuth, E. H., & Covi, L. (1974). The Hopkins Symptom Checklist (HSCL): A measure of primary symptom dimensions. In P. Pichot (Ed.), *Psychological measurements in psychopharmacology*. Basil, Switzerland: Karger.

Emerson, R. W. (1940). *The selected writings of Ralph Waldo Emerson* (B. Atkinson, Ed.). New York: Modern Library.

Fitchett, G., Rybarczyk, B. D., DeMarco, G. A., & Nicholas, J. J. (1999). The role of religion in medical rehabilitation outcomes: A longitudinal study. *Rehabilitation Psychology, 44*, 333-353.

Fry, P. S. (2000). Religious involvement, spirituality and personal meaning for life: Existential predictors of psychological wellbeing in community-residing and institutional-care elders. *Aging and Mental Health, 4*, 375-387.

Genia, V. (1998). Religiousness and psychological adjustment in college students. *Journal of College Student Psychotherapy, 12,* 67-77.

Hann, D., Winter, K., & Jacobsen, P. (1999). Measurement of depressive symptoms in cancer patients: Evaluation of the Center for Epidemiological Studies Depression Scale (CES-D). *Journal of Psychosomatic Research, 46,* 437-443.

Idler, E. L., & Kasl, S. V. (1997). Religion among disabled and nondisabled persons, I: Cross-sectional patterns in health practices, social activitiesd, and well-being. *Journals of Gerontology: Series B. Psychological Sciences and Social Sciences, 52,* S294-S305.

Impara, J. C., & Plake, B. S. (Eds.), (1998). *The 13th mental measurement yearbook.* Lincoln, NE: University of Nebraska Press.

Kierkegaard, S. (1843, 1849/1954). *Fear and trembling, and the sickness unto death.* Garden City, NY: Doubleday Anchor Books.

Kierkegaard, S. (1962). *Works of love.* New York: Harper, Row.

King, L. A., King, D. W., Fairbank, J. A., Keane, T. M., & Adams, G. A. (1998). Resilience-recovery factors in post-traumatic stress disorder among female and male Vietnam veterans: Hardiness, postwar social support and additional stressful life events. *Journal of Personality and Social Psychology, 74,* 420-434.

Kobasa, S. C., Maddi, S. R., Puccetti, M. C., & Zola, M. A. (1986). Effectiveness of Hardiness, exercise and social support as resources against illness. *Journal of Psychosomatic Research, 29,* 525-533.

Koenig, H. G., Cohen, H. J., Blazer, D. G., Pieper, C., Meador, K. G., Shelp, F. et al. (1998). The relationship between religious activities and blood pressure in older adults. *International Journal of Psychiatry in Medicine, 28,* 189-213.

Maddi, S. R. (1970). The search for meaning. In M. Page (Ed.), *Nebraska symposium on motivation.* Lincoln, NE: University of Nebraska Press.

Maddi, S. R. (1986). Existential psychotherapy. In J. Garske & S. Lynn (Eds.), *Contemporary psychotherapy* (1st ed.). New York: Merrill Publishers.

Maddi, S. R. (1990). Issues and interventions in stress mastery. In H. S. Friedman (Ed.), *Personality and disease.* New York: Wiley.

Maddi, S. R. (1997). Personal Views Survey II: A measure of dispositional hardiness. In C. P. Zalaquett & R. J. Woods (Eds.), *Evaluating stress: A book of resources.* New York: University Press.

Maddi, S. R. (1999). The personality construct of hardiness, I: Effects on experiencing, coping, and strain. *Consulting Psychology Journal, 51,* 83-94.

Maddi, S.R. (2001). Creating meaning through making decisions. In P. T. P. Wong & P. S. Fry (Eds.), *The human quest for meaning.* New York: Erlbaum.

Maddi, S. R. (2002a). The story of hardiness: Twenty years of theorizing, research, and practice. *Consulting Psychology Journal, 54,* 173-185.

Maddi, S. R. (2002, June). *Existential courage and searching for meaning*. Keynote address at 8th International Conference on Motivation, Moscow.

Maddi, S. R., & Hess, M. (1992). Hardiness and success in basketball. *International Journal of Sports Psychology, 23*, 360-368.

Maddi, S. R. & Hightower, M. (1999). Hardiness and optimism as expressed in coping patterns. *Consulting Psychology Journal, 51*, 78-86.

Maddi, S. R., & Khoshaba, D. M. (1994). Hardiness and mental health. *Journal of Personality Assessment, 63*, 265-274.

Maddi, S. R., & Khoshaba, D. M. (1998). *Personal Views Survey III manual*. Newport Beach, CA: Hardiness Institute.

Maddi, S. R., & Kobasa, S. C. (1984). *The hardy executive: Health under stress*. Homewood, IL: Dow Jones-Irwin.

Maddi, S. R., Khoshaha, D. M., & Pammenter, A. (1999). The Hardy Organization: Success by turning change to advantage. *Consulting Psychology Journal, 51*, 117-124.

Maddi, S. R., Wadhwa, P., & Haier, R. J. (1996). Relationship of hardiness to alcohol and drug use in adolescents. *American Journal of Drug and Alcohol Abuse, 22*, 247-257.

Maddi, S. R., Brow, M., Khoshaba, D. M., & Vaitkus, M. (2003). *The relationship of hardiness and religiosity to depression and anger*. Unpublished manuscript.

Matthews, D. A., McCullough, M. E., Larson, D. B., Koenig, H. G., Swyers, J. P., & Milano, M. G. (1998). Religious commitment and health status: A review of the research and implications for family medicine. *Archives of Family Medicine, 7*, 118-124.

McCullough, M. E., Hoyt, W. T., Larson, D. B. Koenig, H. G., & Thoresen, C. (2000). Religious involvement and mortality: A meta-analytic review. *Health Psychology, 19*, 211-222.

McIntosh, D. N., Silver, R. C., & Wortman, C. B. (1993). Religion's role in adjustment to a negative life event: Coping with the loss of a child. *Journal of Personality and Social Psychology, 65*, 812-821.

Meyer, M. (1986). *The secret teachings of Jesus: Four Gnostic gospels*. New York: Vintage Books.

Moos, R. H. (1979). Socio-economic perspectives on health. In G. S. Stone, F. Cohen, & N. E. Adler (Eds.), *Health psychology*. San Francisco: Jossey Bass.

Nagy, S., & Nix, C. L. (1989). Relations between preventive health behavior and hardiness. *Psychological Reports, 65*, 339-345.

Radloff, L. S. (1977). The CES-D scale: A self-report depression scale for research in the general population. *Applied Psychological Measurement, 3*, 385-401.

Sartre, J. P. (1956). *Being and nothingness*. New York: Philosophical Library.

Schein, R. L., & Koenig, H. G. (1997). The Center for Epidemiological Studies – Depression Scale: Assessment of depression in the medically-ill elderly. *International Journal of Geriatric Psychiatry, 12*, 436-446.

Sherman, A. C., Plante, T. G., Simonton, S., Adams, D. C., Harbison, C., & Burris, S. K. (2000). A multidimensional measure of religious involvement for cancer patients: The Duke Religious Index. *Support Care in Cancer, 8,* 102-109.

Tillich, P. (1952). *The courage to be.* New Haven, CT: Yale University Press.

Wallace, J. M., Jr., & Forman, T. A. (1998). Religion's role in promoting health and reducing risk among American youth. *Health Education and Behavior, 25,* 721-741.

Westman, M. (1990). The relationship between stress and performance: The moderating effect of hardiness. *Human Performance, 3,* 141-155.

Weibe, D. J., & McCallum, D. M. (1986). Health practices and hardiness as mediators in the stress-illness relationship. *Health Psychology, 5,* 425-438.

The Existential Roots
of Mindfulness Meditation

Abstract

Mindfulness meditation is an ancient Buddhist practice that has
recently demonstrated clinical efficacy for many psychological
problems. This paper presents the traditional existential context
of mindfulness meditation. Specific attention is paid to two
practices that are important applications of mindfulness while
confronting our own mortality and when faced with daily hardships. The first is the Nine Charnel Ground Contemplations as
presented within the Buddhist canon. The second are the Lojong
teachings that developed later and were preserved in the Tibetan
tradition. These techniques of practicing mindfulness not only
highlight the existential origins of this ancient practice, but also
point to its spiritually transformative effects in the search for
meaning in suffering and human life.

INTRODUCTION

Recently, the practice of mindfulness meditation has demonstrated clinical
efficacy for the treatment of a variety of psychological problems. Mindfulness
meditation, alone or in conjunction with other psychotherapeutic tools, has
been found to alleviate the symptoms of chronic pain (Kabat-Zinn, Lipworth,
Burney, & Sellers, 1986), depression, including depression relapse (Teasdale, Segal,
Williams, Ridgeway, Soulsby, & Lau, 2000), binge eating (Wiser & Telch, 1999),
and addiction (Marlatt, 2002). Mindfulness meditation has also been shown to

87

benefit the immune system and may even alter the hard wiring of our brains to experience greater contentment (Davidson et al., 2003).

Given the burgeoning of research on how mindfulness meditation can be applied to modern psychological problems, a better understanding of its history and traditional applications may shed light on the often-overlooked existential aspects of this practice. Although mindfulness meditation has recently been applied within a predominantly cognitive-behavioral paradigm, the origins of mindfulness meditation have deep roots in an existential tradition.

Buddhist texts describe mindfulness meditation as among the first techniques taught by the Buddha shortly after attaining enlightenment. From its earliest recorded appearance in the written Buddhist canonical tradition, mindfulness meditation has been seen as a valuable tool in confronting the meaning of human suffering and mortality. Mindfulness is a set of practices that forms the cornerstone of many different Indian and East Asian meditation techniques of different spiritual traditions, but develops a complete articulation in particular in the various schools of Buddhism. Most Buddhist religious and historical texts consider mindfulness meditation to be the foundation of all other meditation practices, ranging from analytical and compassion-based exercises to the more esoteric tantric techniques that later developed in India.

THE TRADITIONAL PRACTICE OF MINDFULNESS

In the Buddhist canon, the practice of mindfulness is presented in the Mahasatipatthana Sutta (Nanamoli & Bodhi, 1995). "Sutta," in the Pali language which the Buddha spoke, or "sutra" in Sanskrit, means "teaching." Popular misconceptions of mindfulness describe the practice as an effort to empty the mind or become undistracted. In fact, mindfulness has been historically described as a way of paying attention to the unending internal narrative of our thoughts, feelings, and physical sensations. By using the breath as an anchor, the practitioner becomes able to focus on the automatic, internal narrative of selfhood, thereby allowing for a deliberate yet spontaneous, self-reflexive disruption in its automaticity. Mindfulness, therefore, to a certain extent uses the tendency towards distractibility itself as an object of focus.

The practice of mindfulness relies on an awareness of the process of diaphragmatic breathing. Particular emphasis is placed on concentrating on inhalation, exhalation, physical posture, and the here-and-now. Although most commonly practiced as a sitting meditation, mindfulness can be practiced in a variety of postures, such as lying down, and through a variety of activities, such as eating or walking.

In mindfulness meditation, there is an attitude of unconditional welcoming toward the continuous supply of distracting narratives, thereby neutralizing the self-referential, secondary emotional processes associated with negative cognitions. Mindfulness can therefore be understood to embody acceptance-based strategies for coping with distress. This unconditional welcoming of inner phenomena eventually becomes applied to external phenomena. That is, in gradually accepting one's own thoughts and feelings, one gradually becomes more compassionate towards others' thoughts and feelings.

THE NINE CHARNEL GROUND CONTEMPLATIONS

The text of the Mahasatipatthana Sutta, following preliminary instructions on mindfulness, encourages practitioners to practice this unconditional welcoming of death and impermanence. The text discusses a set of practices referred to as the Nine Charnel Ground Contemplations which involve practicing mindfulness meditation while observing corpses in nine progressive states of decay in open-air crematoriums that can still be found in South Asia today. The sutta encourages the practitioner, relatively soon after learning mindfulness skills, to instigate this profound contact with death by focusing on these corpses as harbingers of his or her own eventual physical death and decay, as well as embodiments of the transient nature of all existence. Indeed, there are explicit verses that connect the experience of this meditation to one's own eminent death and mortality.

The Buddha himself came to practice mindfulness as an outcome of an existential crisis that he experienced at the age of 29. Prior to that time, he lived in the existential vacuum of a life devoted to sensual pleasures and comfort. He lived sequestered in his father's palace, free from contact with any hardship or suffering. After his first face-to-face contacts with the physical sufferings of illness, old age, and death, he abandoned his opulent lifestyle, compelled to search for the meaning of the presence of suffering in the human condition.

As a wandering ascetic, he began to explore the various spiritual and religious traditions of ancient India. Finally, after years of practicing severe austerities, he sat down under a banyan tree to begin his final meditation, vowing not to end the session until enlightenment or death. Following his enlightenment, the Buddha then began a 45-year period of teaching.

The existential distress that compelled the Buddha to search for the meaning of human life, and the meaning of the ubiquity of suffering within all of our lives, eventually led him to the practice of mindfulness. The Mahasatipatthana Sutta instructs practitioners of mindfulness to follow the same path—to investigate the meaning of human life by contemplating its impermanence. In effect, the practice of mindfulness meditation helps practitioners gain a heightened awareness of each precious moment as a side effect of the search for meaning.

The existential origins of mindfulness, therefore, are twofold. The first key moment is the turning point in the life of the Buddha, his own witnessing of old age, sickness, and death. The practice of mindfulness meditation, more so than his practice of austerities, fills the existential vacuum of the privileged, sheltered life with which he had become profoundly disillusioned. The second occurs in the written instruction and practice of mindfulness which recreates the Buddha's own path of spiritual development in the lives of practitioners, who are encouraged to confront their own inherently impermanent existence by meditating mindfully on the end of life in charnel grounds.

Mindfulness meditation practice diminishes the existential anxiety created by mortality by facilitating a gradual acceptance of uncertainty in the face of an impermanent existence. This acceptance becomes the cornerstone of Buddhism's First Noble Truth, which is discussed at the conclusion of the sutta. Although frequently translated as "life is suffering," the First Noble Truth can be better understood as a declaration of the universality of suffering and impermanence, great and small, in every aspect of our lives.

As an existential tool, mindfulness facilitates an acceptance of suffering and impermanence which gradually unfolds alongside the search for meaning in life. In the Buddhist tradition, the search for meaning is an intimately spiritual journey, in that mindfulness-based acceptance of the inherent impermanence of life and the ubiquity of suffering develops into compassion for others. Thus, the traditional purpose of mindfulness meditation has not solely been for self-improvement. Rather, mindfulness is seen as an essential first step towards greater compassion for all living beings.

The mindful confrontation with the fleeting nature of life and the inevitability of death as instructed in the Nine Charnel Ground Contemplations is meant to facilitate a sense of reverence for life. All the manners of death that bring people to charnel grounds—illness, old age, accident, foul play—illustrate the precarious nature of life. An understanding of how quickly and unexpectedly life can end motivates the practitioner to live ethically and to aspire to a spiritual preparation for death.

The awareness of death generated by this application of mindfulness becomes the ultimate motivator for spiritual development. In becoming intimately familiar with various aspects of death, the preciousness of not only life, but also of each of the precious moments that constitute life, becomes deeply ingrained in the practitioner. The mindful awareness of impermanence is meant to not only facilitate an acceptance of death and impermanence, but also to motivate a search for meaning about the nature of life without providing explicit answers. Mindfulness of death and suffering has traditionally been used to develop a motivation to realize the positive potential of each moment, and to experience life as a valuable opportunity for spiritual enlightenment. For this reason, "precious human life" is the standard term used to refer to our existence in many Buddhist teachings (Gampopa, 1998).

Understood within its existential development, mindfulness meditation is also a powerful spiritual tool for transforming suffering—mental, physical, emotional, and spiritual—into compassion. The practice of mindfulness therefore embodies the goal of not only the Buddhist spiritual tradition, but also of many of the world's religious and spiritual traditions: living a compassionate life in the face of universal uncertainty.

TRADITIONAL MIND TRAINING AND MINDFULNESS

The transformative potential of mindfulness is discussed at length in a set of practices preserved in the Tibetan tradition as the Lojong ("mind-training") teachings (Gyatso, 1999). The Lojong teachings challenge practitioners to reframe hardships and suffering as opportunities for spiritual transformation. These teachings ask us to reframe the difficult relationships, physical discomforts, and even negative emotions that color all of our lives as opportunities to practice mindfulness and compassion. As these difficult moments in our lives emerge, mindfulness reminds us of our capacity to choose our response; we can engage in the automaticity of our normal reactions, or we can use these moments as opportunities for practicing compassion. In effect, these seemingly overpowering experiences of suffering are transformed into the very building blocks of spiritual enlightenment.

In a sense, the Lojong teachings are a more practical application of the Nine Charnel Ground Contemplations. Since we do not have access to charnel grounds, we are encouraged to instead use the here-and-now events of our lives as opportunities for engaging in the mindfulness of impermanence and suffering. Like the Nine Charnel Contemplations, the Lojong teachings advocate applying mindfulness meditation to those experiences in our lives that are the most uncomfortable not only in their traditional, historical setting, but also in contemporary society. Death and suffering remain the most profound mysteries in all of our lives, and mindfulness meditation offers us a tool to transform these experiences into meaningful, spiritual growth.

CONCLUSION

Mindfulness meditation is sure to gain more popularity and applications in contemporary psychology. The long-standing relationship between mindfulness and existentialism offers a rich avenue of exploration. By understanding the traditional existential context of mindfulness meditation, it is hoped that a greater understanding of the inherent transformative capacity of this practice can be conveyed in its current and future applications. Although initially taught to practitioners in the charnel grounds of South Asia, mindfulness can be applied to all of our lives in our relationships and daily hardships. Mindfulness of suffering and death, although seemingly distant from the goals of modern psychotherapy, offers valuable insight and motivation for living a more compassionate and meaningful life.

References

Davidson, R., Kabat-Zinn, J., Schumacher, J., Rosenkranz, M., Muller, D., Santorelli, S. et al. (2003). Alterations in brain and immune function produced by mindfulness meditation. *Psychosomatic Medicine*, *65*, 564-570.

Gampopa. (1998). *The jewel ornament of liberation* (K. Konchog, Trans.). Boston, MA: Wisdom Publications.

Gyatso, T. (1999). *Lojong: Training the mind*. Boston, MA: Wisdom Publications.

Kabat-Zinn, J., Lipworth, L., Burney, R., & Sellers, W. (1986). Four-year follow-up of a meditation-based program for the self-regulation of chronic pain: Treatment outcome and compliance. *Clinical Journal of Pain, 2*, 159–73.

Marlatt, G. A. (2002). Buddhist philosophy and the treatment of addictive behavior. *Cognitive and Behavioral Practice, 9*, 44-50.

Nanamoli, B., & Bodhi, B. (1995). *The middle length discourses of the Buddha: A translation of the Majjhima Nikaya*. Boston, MA: Wisdom Publications.

Teasdale, J. D., Segal, Z. V., Williams, J. M., Ridgeway, V. A., Soulsby, J. M., & Lau, M. A. (2000). Prevention of relapse/recurrence in major depression by mindfulness-based cognitive therapy. *Journal of Consulting and Clinical Psychology, 68*(4) 615-23.

Wiser, S., & Telch, C. (1999). Dialectical behavioral therapy for binge-eating disorder. *Journal of Clinical Psychology, 55*, 755-768.

Approaches to Deepening Personal Meaning

ADAM BLATNER

Abstract

This paper briefly reviews several contemporary trends that help people acquire a greater sense of personal meaning. It will show that psychotherapy has moved beyond Freud's narrow focus on resolving infantile conflicts, and has moved towards Victor Frankl's emphasis on personal meaning and Alfred Adler's concept of social interest. This brief overview will serve the purpose of showing the breadth of meaning-oriented approaches to psychology and psychotherapy.

MEANING-CENTERED PSYCHOTHERAPY AND COUNSELING
Humanistic Psychology

At mid-twentieth century, two forces dominated the field of psychology: behaviorism in academic circles and psychoanalysis in clinical circles. Neither fully addressed the more humanistic capacities of play, spirituality, and other meaning-filled dimensions of life. Thus, a "third force" emerged, led by visionary psychologists such as Abraham Maslow, Rollo May, Charlotte Buhler, James Bugental, and others. They were influenced by existential psychiatrists and psychologists such as Viktor Frankl and Ludwig Binswanger. They addressed such phenomena as "peak experiences," talked about authenticity, and actively considered questions of personal meaning as a factor in psychotherapy (Goble, 1971). Many of their ideas continue to be a source of insight in humanistic and existential psychology.

Transpersonal Psychology and Psychiatry

Out of humanistic psychology emerged another trend, one that extended psychology into the realm of spirituality. (I define *spirituality* as that activity of developing a deeper relationship or sense of connection with the Greater Whole-ness of Being, usually called "God" in Western cultures. I define *religion* as the *social organization* of that spiritual impulse, which sometimes helps channel it, and sometimes unfortunately interferes with this mission.) At the end of the 1960s, the Association of Transpersonal Psychology was founded (Walsh & Vaughan, 1993; Scotton, Chinen, & Battista, 1996). Essentially, it proposed that an exploration of people's spiritual dimension could help them work out their spiritually related personal problems.

Transpersonal psychology quickly moved beyond the challenge of purely clinical concerns—helping individuals or families with personal problems—and became involved with a somewhat larger concern for consciousness expansion, including ecology and social activism. Over the last few decades, a number of organizations and journals have been founded to support this effort, such as the Institute of Noetic Sciences (IONS), *ReVision: A Journal of Consciousness and Transformation*, *The Journal of Consciousness Studies,* and numerous other magazines. There is also a radio program called "New Dimensions."

Another development emerging from this field has been an expansion of philosophical ideas, such as those worked out by Ken Wilber (2000), who has created a model for integrating many seeming opposites, such as science and spirituality. Other areas of academic philosophy have begun to build on these ideas.

Carl G. Jung's Analytical Psychology

By the 1950s, for various reasons, Jung's ideas had not become as well known as Freud's, but around the mid-late 1960s they enjoyed a renaissance. Perhaps no other approach addressed the richness of the psychedelic experience. Once intel-lectuals began contemplating "the farther reaches of human nature," a psychology with a wider scope was needed. Jung's inclusion of many dimensions, spirituality as well as sexuality and all the other archetypes, invited people to think about the more general goals of life (Blatner, 2002).

In the last few decades, a number of writers have become widely known, such as Thomas Moore, James Hillman, and Jean Shinoda Bolen (Bolen, 1990). These writers have addressed the challenges of personal meaning from a variety of fascinating standpoints. One common underlying theme is that life becomes more meaningful when lived in depth and experienced simultaneously at several levels, such as art, philosophy, and social concern, in addition to the immediate problems of survival. Of course, analytical psychology is also an influential element in the aforementioned field of transpersonal psychology.

The Creative Arts Therapies

Using music, dance and movement, art, poetry, sculpture, and drama as vehicles for therapy emerged with the creative efforts of many innovators. By the 1980s, these diverse efforts had become subfields in themselves and interdisciplinary efforts emerged. (Indeed, a related field called "expressive arts therapy" promotes the integration of several modalities.) Also, like many aspects of psychotherapy, the creative arts therapies offered much, not only to sick people wanting to get better, but also to healthy people who want to become healthier and even more resilient. Many of their techniques may be applied in workshops aimed at deepening personal meaning.

Psychodrama

In the mid-1930s, Dr. J. L. Moreno developed an approach which emerged as an alternative to the primarily verbal method (on the couch) of psychoanalysis. Psychodrama utilizes the power of role playing to help people explore their problems in action. This method influenced many other approaches, such as Gestalt therapy, some forms of family therapy, and the encounter group (Blatner, 2000a). At the 2002 Meaning Conference, I gave a workshop that showed how psychodramatic methods were particularly effective in promoting a deeper sense of personal meaning (Blatner, 2002). Psychodrama also at times integrates many of the elements in the creative arts therapies, as well as experiential therapy, narrative therapy, and group therapy.

Group Psychotherapy

This approach began as a treatment of those who were mentally ill; later, various group-oriented methods were applied to helping healthy people as well. Beginning with *T-Groups* in the late 1940s, group work began to be integrated with humanistic psychology in evolving into sensitivity training—some of it used in business—and then into encounter groups. Different support groups have sprung up to help people with life threatening illness, bereavement, and recovery from addiction. Personal meaning was a natural subject for sharing in these settings.

Narrative Therapy

Instead of trying to discover insight into the past, this approach concerns itself with simply clarifying the meanings of stories people tell about themselves. The therapy primarily consists of re-telling or re-authoring the story from a problem-saturated account to a more constructive, life-affirming narrative. The problem with traditional psychodynamic approaches, especially as applied to family work, from which narrative therapy chiefly emerged, was that everyone in the family had a different version of history and it became a fruitless task to seek to discover "what really happened." Narrative therapy's emphasis on co-creating the past helps redirect the family towards a more positive future. It became clear that such artful constructions benefit from an inclusion of people's higher aspirations. The process of identifying and clarifying these values and ideals before weaving them into a more meaningful story is similar to logotherapy (Sarbin, 1986).

Experiential Therapies

Various forms of experimental therapies have emerged, addressing dimensions that had been overlooked in conventional talk therapy. These include body therapies, especially the post-Reichian form of bioenergetic analysis, imagery therapies, and Gestalt therapy. Experimental therapies make people aware of a wider range of their experiences, including their bodily sensations, the feeling of the streaming of bodily energy, and the vividness of imagery evoked by quasi-hypnotic techniques. These and other approaches also help people develop a more holistic sense of personal meaning.

Other Developments

Rehabilitation psychology and occupational therapy have shown increasing interest in the role of meaning in rehabilitation. These fields need to help clients to rise above their trauma and disability and to rediscover a sense of meaning and purpose. Trauma counseling, sexual abuse counseling, and grief counseling are also concerned with issues related to shattered assumptions and loss of meaning. These developments highlight the vital role of meaning of life (Baumeister, 1991) and meaning-centered counseling and therapy (Wong, 1998).

CULTURAL DEVELOPMENTS

From the mid-twentieth century onward, dynamic psychology has increasingly penetrated the fabric of culture, in the humanities, academia, the media, and even in popular cartoons, and has in turn stimulated a more popular resurgence in philosophy. In addition, a number of general developments in the wider culture have added to the wealth of approaches available for the deepening of personal meaning.

Comparative Mythology and Religion

Research deriving from anthropology, history, cross-cultural sociology, and other fields supported a natural emergence of interdisciplinary studies. Religion has moved from being a denominationally biased mode of inculcating the young to a subject of impartial and cross-cultural study. Efforts were made to elucidate the common elements that could be discerned in many, if not all, religions (Walsh, 1999). One impetus to this effort was the influx of Asian influences after the Second World War: Zen Buddhism and the resurgence of Yoga. Tibetan Buddhism, Native American Indian religions, and the mystical streams within the major Western and Eastern religious traditions have also become important players in the therapeutic community and popular culture.

In the early 1980s, the work of the comparative mythologist, Joseph Campbell (who based many of his ideas on Jung's theories), was popularized in a public television series hosted by Bill Moyers. One theme from this series and his then-popular books is that we can all participate in a kind of "hero's journey." Since then, several books on personal mythology have been written in order to elaborate on this general theme (e.g., Feinstein & Krippner, 1988; Keen & Fox, 1989; and Pearson, 1991).

Another effect of the exploration of myths of other cultures is that it brought sharper awareness of the *myths*, i.e., unquestioned assumptions and implicit attitudes of Western culture. Modern culture presumed to be scientific, rational, and beyond the grip of myth, but the combination of cross-cultural studies and dynamic psychology revealed that our own society was riven with a host of norms based on a combination of tradition and the sustaining of familiar power structures—we, too, had our own myths. In our own time of rapidly changing circumstances, international travel and mixing of cultural influences, the impact of new technologies, etc., we are being forced to re-evaluate what seem to be fixed truths, but in actuality relative value systems, and knowing about comparative religions and mythologies help to identify such assumptions, better bringing consciousness to their revision and refinement.

The Human Potential Movement

The human potential movement, which emerged in the 1960s, invited people to explore the frontiers of mind and socially constructive behavior. Beginning primarily at Esalen Institute in California, it soon spread nationally and internationally, with "growth centers" in the late 60s and throughout the 70s, hosting a wide range of workshops relating to psychology, spirituality, body awareness, etc. The *encounter group* was a prominent element for a decade, but then fell out of fashion, transforming into many more focused programs for personal development.

The present positive psychology movement can be considered a continuation of humanistic psychology and the human potential movement. Although positive psychology focuses on scientific research, this movement has inspired large numbers of positive psychologists, life coaches, and happiness coaches who help clients to develop their full potentials and lead happy and successful lives.

New Trends in Spirituality

An increasing percentage of people—more among young adults—has begun to explore nontraditional avenues in religion. Some of these efforts involve rediscovering or recreating greater depth within the mainstream traditions, with a greater emphasis on personal experience and social action, while others try out different, sometimes rather "foreign," spiritual traditions. The activity of finding one's most satisfactory spiritual path has itself become a common phase in the life journey (McLennan, 1999). This incredibly rich trend in contemporary culture deserves to be vividly recognized (Taylor, 1999; Smolley & Kinney, 1999; Drury, 1999). This spiritual renaissance, of course, brings into sharp focus the question of meaning in life.

Another effort has been in the direction of interfaith dialogue. At a recent World Congress of Religion (Barcelona, 2004), a number of leaders in the field of religion met to explore this frontier. Notable in this effort has been the work of the late Brother Wayne Teasdale.

With roots in the human potential movement and new trends in spirituality, the idea of becoming more conscious about a wide range of other issues—political, social, environmental—also relates to our view of the meaning of our lives. The point here is that meaning is not merely a matter of acting for oneself, but also of fostering greater advancement of the species in harmony with all of life.

Vital Aging

With advances in health care, increasing numbers of people are living beyond 70 and doing so with remarkable vitality. A significant cultural trend has been towards addressing the needs of this sector of the population. One aspect of this is the recognition of the need for more meaning in reviewing and living life, and also for contemplating its ending (Schachter-Shalomi, 1997).

A growing theme for seniors—and for others—is that of creating autobiographies, memoirs, or even just collections of stories. New developments in genealogy, the possibilities of creating CD-ROMs, videos, scanning photographs, websites, and desktop publishing, all make it more possible for the sharing and archiving of these family stories.

A combination of the themes of group work and narrative mentioned above can be applied as a form of recreation or community theatre by sharing our stories or dramatizing them. For example, the recent psychodramatic-theatrical innovation called "Playback Theatre" (Fox & Dauber, 1999). Several books have been written about how to write your own memoir. Group work shows some more specific techniques for telling your story. Discovering the depths of meaning in the tapestry of your life is the subject of the workshop I am presenting at this conference.

Thanatology

The study of the dying process, somewhat of a taboo subject before the late 1960s, has become the focus of increased attention. In addition to seeking ways of helping the dying become more comfortable, there has also been a focus on promoting opportunities to experience and review life in order to make its ending a more meaningful experience. The popularity of the recently published and persistently best-selling book, *Tuesdays with Morrie*, (Albom, 1997) reflects the spread of this growing sensitivity to this subject. Recent research on death attitudes has shifted from death anxiety to death acceptance; most of this research focus on the vital role of meaning and spirituality (Wong, 2007).

OTHER ELABORATIONS

A number of other related threads of development also have implications for cultivating and deepening the sense of personal meaning.

Enchantment

Another dimension of meaning is enhanced by the elaboration of imagery and fantasy. In the last forty years these dimensions were given new life by the popularity among older youngsters and many adults of the Tolkien books, *The Hobbit* and *Lord of the Rings*, in the late 1960s, through Castaneda's writings about his Mexican sorcerer-teacher, Don Juan, through the *Dungeons and Dragons* games, and now in the best-selling Harry Potter books. Themes of wizards and magical creatures, dragons and angels, fairies and gnomes have become more prominent in literature and toy stores, television cartoons, and movies.

In many ways, as mentioned above, the early part of the last century was characterized more by a tendency towards demythologization, a tendency to explain phenomena "scientifically," in order to pull away more distinctively from the forces of mere superstition. However, later there came a relative lack in the celebration of personally meaningful images, and as with other aspects of spirituality and the dimensions of imagination and playfulness, the pendulum is swinging back.

Remythologization is emerging, as is reflected in the title phrase of a recently published book (Moore, 1996), *The Re-Enchantment of Everyday Life*. Like romance, a measure of magic adds a kind of sparkle. It involves a cultural rebalancing, a reowning of the magic of the imagination and spontaneity of childhood. The key point is integrating into one's life imagery, poetry, song, ornamentation, and art, and developing personal symbols.

Many Parts of the Self

Another development in the field of psychology has been the emergence of a pluralistic model of mind; that is, instead of thinking of self as one person, a personality with a given set of traits; we are coming to find that many people are not only multifaceted, but actually healthier and more resilient because of it (Rowan, 1990). The postmodern condition can lead to a kind of *identity diffusion*, as Erikson called it, but it can also lead to what I have termed "multiple personality order." The point here is not that there may be a plethora of roles, but rather that the *management* of the employment of those roles can be relatively more or less competent (Blatner, 2000a; Lifton, 1993).

One of the roots of this approach arose from the problem of multiple personality *disorder*; the therapeutic approach is treating each subpersonality with respect, helping each personality fragment to have a voice and to speak for its own needs as a way of negotiating some movement towards integration. This approach was expanded for use with people who were not dissociated so much as merely in conflict among different roles. This is actually an old psychodramatic technique, which became well known when Fritz Perls co-opted it and made it part of Gestalt therapy. The idea of having different parts of yourself talk to each other is fairly simple and, if done correctly, is very useful, not just in therapy, but also as a technique that can become part of ordinary life, as a form of ongoing mental hygiene (Blatner, 2003). The practical implication of a pluralistic model of the mind is that people can begin to celebrate their own multifaceted nature, exulting, as did Walt Whitman in his *Leaves of Grass*, "Do I contradict myself? Very well, then, I contradict myself! I am great! I contain multitudes!"

Ceremonies and Rituals

As an extension of a combination of the arts therapies, drama therapy, and narrative, there have been several books encouraging people to create new ceremonies and rituals to celebrate life transitions in ways that feel more meaningful to all concerned. Such rituals anchor the feeling of meaning in life (Blatner, 2000b).

SUMMARY

The need for personal meaning is being addressed in many ways at this conference; however, a vision gathers strength when it has some sense of how that vision may be implemented. The trends mentioned above include a wealth of methods, techniques, and concepts, all of which offer a rich palette of colors for the individual to create a sense of deepened personal meaning.

People's capacities for deepening their sense of personal meaning has been facilitated by the emergence of a number of trends in contemporary culture. From the fields of psychology, psychotherapy, and comparative religion, and from many grassroots trends, including literature, popular fashions, and the emergence of a new interest in consciousness expansion, a wealth of approaches are now available for integration. For the first time in history, we are capable of considering a new possibility, that of expanding consciousness to a new level of self-awareness and self-reflective behavior. This, in turn, opens us to the possibility that purposeful cultural evolution may be the next step in the evolution of our own species. Considering the theme of personal meaning is an integral element in that creative advance.

This list is meant to be evocative rather than exhaustive; its purpose is to stimulate your thinking about all the emerging trends that also relate to the enriching of the capacity of individuals to seek to live more meaningful lives, or to find meaning at the end of those lives.

References

Albom, M. (1997). *Tuesdays with Morrie*. New York: Doubleday.

Baumeister, R. F. (1991). *Meanings of life*. New York: Guilford.

Blatner, A. (2002). The relevance of the concept of the archetype. Retrieved March 29, 2006, from http://www.blatner.com/adam/level2/archetype.htm

Blatner, A. (2000a). Applied Role Theory. In *Foundations of psychodrama: History, theory, & practice*. New York: Springer.

Blatner, A. (2000b). A new role for psychodramatists: Master of Ceremonies. *International Journal of Action Methods, 53*(2), 86-93.

Blatner, A. (2002). Deepening personal meaning: using dramatic approaches. Retrieved March, 2006, from http://www.blatner.com/adam/psyntbk/persmndr.htm.

Blatner, A. (2003). Not merely players: Applications of psychodramatic methods in everyday life. In J. Gershoni (Ed.), *Psychodrama in the 21st century: Clinical and educational applications* (pp 103-115). New York: Springer.

Blatner, A. (2006). On self-ing as process. Retrieved March 29, 2006, from http://www.blatner.com/level2/self.htm

Bolen, J. S. (1990). *Gods in everyman*. San Francisco: Harper & Row.

Drury, N. (1999). *Exploring the labyrinth: Making sense of the new spirituality*. New York: Continuum.

Feinstein, D., & Krippner, S. (1988). *Personal mythology: The psychology of your evolving self*. Los Angeles: J. P. Tarcher.

Fox, J., & Dauber, H. (Eds.). (1999). *Gathering voices: Essays on playback theatre*. New Paltz, NY: Tustitala Fox.

Goble, F. G. (1971). *The third force: The psychology of Abraham Maslow*. New York: Pocket Books.

Keen, S., & Fox, A. V. (1989). *Your mythic journey: Finding the meaning of your life through writing and storytelling*. Los Angeles: Tarcher.

King, G. A., Brown, E. G., & Smith, L. K. (2003). *Resilience: Learning from people with disabilities.* Westport, CT: Praeger.

Krippner, S. (1990). Personal mythology: An introduction to the concept. *The Humanistic Psychologist, 18*(2), 137-142.

Lifton, R. J. (1993). *The protean self: Human resilience in an age of fragmentation.* New York: BasicBooks/Harper-Collins.

Moore, R. L., & Gilette, D. (1990). *King, warrior, magician, lover: Rediscovering the archetypes of the mature masculine.* San Francisco: Harper & Row.

Moore, T. (1996). *The re-enchantment of everyday life.* New York: HarperCollins.

McAdams, D. P. (1993). *Stories we live by: Personal myths and the making of the self.* New York: Wm Morrow & Co.

McLennan, S. (1999). *Finding your religion: When the faith you grew up with has lost its meaning.* San Francisco: Harper SanFrancisco.

Pearson, C. S. (1991). *Awakening the heroes within.* San Francisco: Harper & Row.

Rowen, P. (1990). *Subpersonalities: The people inside us.* London: Routledge.

Sarbin, T. (Ed.). (1986). *Narrative psychology: The storied nature of human conduct.* New York: Praeger.

Schachter-Shalomi, Z. (1997). *From age-ing to sage-ing.* New York: Warner.

Scotton, B. W., Chinen, A. B., & Battista, J. R. (1996). *Textbook of transpersonal psychiatry and psychology.* New York: Basic Books.

Taylor, E. (1999). *Shadow culture: Psychology and spirituality in America from the Great Awakening to the New Age.* Washington, DC: Counterpoint Publishing.

Schwartz, T. (1995). *What really matters: Searching for wisdom in America.* New York: Bantam.

Smoley, R. & Kinney, J. (1999). *Hidden wisdom: A guide to the Western inner traditions.* New York: Penguin/Arkana.

Walsh, R. (1999). *Essential spirituality.* New York: John Wiley & Sons.

Walsh, R., & Vaughan, F. (Eds.). (1993). *Paths beyond ego: The transpersonal vision.* Los Angeles: J. P. Tarcher.

Wilber, K. (2000). *Integral psychology: consciousness, spirit, psychology, therapy.* Boston: Shambhala.

Wong, P. T. P. (1998). Meaning-centered counseling. In P. T. P. Wong, P. S. Fry (Eds.), *The Human Quest for meaning: A handbook of psychological research and clinical applications.* Mahwah, NJ: Lawrence Erlbaum.

Wong, P. T. P. (2007). Meaning management theory and death acceptance. In A. Tomer, E. Grafton, & P. T. P. Wong (Eds.), *Death attitudes: Existential & spiritual issues.* Mahwah, NJ: Lawrence Erlbaum.

PART TWO

EXISTENTIAL, RELIGIOUS, & NARRATIVE THERAPIES

Hell Is Other People:
A Sartrean View of Conflict Resolution

ERNESTO SPINELLI

Abstract

This paper considers the possibilities and limitations of therapeutic interventions designed to reduce, remove, or resolve conflict from the standpoint of a number of key ideas presented in the work of Sartre. Sartre's (in)famous statement that "hell is other people" is a central aspect of the therapeutic relationship itself, whether viewed from the standpoint of the client or the therapist. Further, Sartre's descriptive notions of being-in-itself, being-for-itself, and being-for-others are reconsidered as useful means with which to investigate the varied disturbances presented by conflict issues. The paper argues that the application of Sartre's ideas leads the practice of psychotherapy away from notions of a dissolution of human conflict and, instead, places such dilemmas within the confines of more adequate possibilities of living with conflict in one's relations with self and others. The presentation concludes with an overview of an innovative training programme at the School of Psychotherapy and Counseling at Regent's College, London, U.K. which provides trainees with a Sartrean-inspired existential approach to mediation and alternative dispute resolution (ADR).

Three people whose names are Garcin, Estelle and Inez have been imprisoned in a single room without windows, furnished with Second Empire furniture in a condition of permanent artificial light and with a door which is shut and usually locked but also at unforeseen moments can be opened. They can never sleep, they have occasional visions of the continuing lives and judgements of those whom they have left behind on earth, they can never blink their eyes, nor can they die.

Garcin is the editor of a pacifist newspaper in Brazil. He is desperate to convince the other two in the room that he died too soon, apparently in an act of cowardice, but that, had he lived longer it would have become evident that he was in fact a hero.

Estelle, a vain and attractive young woman, makes it clear that she is willing to allow Garcin to seduce her, but only in exchange for his overlooking the fact that she murdered her child for the sake of a man's attentions.

Inez, an older woman who is also a lesbian, continually points out to both Garcin and Estelle that they are, respectively, a coward and a murderer. At the same time, she is desperate for Estelle to acknowledge her not only as an object of attraction but of superior attraction to Garcin, something that Estelle is unable—or unwilling—to do.

Garcin and Estelle cannot consummate their passion because Inez is ever-present to taunt and make fun of them. At the same time, Inez wishes that Garcin could simply disappear so that Estelle's need for love and approval will be focused upon her. And Estelle, meanwhile, hunts in vain for a mirror so that she can apply her makeup properly and so ensure the attractiveness of her appearance—which is, for her, the confirmation of her identity.

This circle of mutual anguish, shame, accusation and counter-accusation, denial, and objectification is repeated over and over again throughout Jean-Paul Sartre's (1989) play, *Huis Clos* (which has been translated into English as either *In Camera* or *No Exit*).

At its conclusion, after various individual truths are revealed and confronted, all three characters resign themselves to the truth: "So this is hell... you remember all we were told about the torture-chambers, the fire and brimstone, the burning oil. Old wives tales! There is no need for red-hot pokers. Hell is... other people" (Sartre, 1989, p. 190).

Well, as you may have ascertained by now, it must be said that Sartre's view of human relationships is not exactly optimistic. To be more accurate, it is fundamentally pessimistic. What value might such an outlook that is so closely associated with by now somewhat discredited 1950s-Parisian-Left-Bank-Gitanes-smoking doom-and-gloom intellectuals (so "Old Europe," as George W. Bush would say) have to offer the twenty-first century with regard to issues surrounding conflict resolution in psychotherapy or mediation or in its wider world-arena meaning? Well, as one who has straddled his whole life between "old" and "new" worlds, I want to say: "A good deal, I believe." This talk is my attempt to provide an argument in defense of this assertion.

Sartre's most fundamental assumption rests upon the hypothesis that each of us is faced with a basic and inescapable conflict. This conflict is the continuous tension between what might be labelled as our actuality and our facticity. Sartre's own terms are *being-for-itself* (pour-soi) and *being-in-itself* (en-soi) (Sartre, 1958), but I believe that the terms *actuality* and *facticity* may make it easier to grasp his ideas.

Our actuality is the expression of all that is possible for us to be as human beings. It presents us with the freedom to be as we can be within the wide-ranging limits of our possibilities. Our actuality permits us to transcend the definitions, labels, and habitual stances and attitudes with which we have cloaked ourselves. It is our actuality that offers us the means to remain open to the potential and possibility of our existence. This is all very nice. However, there is a price for this actualising freedom: it is nothing less than the experience of anguish. Anguish of what? Well, most basically, the loss of all substantive meaning. What Sartre is arguing here is that through our actuality we become aware that there is no fixed, reliable, certain objective criterion or value upon which we can base our chosen meaning as to what, how, and who to be. Nothing—no rule, no law, no god, no scientific fact. Nothing outside of our being is responsible for any and all emergent meaning given to our existence. For Sartre, our actualising freedom and choice do not lie at the event level itself—we cannot control, nor truly initiate, events. Rather, our freedom and choice become most apparent when our stance to "what is there," what has emerged at an event level, is to embrace it, accept it, say "yes" to it rather than adopt a stance that pretends and deludes itself into believing that "something else is there for me." Sartre's argument brings to light something that most other approaches have missed: The price of complete actualisation is meaning itself. Psychotherapists have been particularly naïve in taking this implication on board. They have sought to convince themselves and their clients that actualisation and meaning go hand in hand. As usual, it is their clients who have known better. In this Sartrean understanding of actualisation, no meaning remains, or is possible. All is flux, chaos, absurdity.

So what about meaning? Where does meaning exist in the Sartrean view of things? Meaning exists as a property or expression of our facticity. It is through facticity that we approach being from the standpoints of objectivity, necessity, and external or permanent truths, dogmas, facts, meanings. Our facticity continually moves us toward encasing and capturing our actualising freedom—essentialising it through what might be seen as the objectifying realities of life—our bodies, our culture, our place within an historical framework. Our facticity soothes our anguish, removes many of the burdens of actuality, provides us with meaning, or at least the possibility of construing some lasting, externally founded, meaning. But the move toward facticity also has its price: If facticity permits us to escape the anguish of freedom, we are, as a result, brought to the experience of shame that is provoked by our willingness to adopt a servile unfreedom.

As an expression of facticity, being becomes meaningful. All meaning directs us toward facticity: a constructed reality, an interpreted world made up of "self," "others," "scientific laws," "religious truths" and so forth. But for Sartre, our very search for and reliance upon meaning belittles us, and makes us less than the being we are in actuality. It is this awareness, available to us all, that provokes our shame. In embracing facticity, and all the secure, if limiting, meanings that it permits, we deny our actuality. For Sartre, we are nothing pretending to be something. And therein lies the source to all our conflicts.

Sartre is not suggesting that facticity is bad and actuality is good. They both coexist. Even so, while we can speak fairly knowledgeably of facticity, give it defining shape and substance, we cannot speak so directly of actuality since to name it will capture it and place it within facticity. At the same time, if we become aware of our actuality, it is precisely through or via our facticity. Without facticity we would not have the awareness of actuality. We might be actual, but in a preconscious way which is not open to human beings.

However, what is crucial for Sartre is that our very awareness of, and response to, this personal or subjective conflict does not arise as a result of some internalised, isolated, intrapsychic mechanism of tension as might be suggested by Freud and all his subsequent followers. Rather it is an inter-relational consequence. For Sartre, self and other are inextricably bound together in an inescapable relationship. If my life projects are attempts to fulfill my actuality, the presence and demands of others serve to remind me of my facticity.

As such, Sartre argues that the dilemma we all face is that each of us is locked in a continual and unceasing struggle with others. This struggle is no minor thing: It is the basis to each person's being confronted with his or her actuality and facticity.

When two people meet, a struggle begins between each person's desire to be perceived as a transcendent, actualizing, subject and to avoid being captured as a defined and limited factual object. Each person wants the same and fears the same. And each places the outcome of the struggle, be it success or failure, in the hands, or more accurately, in the gaze of the other.

As a way of encapsulating this, Sartre describes a person in a corridor outside a closed door who is irresistibly tempted, whether because of curiosity, jealousy, or vice, to look through its keyhole. As the person bends down he is riveted by what is opened to his gaze (it is another undressing while oblivious to his gaze) and experiences himself as pure actuality—every possibility set by the circumstance is open to the one who gazes. His power, within such a situation, is overwhelming. He is at one with his behavior, the subject of his own story.

But, unfortunately, this situation will not last. Taking on the role of the person peeking through the keyhole, Sartre writes: "But all of a sudden, I hear footsteps in the hall. Someone is looking at me. What does this mean?" (Sartre, 1958, p. 260).

At this moment, the gazing person experiences a rapid shift of perception and finds himself having a far more disagreeable experience. He is now embarrassed, uncomfortable, shamed. What has happened? He has suddenly found himself to be the object of someone else's gaze and is now conscious of the way in which the onlooker sees him. Not only might he come to the conclusion that he looks like a "peeping tom," the other's gaze shows him that he has become one. He has been impaled upon this label and categorisation via the transformative power of the other's opinionated gaze.

So, what happens to the person at the keyhole? This person, we are told, will suffer the objectifying shame of the other's gaze to be sure, but even so, he will later go away and rely upon some form of bad faith—perhaps a lie or self-deception of some sort or other, perhaps the suppression of the event, perhaps a transformation of its experienced meaning into something quite different, perhaps an excuse or other—that will explain away the objectifying experience of the other's gaze. Perhaps he will even convince himself that it was the other all along who had intended to gaze into the keyhole and that his own act had prevented a truly perverse or disgusting or violent scenario from having occurred. As such, he might further convince himself of how wise, or forward thinking, or even heroic, if misunderstood, he actually is. Given the circumstances of such self-other relations, what way out is there? For Sartre, there is none, of course.

The other steals my projects and gives them another meaning. The other rewrites my scripts. The other seeks to rid me of my freedom. Think carefully on this. Is this not what, for many of us, psychotherapy is both for and about? To create new meanings, novel narratives. Fine, but at what price? Could Sartre actually be correct in asserting that the price of such possibly caring acts on the part of "the other" who is the therapist is the client's actualising freedom itself?

That is a scary thought. But let us not worry over psychotherapy for the moment. Sartre's concerns are much wider than this. How do we respond to the other's attempts to reshape and redefine and transform us? Well, in brief, we retaliate, we make attempts to disorient or displace the other by adopting various attitudinal and behavioral stances. Here are some of the most typical and obvious:

First, we might adopt a masochistic stance. In order to be approved of by the other, I must attract the other's attention in such a way that the other experiences me as an object of interest or desire. For instance, I might compose a lecture that the other will find interesting or amusing or befuddling and, thereby, his or her gaze will be distracted from, or miss entirely, some of my other, perhaps more pertinent, actualising projects. Even if I achieve this, however, I become a slave to the other's master. I become a thing—no matter how interesting or wise or attractive, still a thing—for the other and thereby limit my actualising possibilities.

Alternatively, I might adopt a sadistic stance. In order to reduce the power of the other in my project, I can reverse the masochistic scenario and try to ensure that I perceive the other as an object for my wants and desires. Even better, I can try to get the other not just to accept this strategy of objectification, but to actually be grateful for it and beg me for more. Much of psychotherapy utilises this approach to some degree. However, the success of this strategy is unlikely without my resorting to some form of coercion or even, at the extreme, some sort of violence, be it physical, emotional, sexual, or verbal. I might, for instance, create the means whereby I convince the other to attend my talk because in some way or other it will be seen by him or her to be important, desirable, or even necessary to do so. If I can succeed sufficiently, I might also convince the other that it is both valuable and pleasurable for him or her to attempt to make sense of what I say, to view and value me as some expert, some man of wisdom, some superior being. Best of all, if the other experiences confusion by what I say or do, he or she will be convinced that its basis lies in his or her own deficiencies rather than my own. The use of such a strategy by psychotherapists is somewhat obvious. But this strategy, too, will only serve to capture me in that I am forced to concede the other's control of my project in forcing me to adopt such strategies. This is the old "s/he made me do it!" gambit. And further, even if I should succeed and gain the other's acknowledgement of my power over him or her, it remains the unhappy case that the other who now confirms me does not do so willingly, but only as a slave reduced to the condition of being a mere object. This brings me no lasting comfort—as the bully, the rapist, the molester, the tyrant, the chauvinist, the celebrity, and the god will readily testify.

Failing the above, I can adopt an indifferent stance. If I become indifferent to all of my relations with others by denying the possibility of any form of rapport with others, this may succeed in providing me with at least a partial resolution. But no. My very determination to avoid others ties me even more to them. I must now avoid them at all cost. And in order for me to do so, I must be forever out-thinking and outmaneuvering the other, and thereby, all my thoughts, concerns, projects, and behaviors become other-focused, even other-obsessed.

Still, I might now adopt the scapegoat stance. I can attempt to create a view of a persecutory outsider (perhaps the other who disturbs me, or some "other" other who disturbs us both). For instance, let us say that both you and I agree that I have delivered an excellent and stimulating talk. Much to our chagrin, we come upon yet another who takes a very different view on the matter. For him or her, the talk is boring, or inadequate or dangerous or heretical in some fashion or other. In such circumstances you and I might join together in order to maintain our differing projects and seek to find the means to dismiss this alien other. We might argue that he or she misunderstands, is incapable of understanding, is a representative of another approach which remains closed-minded to this one, is pathetic, or dangerous, or sick. In this way you and I can attribute all manner of qualities, including that of evil, to the outsider and create a false sense of harmony and social community. You and I are now joined in a mutual exercise of limiting the power of the scapegoated other, or even seeking to eradicate the scapegoat's existence. (Think of current propaganda surrounding—you name it: Israelis, Palestinians, terrorists, Communists, Fascists, unwanted immigrants, the Axis of Evil, and so forth—and it becomes obvious how common this stance remains.) But this creation of a social actualization project diminishes or compromises or eradicates or obscures any private project each of us may have had and which each may still be attempting to maintain. It is bad faith at a societal level.

Or, as an almost last resort, I might fall in love with one other. In love, each lover wants two possibilities: to be the provider of the beloved's freedom and, in turn, to be provided freedom by the beloved. The lover must be secure in the gaze of the beloved. And, in turn, the beloved must be secure in the gaze of the lover. But how? The sad paradox is that in this strategy the very opposite to what is intended comes into being.

To achieve the desired outcome, each, lover and beloved alike, paradoxically abdicates his or her freedom and demands the abdication of the other's freedom. "You can be free," each says to the other, "but only insofar as that freedom rests upon your acknowledged wish to be bound to and by me. It is I, not you, who determines the confines and boundaries of your freedom."

Each lover must become an ever-fascinating, ever-desirable object designed to seduce the beloved into retaining an abiding interest surpassing that which might arise from the gaze of any alternate, competing, other. And this cannot succeed. The beloved will begin to love the object that I have become and not me. I will begin to love the object that my beloved has become and not him or her.

If my falling in love provided me with an initial sense of an actualising freedom potential, the experience and struggle of my remaining in love, and of the beloved's remaining in love with me, is one of ever-increasing, and demanding, containment and restriction, a captured facticity rather than an uncertain actuality.

When I take the other's freedom as my end, the other becomes an object by the mere fact that I make it my goal to be the provider of his or her freedom. If I act for the other's benefit in order to realise the other's freedom, I am forcing the other to be free on my terms—even if I am acting from a stance of comfort and reassurance rather than coercion or force. Again, this might be something for the therapist who is so keen to free up or improve the life experience of clients to consider with some degree of caution and humility.

And if, as a final strategy, I hate the other? Hate implies the recognition of the other's freedom in that he or she does not act, or is not, how I want him, her, or them to be. To hate is to be reminded of my own lost possibilities, my own loss of actualising freedom, the power of the other over me.

And what is the felt experience of all these failed attempts? Anguish, shame, self-deception, disgust of others and of self. Every human enterprise may begin with the best of intentions but will eventually turn into its opposite. What begins as an attempt at actualising freedom becomes the facticity of oppression. If we stay with Sartre's argument, what implications might there be for conflict resolution, whether in the form of psychotherapy, coaching, or mediation and be it between individuals, organizations, or nations?

If Sartre is correct, then it must also be the case that inter-relational conflict is inevitable. The other—be it the psychotherapist or client, coach or coachee, confronting or confronted parties in a mediation caucus—remains inescapably my antagonist. The various strategies that are adopted in any such instances reveal themselves to be all too reminiscent of the more general strategies summarized before.

Is there truly no way out? Well, Sartre certainly pondered a great deal on this and in his later writings he became more willing to consider a potential alternative relationship which, fraught with peril as it was, nonetheless permitted the possibility of an alternative possibility.

Sartre's beginning of a possible solution comes from Heidegger's insight that "by 'others' we do not mean everyone else apart from me—those against whom the 'I' stands out. They are rather…. those among whom one is too" (Heidegger, 1962, p. 154). Heidegger's insight was that one's very sense of "I"—or more generally speaking, one's sense of self—is also an expression of "other-ness." Who I say I am is also a statement about who I am not; no real separation between the two exists. For Sartre, too, others are the way through which we perceive our own existence. Our experience of being the object of someone else's gaze brings us to our own awareness of ourselves as agent.

This novel stance of being-for-others emerges as the result of a conscious being's ability to consider the world as it is perceived by another such being. Being-for-others rests upon the acceptance of a mutuality of being between beings. Through it we each come to recognize our inescapable reliance upon others for our very sense of self, our very ability to recognize actuality and facticity. But make no mistake: For Sartre, "conflict is the original meaning of being-for-others" (Sartre, 1958, p. 364).

The move toward a being-for-others is not through the abdication or denial of conflict, but rather it is through the very acceptance of its inevitability and via the mutual embracing of its possibilities. A recent, if admittedly uncommon instance of this understanding is, I would argue, the series of "Truth and Reconciliation" hearings carried out in South Africa.

So, with all the above in mind we can now ask: How might an attempt at conflict resolution along Sartrean lines begin to look? A few years ago, The School of Psychotherapy and Counseling, under the impetus of a senior member of its faculty, Dr. Freddie Strasser, developed a mediation and dispute resolution program based upon Sartrean and more general existential principles. As its basic stance, the now highly successful program takes the view that disputes between separate or competing parties are also equally and simultaneously present within the worldview of each participant.

Therefore, one of the fundamental focus points in this approach to mediation is that of considering, exploring and unraveling each party's various self-focused and other-focused relations and motivations in order to then place these face-to-face so that each other's views, beliefs, values, and attitudes can be considered from the standpoint of their impact upon, and challenges to, each party's intended and thwarted aim or project. In turn, the discerned conflicts illuminated through this analysis can then be examined in light of the interpersonal dispute that has led the parties involved to the point of other-focused disagreement and antagonism between them.

This focus upon inter-relational issues permits each party to gain a more accurate awareness of the complex and contradictory structure that makes up his or her values, motivations, beliefs, and behaviors. More often than not, the inadequate awareness and understanding of one's varying motivations allows his or her competing concerns and interests to remain unclear and unseen. As well, this focus also permits each party to consider one's own varying motivations in the light of the other party's own set of conflicting stances. Not surprisingly, what often occurs is that, via the process of mediation, both parties may well discover that their difficulties and differences may rest upon all-too-similar foundational values, beliefs, and projects that are shared by both. Considered broadly, for instance, what is being suggested here is that while the worldviews of fundamentalist Christians and fundamentalist Muslims might initially seem to be in direct opposition to one another, more careful analysis might well actually reveal the source of mutual conflict to be as much (if not more) an expression of shared assumptions in their worldviews as they might be about the divergences between them.

As a more day-to-day example of what is being argued, let me present the following brief vignette of a mediation meeting with a married couple engaged in an acrimonious divorce dispute. In the course of discussion, the couple defined their primary presenting problem as being their inability to develop a satisfactory sexual relationship. The caucus session revealed that the sexual concerns, while undoubtedly real and relevant to them, also served to hold and express a far wider area of concern that had remained obscured. It emerged that each partner felt the other to be overwhelmingly and oppressively powerful in the relationship and that each party experienced major difficulties in maintaining his or her own sense of self-esteem while in the presence of, or while relating with, his or her spouse. These wider interpersonal issues were most clearly exemplified in their sexual relations. But their sexual problems, in themselves, were not causes to their conflict; rather they could now be seen as consequences and expressions of far wider worldview issues. In fact, it could now be seen by the couple that, rather than be at odds with one another, they were actually much more in agreement with each other with regard to their shared experiences of being themselves in the presence of the other. The recognition of this agreement permitted each to be more willing to consider how he or she "became" this oppressively powerful person to the other. Further, this same insight provoked each to question whether the way of engaging with the other that each adopted succeeded in addressing the most important elements of the complex worldview which each sought to embody.

If participants are better able to reveal their worldviews in a far more accurate and widely encompassing fashion, and through this to face their own sets of demands and vulnerabilities, then this in turn may permit an antagonistic attitude to be replaced by a mutually created and mutually responsible working alliance through which both sides may find some partial way to their own wants via the acknowledgement of the other's stance.

This approach to conflict resolution interprets "resolution" as a "living with conflict," not "living without or beyond conflict." This attempt provokes a novel experience: cooperation with one another not because we have eradicated the conflict between us, but rather because our attempt at "being for" one another arises through the mutual recognition of the inevitable conflict between us. It is a "fallen" sort of cooperation and resolution, to be sure: incomplete, always uncertain, and constantly straining to undo itself. In short, it could be seen as a sort of fun-house-mirror image of the pivotal Christian message: "Don't do to others what you do not want done to yourself—for to do so is to do it to yourself."

Now, let me consider some of the more immediate implications for psychotherapy were we to take seriously the notion of conflict presented by Sartre. Sartre saw that our most typical resolution to the inevitable conflict between actuality and facticity is the act of self-deception—we lie to ourselves, continuously. But, as ever, Sartre takes a different spin on this dilemma. He argues that the lie is the behavior of transcendence. That is to say, the fact that we can lie and that we can know that we lie, brings us to the awareness of our actualising possibilities.

In one sense, it is our recognition of the "lies" that infuse our lives that first brings us to psychotherapy and which, in turn, becomes the narrative focus of psychotherapy. Psychotherapy then, viewed in this Sartrean sense, is no longer about the eradication of our lies (as expressed in terms such as "symptoms," "disorders," "dilemmas," and so forth) but rather becomes the investigation of how these very lies serve our project and illuminate its previously unforeseen actualising possibilities.

So, how might a psychotherapy that acknowledges all such begin to look? Well, it would be a psychotherapy that insisted that the focus of psychotherapy would not be a dominating gaze by the psychotherapist upon the client's problems and concerns—as if the client were nothing but these. Rather, the psychotherapist might seek to find the means to provoke the client to attend to his or her own concerns through reflection upon "what is there" between that client and the therapist. As a way of doing psychotherapy, it remains manipulative, to be sure. But it is a manipulation that requires the therapist as well to somehow become the focus of his or her own gaze through the awareness of the client's gaze. The term *transference* only begins to capture the minutest, and least significant, aspects of this process. In essence, it is a move by each participant toward the acknowledgement and embracing of the otherness of the other as it presents itself, without desire or intent to direct any impact, alteration, or amelioration of that otherness.

This sort of psychotherapy would be one that acknowledges that the therapeutic relationship, like all others, remains grounded in conflict and competing strategies. What might distinguish it, then, is not the lack of such, but rather its active and unstinting recognition of this given and the willingness—at first on the part of the psychotherapist, and subsequently, via reflection, by the client as well—to struggle to face such honestly and openly from a "for-the-other" focus.

This attempt at being-for-others that is shared by psychotherapist and client alike and avoids any preimposed focus or aim, is transformative. These transformative possibilities only emerge spontaneously during and through the meeting.

Perhaps the following quote by Vaclav Havel (1999) begins to capture something of the ineffable meaning being hinted at:

> There are no exact guidelines. There are probably no guidelines at all. The only thing I can recommend… is a sense of humour, an ability to see things in their ridiculous and absurd dimensions, to laugh at others and at ourselves, a sense of irony regarding everything that calls for parody in this world. In other words, I can only recommend [the] awareness of all the most dangerous kinds of vanity, both in others and ourselves…. Those who have retained the capacity to recognise their own ridiculousness or even meaninglessness cannot be proud. [The] enemy [to this stance] is the person with a stubbornly serious expression and fire in his eyes. (p. 41)

So just how many therapists do you know who might fit that last description?

So, to conclude: Sometimes the world seems a very bleak place indeed whether because of personal circumstances or those of the more international variety. It is in those moments, I believe, that our willingness to embrace our human existence is truly tested and we are confronted with the full brunt of our own, and the world's, imperfection. I do not know about you, but in my own life I have found that as painful as they are, such moments also permit a certain numinous transcendence, an inkling of my actualising possibilities. Perhaps that is just some self-protective movement; I cannot say. But, whatever, I have found myself sustained by such. Among those things that have sustained me, I count the work of Sartre. I hope that, through this discussion, I have not done too much damage to his ideas. I also hope that, in some mutually acknowledging way, I have provoked you to consider, or reconsider, your ideas surrounding conflict and its resolution. I hope that some hint of your own struggle with actuality and facticity may have been illuminated, even if only momentarily and without the removal of its undoubted uncertainty. I leave you with one final Sartrean-inspired sermonette: "Even if Hell truly is other people, do not forget that the voice that welcomes you to enter therein can only be your own."

References

Havel, V. (1999). The first laugh. *New York Review of Books, 46*(20), 80-100.

Heidegger, M. (1962). *Being and time* (J. Macquarrie & E. Robinson, Trans.). Oxford, U.K.: Blackwell.

Sartre, J. P. (1958). *Being and nothingness.* (H. Barnes, Trans.). London: Routledge.

Sartre, J. P. (1989). *No exit and other plays.* (K. Black, Trans.). New York: Vintage Books.

What "Expert" Therapists Do:
A Constructive Narrative Perspective

DONALD MEICHENBAUM

We each spend a great deal of time, money, and effort in search of excellence. We attend concerts, dance recitals, and athletic events in the hope of catching a stellar performance. We have favorite restaurants where the chef has a "perfect touch." We delight in our favorite novelist, singer, or actor. We try to hire experts to help us with our computers, our taxes, our cars, and our health, and when in distress we may seek the assistance of an expert therapist.

Psychologists have studied many types of experts and compared them to their less accomplished and novice colleagues (See Meichenbaum & Biemiller, 1998, chap. 2, for a review of this literature).

This paper is designed to consider the factors that contribute to an "expert" therapist. For a moment, consider who is the best psychotherapist in your community besides yourself. If you, or a family member, or a friend, needed counseling, to whom would you go for help? Moreover, if you had an opportunity to watch this nominated therapist conduct therapy, exactly what would you see him or her do? Before reading on, take a moment and generate a list of the attributes and activities that you think an expert therapist would evidence and engage in.

The literature on expertise is fascinating as it highlights that experts differ from both novices and experienced non-experts in three areas, namely:

- Knowledge differences that include declarative ("knowing about things" or "knowing that"), and conditional or strategic knowledge ("knowing when, where, why, if-then rules").

- Strategy differences (plans for solving problems and achieving goals) and the ability to monitor implementation and adjust accordingly.

- Motivational differences that contribute to commitment and persistence.

We can now turn to how these concepts apply to expert psychotherapists.

117

In your list of features that characterize the best therapist in your town, you might have included that the expert therapist should achieve favorable outcomes. In the same way that you may wish to know the results of a surgeon you choose, hopefully one with a good track record, you would expect the expert therapist to also have a deservedly favorable reputation for the positive outcomes he or she helped to nurture.

The literature on psychotherapy provides some guidance on what we should look for in the expert therapist's repertoire. First, and foremost, if you wish to become an expert therapist who achieves favorable treatment outcomes on a regular basis, then the most important skill you need in your therapeutic repertoire is the ability to choose your patients carefully. You want to delimit your practice to the proverbial YAVIS patient (young, attractive, verbal, intelligent, and successful) who has a circumscribed nonpsychotic Axis I Disorder with no comorbid problems and no history of victimization. It would help if the patient also has good coping skills and nurturing social supports. In short, the literature indicates that patient characteristics account for most of the variance outcome. But for many therapists, they do not have the option or penchant to only work with YAVIS-like patients. Then what are the other sources of variance that contribute to treatment outcomes? These include: (a) relationship factors, (b) therapist characteristics, and (c) specific intervention procedures. How do these features show up as you watch your nominated expert therapist go about the business of healing?

CORE TASKS OF PSYCHOTHERAPY

The following core tasks of psychotherapy are designed to capture the complex processes of therapy. Because of space limitations, these are enumerated in point form. Elsewhere, I have discussed in detail how to implement each of these core tasks of psychotherapy (Meichenbaum, 1994, 2002).

- Develop a therapeutic alliance that is nonjudgmental, empathic, and supportive. The therapy relationship makes substantial and consistent contributions to psychotherapy outcome, independent of the specific type of treatment (Norcross, 2001; Ahn & Wampold, 2001; Wampold, 2001).

- Educate patients about the nature of their presenting problems (e.g., symptom features and course of their disorder, relapse symptoms, etc.). This educational process is not a didactic lecture, but arises from a Socratic dialogue and from various discovery procedures such as patient self-monitoring, feedback, and a collaborative case conceptualization that is individually tailored to the patient.

- Nurture the patient's hope by engaging in collaborative goal setting and by ascertaining both past and present examples of strengths and resilience. Adopt a strengths-based perspective.

- Help patients develop and implement a flexible coping repertoire, bolstering intra- and inter-personal coping skills. Build in generalization procedures. Do not train and hope for transfer. Follow specific generalization training guidelines (See Meichenbaum, 2002).

- Ensure that patients take credit and make self-attributions concerning the changes that they have brought about. Ensure that patients view the "data" that results from performing in vivo personal experiments as "evidence" that unfreezes their beliefs about themselves, the world, and the future.

- Address issues of relapse prevention; e.g., warning signs, high-risk situations like anniversary events, coping with lapses.

- Employ a flexible repertoire in customizing both relationship stances and specific intervention methods to the individual patient and condition.

- In approximately one-half of clinical cases where there is a documented history of victimization, the expert therapist also needs to ensure patient's safety and address the clinical sequelae of trauma exposure and comorbid problems.

- Help patients do memory work of trauma resolution and reintegration. The focus is not on merely retelling the details of the traumatic event, but instead examining what patients did to survive (focus on the "rest of the story"), and also focus on the conclusions and implications they draw as a result of having experienced the trauma.

- Help patients find and construct meaning (salvaging something positive from the trauma) that gives a sense of purpose, mastery, control, and acceptance. Use patients' already existing belief systems; e.g., religion, communal rituals.

- Ensure that the patients reconnect with others who encourage them to adopt active roles in multiple domains, rather than delimit special contacts to only other victims.

- Ensure that victimized patients develop skills and a sense of efficacy on learning ways to avoid revictimization.

A SEARCH FOR CHANGE MECHANISMS

The "expert" therapist is also curious in searching for the nature of the mediators and moderators that contribute to change. How do the implementations of these core tasks of psychotherapy foster and nurture change? A constructive narrative perspective provides an heuristically valuable framework to answer this question. A beginning point is the recognition that people are storytellers. They offer accounts that are designed to make sense of their world and their place in it. They construct narratives that include descriptions of events and of their and others' reactions to those events.

As Howard (1999, p. 190) observed, "We are lived by the stories we tell. Beware of the stories you tell yourself, for you will surely be lived by them." The observation that people tell stories, or actively construct personal realities, is not new. From the philosophical musings of Immanuel Kant to those of Jean-Paul Satre, from the psychological writings of Wilhelm Wundt to those of George Kelley, there is a long tradition of the importance of story telling or the creation of personal meaning. Common to this tradition is the view that individuals do not merely respond to events, but that they respond to their interpretations of events.

Perhaps it is possible that the core tasks of psychotherapy operate by changing the nature of the stories or narratives that individuals offer themselves and others. The change in the stories that individuals offer may represent a "final common pathway" of behavioral change.

As an example, consider the stories individuals who have been victimized might offer themselves and others. Epidemiological studies indicate that while three-quarters of individuals will experience traumatic events during the course of their lives, only approximately 10% to 25% will evidence a lifetime instance of PTSD. While the nature of the traumatic stimulus, the response to victimization, vulnerability, and recovery factors have each been implicated in influencing the post-trauma adjustment process, the present focus is on whether these variables are mediated through the narratives that individuals offer themselves and others.

Meichenbaum and Fitzpatrick (1993) and Meichenbaum and Fong (1993) compared the nature of the narratives of those individuals who continued to have difficulties following experiencing a traumatic event versus those who were able to continue functioning, in spite of the trauma exposure. Those individuals with lingering distress tend to:

- Evidence more intrusive ideation and are less likely to resolve their stories and integrate their traumas.

- Dwell on injuries and death and continue to search for an explanation and fail to find satisfactory resolution (i.e., they continually try to answer "why" questions for which there are no acceptable answers).

- Engage in "undoing" activities or what has been called *contrafactual* thinking ("what if" or "only-if" thinking).

- Make comparisons continually between life as it is, compared to what it might have been or what it was.

- See themselves or others as blameworthy and are caught up with preoccupying thoughts of revenge.

- See themselves as "victims" and as being "at-risk" with little expectations or hope that things will improve or change.

Moreover, mere words or descriptive accounts of the traumatic event often feel inadequate to describe the horror of what they have experienced and the perceived negative implications for the future. In order to capture and convey the "emotional pain", the traumatized individual becomes a poet (of sorts) and uses metaphorical descriptions such as: (a) "I am a prisoner of the past," (b) "I am soiled goods," (c) "I am on sentry duty all of the time," and (d) "I stuff my feelings." See Meichenbaum (1994) for a collation of the variety of metaphors that patients offer to describe their PTSD symptomatology of hypersensitivity, psychic numbing, intrusive ideation, sense of personal loss, and the implications for their lives.

Consider the impact of individuals telling others and themselves that they are "prisoners of the past," or that they are "soiled goods." The use of such metaphorical descriptors, either by individuals, families, communities, or even nations, can readily influence how they appraise events, the world, and their future. As Janoff-Bulman (1992) and McCann and Pearlman (1991) highlight, traumatic events, such as those of September 11, 2001, can affect an individual's (as well as a nation's) core beliefs concerning safety and trust and the resultant stories they tell. These stories, in turn, can influence the adjustment process, which, in turn, can confirm one's beliefs that strengthen the story line, and thus, the process continues.

What can be done to break this cycle? What naturally occurring socially supportive activities (religious or communal) and what therapeutic procedures can help traumatized individuals alter their stories so they come to find benefits, co-construct meaning, and marshal their strengths? These important tasks are underscored by the treatment literature for traumatized individuals as follows:

- Assimilate their traumatic experiences (Janet).

- Fabricate a new meaning (McCann & Pearlman).

- Develop a healing theory (Figley).

- Re-story their lives (Epston & White).

- Restructure and conclude the trauma story (Herman).

- Come to terms with or resolve their hurt (Thompson).

- Rebuild shattered assumptions (Janoff-Bulman).

- Develop a new mental schema and seek completion (Horowitz).

- Acknowledge and work through memories (Courtois).

- Reconstruct the self and provide new perspectives about the past (Harvey).

- Develop their own voices and not repeat the voice of the perpetrator (Meichenbaum).

Whatever the particular coin of phrase, each of these authors is calling for victimized patients to tell their stories differently. Patients often enter treatment with an account that reflects a sense of victimization, demoralization, helplessness, and hopelessness. They feel victimized by their circumstances, by their feelings and thoughts, and by the absence of support from others. This is especially true if they have a prior history of victimization. (Note that 35% of female victims have such a prior history of repeated victimization.)

Research indicates that therapy can help individuals both alter their narratives by distinguishing threatening and nonthreatening features of trauma and lead to fewer disorganized thoughts (see Foa et al., 1995; van Minnen et al., 2002). As Harvey and Bryant (1999) and Pennebaker (1993) and Pennebaker and Francis (1996) highlight, engaging in more coherent, insightful causal thinking can lead to more positive outcomes and improved health changes.

The various core psychotherapeutic tasks are designed to foster these narrative and behavioral changes as patients alter their accounts from one in which they view themselves as being "victims" to becoming "survivors." For example, in one case the patient initially viewed herself as a "stubborn victim" and over the course of treatment she began to view herself as a "tenacious survivor" based on her history of coping efforts and the variety of personal experiments she was able to perform successfully. In another case a patient was able to transform the emotional pain that she felt at the death of her daughter into a "gift" that she was able to share with others (see Meichenbaum, 2001). The Melissa Institute for Prevention of Violence and Treatment of Victims that I direct, grew out of the tragic murder of Melissa. Her parents, relatives and friends came together to transform their pain into hopefully some good that would come from this tragic loss. If they could help prevent one more such death, then perhaps Melissa did not die in vain. As Viktor Frankl observed (as cited by Mahoney, 1997):

The meaning is always there, like barns full of valuable experiences. It may be the deeds we have done, or the things we have learned, the love we have had for someone else, or the suffering we have overcome with courage and resolution. Each of these brings meaning to life. Indeed, to bear a terrible fate with dignity is something extraordinary. To master your fate and use your suffering to help others is for me the height of all meaning. (p. 32)

Such gifts to others are the basis for new "stories." Expert therapists help individuals engage in meaning-finding activities that transform pain and bolster coping. How expert therapists go about implementing the core tasks of psychotherapy to achieve these objectives of resilience is a story yet to be fully told.

References

Ahn, H., & Wampold, B. E. (2001). Where oh where are the specific ingredients? A meta-analyses of component studies in counseling and psychotherapy. *Journal of Counseling Psychology, 48,* 251-257.

Foa, E. B., Molnar, C., & Cashman, L. (1995). Change in rape narratives during exposure therapy for posttraumatic stress disorder. *Journal of Traumatic Stress, 8,* 675-690.

Harvey, A. G., & Bryant, R. A. (1999). A qualitative investigation of the organization of traumatic memories. *British Journal of Clinical Psychology, 38,* 401-405.

Howard, G. S. (1991). Cultural tales: A narrative approach to thinking, cross-cultural psychology and psychotherapy. *American Psychologist, 46,* 187-197.

Janoff-Bulman, R. (1992). *Shattered assumption: Toward a new psychology of trauma.* New York: Free Press.

Mahoney, M. (1997). Viktor E. Frankl, 1905 - 1997. *Constructivism in the Human Sciences, 2,* 31-32.

McCann, L., & Pearlman, L. A. (1991). *Through a glass darkly: Understanding and treating the adult survivor through constructivist self-development theory.* New York: Brunner/ Mazel.

Meichenbaum D. (1994). *Treating adults with post-traumatic stress disorder: A clinical handbook.* Waterloo, ON: Institute Press.

Meichenbaum D. (2002). *Treating individuals with anger control problems and aggressive behavior: A clinical handbook.* Waterloo, ON: Institute Press.

Meichenbaum, D. (2001). Cognitive-behavioral treatment of posttraumatic stress disorder from a narrative constructivist perspective: A conversation with Donald Meichenbaum. In M. F. Hoyt (Ed.), *Interview with brief therapy experts.* Philadelphia, PA: Brunner Rutledge.

Meichenbaum, D., & Biemiller, A. K. (1998). *Nurturing independent learners: Helping students take charge of their learning.* Cambridge, MA: Brookline Books.

Meichenbaum, D., & Fitzpatrick, D. (1993). A constructivist narrative perspective on stress and coping: Stress inoculation applications. In L. Goldberger & S. Brezntz (Eds.), *Handbook of stress: Theoretical and clinical aspects*. New York: Free Press.

Meichenbaum, D., & Fong, G. (1993). How individuals control their own minds: A constructive narrative perspective. In D. M. Wegner & J. W. Pennebaker (Eds.), *Handbook of mind control*. New York: Prentice Hall.

Norcross, J. C. (2001). Purposes, processes and products of the task force on empirically supported therapy relationships. *Psychotherapy, 38*, 315-356.

Pennebaker, J. W. (1993). Putting stress into words: Health, linguistic and therapeutic implications. *Behavior Research and Therapy, 31*, 539-548.

Pennebaker, J. W., & Francis, M. E. (1996). Cognitive, emotional and language process in disclosure. *Cognition and Emotion, 10*, 601-626.

van Minnen, A., Wessel, I., Dijkstra, T., & Roelofs, K. (2002). Changes in PTSD patient's narrative during prolonged exposure therapy: A replication and extension. *Journal of Traumatic Stress, 15*, 255-258.

Wampold, B. E. (2001). *The great psychotherapy debate: Models, methods and findings*. Mahwah, NJ: Erlbaum.

Religious Discourse in Psychotherapy

ALVIN C. DUECK AND KEVIN REIMER

Abstract

Religious language in psychotherapy has been the occasion of much controversy. On the one hand there are those who argue vigorously for its presence in therapy while others argue just as strongly for its exclusion. This paper explores the role of religion in therapy from a cultural anthropological perspective. We assert that religion is, like ethnicity, a social phenomenon. The religious client has the right to have his/her religion respected, validated, affirmed, and resourced in the process of healing. Failure on the part of the therapist to validate the religious tradition of the client may undermine the therapeutic alliance, diminish the client's willingness to disclose deeper issues of significance, increase absenteeism, and lead to generalized resistance. This paper explores concrete ways in which the therapist can appropriately address religious issues and create a psychotherapeutic culture in which clients feel free to use religious language.

American psychotherapy is experiencing a gradual awakening to the essentialist limitations of its own pretexts. Long indifferent to the implicit Westernization of its clients, the field stirs with a growing realization that for non-Westerners, therapy may reinforce feelings of alienation, confusion, and internal fragmentation. After years of impassioned appeals from cultural psychologists, such as Kenneth Gergen, American psychotherapists are faced with a troubling possibility (Gergen, Gulerce, Lock, & Misra, 1996). Western psychotherapeutic paradigms may serve as a form of psychological imperialism when exported to developing countries. Not coincidentally, this complaint is increasingly common among ethnoreligious

125

groups in this country who find that American psychotherapy does not speak their language, meet their needs, or respect their religious heritage. One step toward intercultural sensitivity is the recognition of difference. Each culture develops its own understanding of identity, pathology, and healing. To foist our view on other cultures is an act of imposition. It is our contention that a process of imposition is already well under way here in the United States, and as a result, American clients from ethnoreligious groups tend to avoid therapy or find its ideology alien.

While ethnic particularity continues to occupy a prominent place in American psychological literature, the religious question has been largely divorced from its ethnic referent, and is consistently relegated to the furthest margins of psychotherapeutic practice. The silencing of an integrated, ethnoreligious voice has contributed to a feeling of disempowerment for clinicians and clients alike. In the main, psychotherapists continue to avoid religious issues. Whereas the field lately demonstrates a willingness to entertain generic spirituality in therapy, particular beliefs and potentially exclusive religious practices are pointedly sidestepped. In a therapy of reduced ethnoreligious sensitivity, the clinician's silence regarding cherished issues of religious faith and ethnic identity may be experienced as invalidation by the client.

Tensions over the place of particularity in therapy are representative of a larger, politicized debate between those who believe that ethnoreligious language has no place in public conversation and those who think it does. Recent contestants in the struggle freely associate their positions with illustrious political figures of the past, usually in the service of democratic ideology. Rorty (1999) takes the view that religion has no place in public discourse. Following Jefferson's model for an Enlightenment democracy, Rorty allows only for a privatized religion excluded from public exchange. Rorty contends that religious language cannot be understood in the public square and only serves to heighten the cacophony of voices therein. The language of religion in public is an effectual conversation stopper. Religious issues are relegated to the interior space of the personal, much the same as one's hobbies or musical tastes. Rorty's secular public converses in a common language about shared issues of interest for the greater good. The achievement of universal imperatives for justice and freedom are best actualized where differing viewpoints agree on a common language that makes commensurability possible.

A chorus of voices opposes Rorty's argument (Audi & Wolterstorff, 1997; Mouw & Griffioen, 1993; Yoder, 1994). These philosophers, political theorists, and ethicists cite the example of religious justification for abolishing slavery as a counterpoint to the exclusion of religion from public life. Ethnoreligious particularity became publicly familiar through the civil rights movement in the 1960s. Martin Luther King's speeches were replete with religious allusions that mobilized civic change and charted a course toward moral reparation. Religious images in King's speeches were imbued with the ethnic struggles of the African people in the United States, creating layers of meaning that were co-constructive. Carter (1994) maintains that, in general, religious language has been trivialized in public debate with serious and lasting consequences. The splitting off of the religious in politics (similar to implicit prohibitions for psychotherapists) hinges on the idea that religious justifications are an imposition, discrete belief systems that must be separated from issues of ethnic particularity.

Just as the language of virtue has been neglected in psychotherapy (Dueck & Reimer, 2003), in this essay we maintain that there is mutual reinforcement between the trivialization of religion in public debate and the silencing of the religious voice in psychotherapeutic conversation. In the world of mental health, critical interaction over issues of ethnoreligious particularity lags far behind the debate in the public square. We are morally compelled to recover this lost ground. In the same manner that the ethnoreligious person has the right to express his or her convictions in the public square, so also the ethnoreligious client has the right to expect that his or her convictions will be deeply respected and integrated into the psychotherapeutic process. It may be that the rich heritage of symbol, tradition, community, narrative, and religion of the ethnic client is difficult to graft into a scientist-practitioner model of psychotherapy that focuses on the universal rather than the particular. Nevertheless, the hard work of ethnoreligious integration into psychotherapy arises from an emerging awareness of implicit risk within the status quo. Beyond the question of ethnoreligious imposition by the clinician, we perceive a sizeable danger in the imposition of universality in the therapeutic relationship. The hegemony of Western models for ethnicity and religiosity in psychotherapy must be qualified and reinterpreted in order to obviate the potentially toxic effects of this imposition. The danger of requiring a common language in public parallels the danger of imposing an ideology of universality in the therapeutic relationship. The imposition of a common language in public debate or in psychotherapy is an act that violates differences represented by the religious citizen or client.

Frictions between particularity and public access are therefore common to both the political and psychotherapeutic arenas. Consequently, we make a distinction between thin and thick discourse and regard each as useful (Geertz, 1973; Walzer, 1994). We will begin our discussion with an analysis of thin discourse, the language of consensus, applicable across cultures and comprehensible to each. Thinness is reflected in a commitment to scientific generalizations that are acontextual, ahistorical, and perceived as being interculturally sensitive. Religion is thinly framed in terms of morality common to humanity. This position is represented by individuals such as Rorty (1999), Rawls (1972), Kohlberg (1984), and Freud (1961). Thickness weighs in as a commitment to particularity that is unique and historical, grounded in a local community of linguistic distinctives. Here the representatives are Carter (1994), Walzer (1994), Sandel (1982), Hauerwas (1999), Wittgenstein (1958), MacIntyre (1990), and Jung (Jung & Jaffae, 1963).

Within each of these forms of discourse we intend to examine the avoidance or legitimation of ethnoreligious dialogue in American psychotherapy. We are at pains to outline the contours of a thick psychotherapy, believing at the same time that thinner scientific modes of discourse are on occasion useful. Accordingly, we propose a religion-accommodating approach to psychotherapy that is respectful of differences and places greater weight on mutuality in conversational exchange. We contend that thin approaches to psychotherapy, functioning as they do with a preordained script, are vulnerable to the charge of imposition of an Enlightenment ethos on the client. To avoid charges of cultural generalization we require models of psychotherapy that take seriously the thick nosology of ethnoreligious clients, modulating between thick and thin discourse where appropriate.

THIN DISCOURSE, THINNER THERAPEUTIC IMPERATIVES

Research findings on ethnoreligious issues in psychotherapy are limited by their own positivistic scope, making broad inferences risky without due attention to the cultural contexts of ethnoreligious being. For our purposes, epistemology, morality, self, and psychotherapy all have a stake in a landscape of ethnoreligious experience and the ensuing conversation over its thin and thick constituents.

The thin emphases of the democratic West are used as a foil in the cultural anthropology of Geertz (1973). Based on the work of Gilbert Ryle, Geertz proposes an exchange between thick and thin in social discourse. A thick understanding of culture assumes that a society develops symbolic systems of meaning that serve as the context of speech and action. Structures of meaning are layered, where symbolic interpretation is not universal but instead remains particular to a given culture. Culture is not defined by the application of universal laws to specific communities. Instead, Geertz notes that "it may be in the cultural particularities of people—in their oddities—that some of the most instructive revelations of what is to be generically human are to be found" (Geertz, 1973, p. 72). Geertz's vision for thick ethnoreligious particularity effectively exposes an agenda of Western thinness implicit even to the anthropological task. Thinness may obscure or even obliterate the integrity of local knowledge. Geertz worries that the unique symbolism of religious structures in tribal peoples will be minimized as a cultural accident in the West. Indeed, thin knowledge is easily transposed into moralities that lack cultural narrative, potentially dehumanizing diverse views of human experience that constitute the greatest single contribution of a people group (Geertz, 1983; Lyotard, 1984). Geertz's emphasis on local knowledge is a call to reexamine themes that may, ironically, mask the narrative contribution of Western culture to its neighbors in the developing world, or by extension, the value bestowed upon human dignity in the therapeutic relationship.

Thin Morality

In thin traditions morality is a matter of rules that guide the process of becoming virtuous. Morality requires that ordinary persons in all places agree regarding the duties necessary for the survival of society, and do so independently of religious faith. By definition, rules are indicative of universal human experience, whereas religious faith adds nothing to what is already known. Thinly speaking, moral theory is assumed to be able to correct the distortions of particularist and provincial religions. Non-Western traditions are treated as superstitious and primitive given their commitment to rules of taboo.

Modern moral philosophy has sought to provide a foundation for thin minimalism and to build a superstructure on this foundation. Minimalism, it was hoped, would supply a few generative rules that guide the construction of complex moral structures. A thin view of equality, though useful, appears to be incapable of addressing the complexity of distributing social goods. Walzer (1994) argues that a thin morality is simply one that reiterates the common features of thick moralities. The hope that universal morality will apply to all cultures fails to reflect our moral experience and pays too high a price for its imposition on thick local cultures. Walzer (1994) comments:

> The hope that minimalism, grounded and expanded, might serve
> the cause of a universal critique is a false hope. Minimalism makes
> for a certain limited, though important and heartening, solidarity. It
> doesn't make for a full-blooded universal doctrine. So we march for
> a while together, and then we return to our own parades. The idea of
> a moral minimum plays a part in each of these moments, not only
> in the first. It explains how it is that we come together; it warrants
> our separation. By its very thinness, it justifies us in returning to the
> thickness that is our own. The morality in which the moral minimum
> is embedded, and from which it can only temporarily be abstracted,
> is the only full-blooded morality we can ever have. In some sense,
> the minimum has to be there, but once it is there, the rest is free. We
> ought to join the marchers in Prague, but once we have done that, we
> are free to argue for whatever suits our larger moral understandings.
> There is one march, and there are many (or, there are many marches,
> and sometimes there is one). (p. 11)

Within a thin view of culture, knowledge and morality appear to be connected by a thread of implicit commensurability between all peoples. Thin perspectives are built on a foundation that is assumed to be interculturally viable and universally rooted in human experience. Hence, the moral prescriptions derived from this encyclopedic morality of the minimum will not be an imposition, but rather a basis for freedom and individual expression.

The Self in Thin Relief

Thin descriptions of the self tend to assume an organization of personality in universal terms—an essential structure of human nature. Examples abound in the psychological literature. Freud believed his model of the self (superego, ego, and id) was universal, as did Jung with his vision of the collective unconscious. Behaviorists assume that shaping of behavior occurs regardless of culture. Thin theories of personality might also include transcultural stages of moral development. Kohlberg generalized his stages of moral development to all cultures, as did Piaget before him in the cognitive and developmental spheres. A pervasive minimalism appears to be implicit to the Western view of human nature as naturalistically consistent in time and space.

Walzer (1994) engages this esteemed tradition by extending his view of thinness to the self. He begins with the assumption that the self is plural and that this plurality reflects the democratic prerogatives of Western culture. Inner plurality includes an internalization of various roles, names, and values that are held more publicly. In a pluralist culture, the social roles (citizen, parent, professional) played in any given day are represented internally. The names for these varied identities include father, mother, deacon, parishioner, accountant, clerk, and many others. Inner personalities associated with these roles may also reflect one's moral ideals, principles, and values (Dueck, 1995).

The thin self for Walzer is not circular, but rather linear and hierarchical. One voice dominates, a kind of "executive" appointed with the mandate to manage and consolidate plural voices. The executive functions as a single critical "I," at times repressing or ignoring the other selves. Thin descriptions for Walzer tend to be hierarchical and utilitarian—the upper layers of the human psyche determine lower layers, commending reason over will and personality over biology. This perspective raises an additional issue regarding the relationship of internalized selves to each other, when some are more particular and others are more general. Thick particularity suggests that the self, or the various selves presented in Walzer's democracy, is nuanced, particular, and ethnically unique. Some internal selves may represent disembodied value positions. It may be that just as ethnic individuals feel embarrassed in the presence of the individuals from the dominant culture, so also thick internal selves are considered negatively by selves that represent the ideological strains of the dominant Enlightenment culture. As such, the self lives between the two worlds of universal and particular experience that define external relationships. The ambivalence associated with this tension carries a significant burden for the integrity of the psychotherapeutic process.

Thin Psychotherapy

It is not lost on us that issues of plurality in psychotherapy reflect a cultural commitment to pluralism, centrally implicating the public square in the private sphere of therapy. The nature and content of the debate about public religiosity may be found in the therapist's response to a client's ethnoreligiosity. The potential ramifications for Rorty's vision of public debate are clearly outlined by Walzer (1994):

> In the psychoanalytic tradition, it is the instincts that are universal, while the critical standards by which the instincts are judged are always the standards of a particular culture. The id is the old Adam, and "in Adam's fall/we perished all." The superego, by contrast, is a human artifact, a social creation, different in different times and places, enforcing different rules and regulations, with different degrees of rigor and zeal. But these differences make only a marginal difference, for the function of the superego is determined not by its own particularist content but by the universal id, which is always there and always in need of repression. The philosophical view reverses the terms of this argument. Now it is the castigated self that is various in form and parochial in content, the product of this or that local history, while the critical "I" is in touch or at least aspires to be in touch with universal values. Self-criticism for the philosopher is much like social criticism (for the philosopher); it is a kind of reflection in tranquility, a scrutiny of the self sub-specie aeternitatis. I step back, detach myself from my self, create a new moral agent, let's call him superagent, who looks at the old one, me, as if I were a total stranger. Superagent studies me as one among the others, no different from the others, and applies to all of "them," including me, [and] objective or universal moral principles. (pp. 89-90)

It is therefore possible for one voice to dominate internal discourse. Modern psychotherapists in most cases give priority to the thin discourse of the Enlightenment morality. We would not deny a voice to the therapist or the internalized therapist who takes a universal perspective. Such a voice is concerned about the effects of an agent's actions on all humanity. However, an internalized voice as powerful as that of the clinician may serve to undermine or suppress the voices of ethnoreligious particularity within the client self. It is the clinician's voice that risks colossal imposition of cultural universality upon the client, with the concomitant hazard that the therapeutic relationship itself becomes a process of enculturation rather than the liberation so assiduously sought within the foundationalist model. Following Carter's (1994) description of the nature of conversation in the public square, the inner voice that speaks for particularity may well feel slighted and discouraged to speak. A model of public debate that legitimizes thick discourse would imply that, internally, all uniquely particular reasons for an action would also need to be considered and given an opportunity to speak. Insofar as the therapy is successful, one arrives at a historically and morally departicularlized self.

THICK DISCOURSE, THICKER THERAPEUTIC IMPERATIVES

In contrast to the thin perspectives described above, we embrace ethnoreligious particularity. We do not begin with religion in general because religions don't function "in general." Religious communities have histories, memories, rituals, and symbols that differ by tradition. To assume religion is generic or universal seems to be a prevalent perspective, but is potentially hazardous for the departicularized self. For us, religion is not an invisible entity common to all humanity. Rather, it is the expression of a particular confession made by a visible, historical community.

We now present a counterpoint to thinner views of culture, the self, morality and psychotherapy. We begin with an assessment of the effect of mismatching thick and thin therapists and clients. We then follow the same pattern of defining the nature of thickness, assessing the problems of thin universality and exploring a maximalist ethic for a religion-accommodating psychotherapy.

The emergence of thick and thin forms of discourse suggests that thin language is a consequence of difficulties intrinsic to communication between thick cultures. When a fundamentalist Christian, agnostic, Muslim, and secular Jew meet to converse in the public square, each is pressed to speak in a language that all will understand, compromising the uniqueness of their individual languages. In their ethnic embarrassment, these individuals may downplay their particularity for the sake of public acceptance and because the demands on the hearer are considerable. The sensitive therapist is faced with a similar situation. The therapeutic mandate to heal includes not only using the technical means to achieve this goal, but also to legitimate the deepest, most intimate features of an individual's narrative. Without this commitment, mental health becomes a structured arrangement of managed interventions impervious to the thick differences a client may bring to the therapeutic conversation.

What preliminary data are available to suggest that a mismatch of thick and thin discourse does, in fact, affect therapeutic outcomes? Theoretically, it is conceivable that the exclusion of ethnoreligious particularity will undermine the therapeutic alliance, diminish the client's willingness to disclose deeper issues of therapeutic significance, or keep those disclosures at a superficial level. Additional complications might include client resistance to interventions, absenteeism, premature termination of therapy, or even a diminished ability for the client to imaginatively engage with intervention strategies. In fact, some of these outcomes are already evident in the psychotherapeutic research literature.

Using an *emic-etic* distinction, Thompson, Worthington, and Atkinson (1994) linked Black female clients with Black or White female therapists who in turn were asked to use verbal statements that were either culturally unique or universally applicable to humanity. The emic approach begins with the cultural reality of the client whereas the etic posture ignores cultural particularity and focuses on what the client shares with humanity. Outcome measures in the study included the number and depth of self-disclosures of the clients and ratings of satisfaction with the clinician (perceived counselor credibility and willingness to self-refer). Using 20 items of the interpersonal, education, and training subscales of the Cultural Mistrust Inventory (CMI), the researchers divided clients into high and low levels of racial mistrust. Clinicians underwent an intensive training period geared toward increasing their levels of awareness of Black clients. The etic, universal model of psychotherapy used in the study, emerged out of Rogerian counseling interventions that focus on general themes of human emotion rather than the contexts affiliated with feelings. Clinicians were instructed to make three cultural content statements such as, "Tell me how your feelings of loneliness reflect your experiences as a Black student on this campus," or three universal content statements including, "As a student here, you've encountered some difficulties in your effort to make friends," during the course of therapy. Participants exposed to the cultural content condition indicated a greater willingness to make positive use of the therapist than did the participants exposed to the universal content condition. Moreover, participants disclosed more intimately in the cultural content condition than in the universal content condition.

The literature also suggests that ethnoreligious clients tend either to avoid psychotherapy, refrain from raising religious issues, or translate their personal problems into thin psychological language in order to communicate with the clinician (Larson, Hohmann, Kessler, & Meador, 1988). One well-known American psychotherapist responded to the first author's question regarding the presence of religious issues in psychotherapy by noting that "it never comes up." Religious individuals tend naturally to construe their concerns in religious language. However, when in the strange, seemingly "public" environment of psychotherapy, they may adapt by using neutral language for personal problems, often parroting psychological terminology such as "self-worth," "personal choice," and "depression." Shafranske (1991) reported the case of a successful Roman Catholic professional who lost his faith and reported it as a loss of a vitality to live.

It may be that ethnoreligious clients sense a therapeutic ideology that is different from their own religious tradition. The disparity in religiosity of the American psychological community and the general public is enormous with some 72% of the general population claiming some form of religious faith as compared to only 29% of mental health professionals (Bergin & Jensen, 1990). In fact, a substantial minority of psychologists view religion as irrational and many more continue to view it as an illusion (Ellis, 1990). Post (1992)has pointed out that in the Diagnostic and Statistical Manual of Mental Disorders (version 3), religion is portrayed negatively, where all 12 references to religion in the Glossary of Technical Terms are associated with psychopathology.

Tradition is not a popular basis for reflecting on the nature of conversation in the public square, carrying as it does the historical freight of its forebears. One has only to recall the crises in Rwanda, the Balkans, Nazi Germany, and Northern Ireland to be reminded of the bigotry and ethnic cleansing conducted in the name of tradition. Despite this, MacIntyre (1990) calls for a refurbished notion of tradition as an alternative to thinly universal knowledge. Traditions must be evaluated in terms of strengths and weaknesses, and should be assessed from within according to their presuppositions and commitments rather than from external vistas. What the traditionalist refuses to do is to make the morally particular into the rationally universal. It is in this last case that the contemporary emphasis on individual rights is confused with human nature.

A Thicker Morality

MacIntyre's (1984) argument is reminiscent of his effort to restore an Aristotelian ethic to a place where human *telos* is central to moral discourse. It is from within this teleological orientation that the traditionalist critiques the universalist for assuming fragments to be wholes. Modern moralities are fragments wrested from traditions, leaving moral debate in an unresolved state until the fragments are restored to the wholes from which they received their parts (Hauerwas, 1983). In the traditionalist perspective, moral rules are integral to the life of the community, and are given not to the oppression of rival traditions but to the longevity of the community and its telos.

Walzer (1994) underscores the salience of thick moral discourse in understanding and supporting thinner forms of morality. He begins with the community that has already forged a history and a set of shared meanings. Thick morality is therefore "richly referential, culturally resonant, locked into locally established symbolic system or network of meanings" (Walzer, 1994, p. xi). This is the language of a teleologically-oriented thickness that engages in thin dialogue, not at the expense of its own identity, but on behalf of the other. When a form of justice that crosses cultures becomes necessary, moral minimalism is invoked. Conversely, when the justice needed is local, a more thickly nuanced morality of justice can serve as the basis of discussion. The relationship of thick-to-thin moralities is such that within every thick, particularist morality, there are the makings of a thin and universalist morality, even if that universality is never realized. Definitions of justice for Chiapas Indians in Mexico, Kosovar Albanians in the Balkans, and Soweto Blacks in South Africa are necessarily thicker than those of the United Nations or other international interests with a stake in their struggles. Similarly, when Czech citizens debate their health care system, the justice defined is less universal and more a reflection of local history and culture than when the people parade with placards on CNN.

Making Space for the Thick Self

If we begin with a thicker view of discourse and of morality, what then are the implications for the self and the psychotherapeutic process? What if the self is nurtured within a community of teleological thickness? Walzer (1994) states:

> The order of the self is better imagined as a thickly populated circle,
> with me in the center surrounded by my self-critics who stand
> at different temporal and spatial removes (but don't necessarily
> stand still). Insofar as I am receptive to criticism, ready for (a little)
> castigation, I try to draw some of the critics closer, so that I am more
> immediately aware of their criticism; or I simply incorporate them, so
> that they become my intimate worriers, and I become a worried self.
> I am like a newly elected president, summoning advisors, forming
> a cabinet. Though he is called commander-in-chief, his choices in
> fact are limited, his freedom qualified; the political world is full of
> givens; it has a history that pre-dates his electoral triumph. My inner
> world is full of givens, too, culturally bestowed or socially imposed—I
> maneuver among them insofar as their plurality allows for the
> maneuvering. My larger self, my worried self, is constituted by the
> sum of them all. I am the whole circle and also its embattled center.
> This at least is the thick view of the self. (pp. 98-99)

Walzer suggests that the thin self needs a thick, pluralist, democratic correction. He would prefer that the entire community of selves have a voice and that democratic rules govern the discussion rather than the hegemony of a single voice.

As in social and political conflicts, there are many internal critics who are engaged in the internal debate. However, he also writes:

> I am not, nor is any one of my self-critics, the sovereign director of these critical wars. The critics that crowd around, speaking for different values, representing different roles and identities, have not been chosen by me. They are me, but this "me" is socially as well as personally constructed; it is a complex, maximalist whole. I am urged to conduct myself, let's say, as a good citizen, doctor, or craftsman; or I am condemned for not conducting myself as a faithful American, Jew, black, woman, or whatever. Many external "causes" are represented in my critical wars, and the representatives come from and still have connections outside. They have been internalized, in the common phrase, and, if I am lucky, naturalized-adapted to their new environment (my mind and heart) and to the requirements of competitive coexistence. None of them aspires, if I am lucky, to the part of superego or superagent, aiming at singular and absolute domination. (Walzer, 1994, p. 96)

We agree in principle with Walzer's plural understanding of the self but would modify his overly democratic reading of the nature of the internal selves and the governance of their conversation. What is not clear to us is how consensus is realized within the internal community. To Walzer's use of American democracy, we prefer the model of the congregation. We suspect that the ordering of the self might reflect the harmony of a congregation that inclusively listens to its members, empowers the weak to speak, affirms giftedness, waits patiently for consensus to emerge, and does all from within an eschatological telos that is the incarnate gift of God (Dueck, 1995). As a consequence, we propose that the thickness of the internal conversation is a gift. It is this inner conversation that is thick with ethnoreligious reference. Such a conversation will fire the imagination or condemn the guilty self in a way that thin morality can never approach. Rather than the bully pulpit of a single, fanatically religious voice in the inner congress of selves, multiple voices of expectation and experience are mediated within the self into representations that can be translated into behavior and speech in the public square.

RELIGION-ACCOMMODATING PSYCHOTHERAPY

In another context we have outlined an approach we refer to as tradition-sensitive psychotherapy (Dueck & Reimer, 2003). This model assumes the following:

- Tradition-sensitive, multicultural therapy involves first and foremost a validation of ethnoreligious particularity.

- Therapy with ethnoreligious clients can be modeled after cross-cultural models as is apparent in premodern shamanic rituals where the shaman's diagnosis and treatment function within the context of the ethnoreligious perspective of the community (Eliade, 1964).

- The clinician assumes that there is no transcendent position that permits assessment of rationality or normality for any client independent of conversation, nor does tradition-sensitive therapy appeal first to transcultural ideals.

- The therapist begins with the client's particularity, granting special attention to his or her embeddedness in a preexisting historical community.

- In the tradition-sensitive approach to psychotherapy the therapist begins with the local meanings the client brings regarding justice, truth, and the good.

- It recognizes the client's unique narrative, his or her developed traditions and symbols, and the unique language and grammar needed to articulate these differences.

- Therapy is not a conversation with a predetermined script or theory about how healing should occur independent of the client's shared world of meanings.

- Change is a consequence of the conversation rather than a preordained script.

- Thin interventions are often thickly driven by an ideology that may differ from that of the ethnoreligious client.

- Therapy capable of accessing the social network of the client and its thick cultural heritage will manage the pain of human experience from within local narratives.

Several studies reflect this commitment to ethnoreligious sensitivity to the client population. Propst, Ostrom, Watkins, and Dean (1992) utilized two versions of cognitive behavioral therapy—one religious and one nonreligious. Patients were all diagnosed as having nonpsychotic, nonbipolar depression and all 59 patients were religious. A control group was included as well as a group that received standard pastoral counseling. The results indicated that those patients receiving religious cognitive therapy or pastoral counseling scored lower on measures of depression, a difference that persisted when measured again after three months and two years. Furthermore, there was greater social adjustment and reduced general symptomatology for religious individuals receiving religious cognitive therapy. In addition, individuals in the pastoral counseling treatment condition significantly improved as measured by the Beck Depression Inventory. Propst and her group reasoned that there might be a clash in cultural values between traditional cognitive therapy that associates personal autonomy and self-efficacy with religious individuals who value dependence on a divine being.

Using an inpatient population of clinically depressed Christian adults, Hawkins, Tan, and Turk (1999) found that when a client group received a Christian form of cognitive-behavioral treatment, better outcomes were obtained than when the same population was provided with cognitive-behavioral treatment alone. We believe that with thick ethnoreligious clients, thinner interventions are less effective than thicker modes because the latter respectfully taps into the resource-rich nature of the ethnoreligious identity of the client population. This study raises the question of replicability across other religious groups, along with the use of other treatment modalities and diagnoses.

If ethnic clients are better understood by tradition-sensitive therapists, then improved therapeutic outcomes are implied by matching the two. Sue, Fujino, Hu, and Takeuchi (1991) found that ethnic match had a significant impact on therapy. Using a large sample (13,439) of Asian-American, African-American, Mexican-American, and Caucasian clients in a database of the Los Angeles County Department of Mental Health, the researchers obtained positive outcomes as measured on the Global Assessment scale, and premature termination when match occurred on ethnicity, gender, and language. Results were not consistent across all ethnic groups.

As is the case with ethnic similarity and dissimilarity, religious similarity of client and therapist affect variables that are related to therapeutic outcomes, including pre-therapy expectations and trust. Dougherty and Worthington (1982) found that when religious clients were presented with a case and four religious treatment plans, they tended to prefer the religious treatment closest to their own religious beliefs. Participants also indicated a reluctance to use secular therapists. Worthington (1988) suggests that highly religious clients prefer therapists with similar religious values to themselves. Highly religious persons were described as granting significant importance to Scripture or sacred writings, religious leaders, and possessing a primary religious group. More religious persons, he argues, use more religious schemata in interpreting the world. After reviewing the literature, Worthington and his colleagues concluded that highly religious Jews, Mormons, Protestants, and Roman Catholics usually prefer therapy with religiously similar therapists.

CONCLUSION

We have attempted to make a place for thick and thin discourse in the context of psychotherapy, laying out a project of religion accommodation for the contemporary therapist. The religion-accommodating posture will require more effort on the part of the therapist to create a common language in situ rather than assume it a priori. We can hope for the emergence of ethnically and religiously indigenous psychologies at home and abroad that co-inform and intersubjectively influence the other. It is just such a therapy that is inclusive of the margins, focusing as it does on the interpretation of actions within a cultural context, sensitizing people to a range of actions that are culturally intelligible and given to transformation.

References

Audi, R., & Wolterstorff, N. P. (1997). *Religion in the public square: The place of religious convictions in political debate, point/counterpoint.* Lanham, MD: Rowman & Littlefield.

Bergin, A. E., & Jensen, J. P. (1990). Religiosity of psychotherapists: A national survey. *Psychotherapy, 27,* 3-7.

Carter, S. L. (1994). *The culture of disbelief: How American law and politics trivialize religious devotion.* New York: Anchor.

Dougherty, S. G., & Worthington, E. L. (1982). Preferences of conservative and moderate Christians for four Christian counselors' treatment plans. *Journal of Psychology & Theology, 10,* 346-54.

Dueck, A. C. (1995). *Between Jerusalem and Athens: Ethical perspectives on culture, religion, and psychotherapy.* Grand Rapids, MI: Baker.

Dueck, A. C., & Reimer, K. (2003). Retrieving the virtues in psychotherapy: Thick and thin discourse. *American Behavioral Scientist, 46,* 1-15.

Éliade, M. (1964). *Shamanism: Archaic techniques of ecstasy.* London: Routledge & Kegan Paul.

Ellis, A. (1980). Psychotherapy and atheistic values: A response to a E. Bergin's "Psychotherapy and religious values." *Journal of Consulting & Clinical Psychology, 48,* 635-39.

Freud, S. (1961). *Future of an illusion.* London: Hogarth Press.

Geertz, C. (1973). *The interpretation of cultures.* New York: Basic.

Geertz, C. (1983). *Local knowledge: Further essays in interpretive anthropology.* New York: Basic.

Gergen, K. J., Gulerce, A., Lock, A., & Misra, G. (1996). Psychological science in cultural context. *American Psychologist, 51,* 496-503.

Hauerwas, S. (1983). *The peaceable kingdom: A primer in Christian ethics.* Notre Dame, IN: University of Notre Dame Press.

Hauerwas, S. (1999). *After Christendom? How the church is to behave if freedom, justice, and a Christian nation are bad ideas.* Nashville, TN: Abingdon.

Hawkins, R. S., Tan, S., & Turk, A. A. (1999). Secular versus Christian inpatient cognitive-behavioral therapy programs: Impact on depression and spiritual well-being. *Journal of Psychology & Theology, 27,* 309-18.

Jung, C. G., & Jaffae, A. (1963). *Memories, dreams, reflections.* New York: Vintage.

Kohlberg, L. (1984). *Essays on moral development* (Vol. 2). San Francisco: Harper & Row.

Larson, D. B., Hohmann, A. A., Kessler, L.G., & Meador, K. G. (1988). The couch and the cloth: The need for linkage. *Hospital & Community Psychiatry, 39,* 1064-69.

Lyotard, J. (1984). *The postmodern condition: A report on knowledge.* Minneapolis, MN: University of Minnesota Press.

MacIntyre, A. C. (1984). *After virtue.* Notre Dame, IN: University of Notre Dame Press.

MacIntyre, A. C. (1990). *Three rival versions of moral enquiry: Encyclopedia, genealogy, and tradition.* Notre Dame, IN: University of Notre Dame Press.

Mouw, R. J., & Griffioen, S. (1993). *Pluralisms and horizons: An essay in Christian public philosophy.* Grand Rapids, MI: Eerdmans.

Post, S. G. (1992). DSM-III-R and religion. *Social Science & Medicine, 35,* 81-90.

Propst, L. R, Ostrom, R., Watkins, P., & Dean, T. (1992). Comparative efficacy of religious and nonreligious cognitive-behavioral therapy for the treatment of clinical depression in religious individuals. *Journal of Consulting & Clinical Psychology, 60,* 94-103.

Rawls, J. (1972). *A theory of justice.* Cambridge, MA: Harvard University Press.

Rorty, R. J. (1999). *Philosophy and social hope.* London: Penguin Books.

Sandel, M. (1982). *Liberalism and the limits of justice.* New York: Cambridge University Press.

Shafranske, E. P. (1991). The dialectic of subjective historicity and teleology: Reflections on depth psychology and religion. In H. N. Malony (Ed.), *Psychology of Religion: Personalities, Problems, Possibilities.* Grand Rapids, MI: Baker.

Sue, S., Fujino, D. C., Hu, L., & Takeuchi, D. T. (1991). Community mental health services for ethnic minority groups: A test of the cultural responsiveness hypothesis. *Journal of Consulting & Clinical Psychology, 59,* 533-40.

Thompson, C. E., Worthington, R., & Atkinson, D. R. (1994). Counselor content orientation, counselor race, and black women's cultural mistrust and self-disclosures. *Journal of Counseling Psychology, 41,* 155-61.

Walzer, M. (1994). *Thick and thin: Moral argument at home and abroad.* Notre Dame, IN: University of Notre Dame Press.

Wittgenstein, L. (1958). *Philosophical investigations.* New York: MacMillan.

Worthington, E. L. (1988). Understanding the values of religious clients: A model and its application to counseling. *Journal of Counseling Psychology, 35,* 166-74.

Yoder, J. H. (1994). *The politics of Jesus: Vicit agnus noster* (2nd ed.). Grand Rapids, MI: Eerdmans.

Existential Implications
of Becoming an Orphan at Midlife

ALAN POPE

Abstract

Based on an empirical phenomenological study of personal transformation in the midlife loss of one's last living parent, this paper explores the deeper existential meanings of this experience. The unique nature of the relationship to the deceased, combined with a crossing of the generational line, provides the principal meanings against which this experience unfolds. Contrary to conventional theory, personal transformation ensues largely as a function of the bereaved orphan's attempts to "hold on" to the deceased parent. The psychological benefits of this process are detailed. In addition, this event opens onto a deepened sense of existential responsibility and commitment that serves a number of psychological functions revolving around a deepening sense of care toward others. It is concluded that the midlife loss of a last living parent can deepen maturity and accelerate ongoing developmental processes.

The loss of one's last living parent at midlife is a normative phenomenon that has received relatively little attention in the bereavement literature (Moss & Moss, 1983-84). Many reasons have been cited for this dearth of attention (Moss & Moss, 1989), but one escaping notice is that this experience has the capability of plunging the individual into existential depths that, until recently (see Wong, 2004), conventional forms of research have shied away from directly investigating. While quantitative, experimental studies have concentrated on the emotional impact of the death of a parent, often with conflicting results (e.g., Owen, Fulton, & Marcusen, 1982-83; Sanders, 1979-80; Littlewood, 1992; Horowitz, Krupnick, Kaltreider, Wilner, Leong, & Marmar, 1981; Scharlack, 1991; Umberson & Chen, 1994), some studies have suggested that losing one's parent can lead to significant developmental gains (e.g., Scharlack & Fredricksen, 1993). When researchers have adopted qualitative, phenomenologically oriented empirical approaches, they have concluded that personal growth is a foundational aspect of mourning a lost parent (Hogan, Morse, & Tason, 1996; Cochran & Claspell, 1987; Kessler, 1987).

This paper is based on an empirical phenomenological study in which I conducted in-depth interviews with four individuals for whom being orphaned at midlife was experienced as personally transforming. In conducting a rigorous phenomenological analysis based on procedures developed at Duquesne University (Giorgi, 1975; Fischer, 1974; Wertz, 1985; Giorgi & Giorgi, 2003), this study uncovered 74 interrelated themes articulating the explicit and implicit meanings of this experience as lived by the participants. These themes were organized into a generalized structural narrative, ranging from the early experiences of caring for a dying parent to an eventual reorganization of self in the months and years following the parent's death. While previous studies using quantitative approaches have yielded valuable behavioral descriptions of the mourning process, the pattern of lived meanings revealed by this study sheds light on a deeper level of existential meanings implicit in the experience.

THE PRINCIPAL MEANINGS OF THE DEATH OF THE LAST LIVING PARENT

Without recourse to phenomenological investigation, brief reflection suggests two significant meanings inherent in the death of one's last living parent: (a) the loss of the physical presence of one's caregiver since birth, the longest, most intimate, and potentially most caring and conflicted relationship of one's life—one that is steeped in archetypal significance (e.g., Neumann, 1993; Samuels, 1986); and (b) the crossing of the generational line, and hence being next in line to die. These two meanings distinguish this particular experience from other bereavement contexts, and, I suggest, are central to its unique transformational potentials. The complexity and significance of this relationship, conjoined with a heightened sense of one's own personal mortality, motivate many of the dynamics through which surviving adult children seek to accommodate this loss in their psychic and worldly lives. In the process of making this accommodation, this study made abundantly clear that it is the ongoing relationship to the deceased parent that is the driving force behind the personal transformation that occurs.

THE CONTINUING RELATIONSHIP: THE TRANSFORMATIONAL IMPACT OF "HOLDING ON"

Freud's (1957) mechanical view that healthy, normal grieving entails deca-thecting all libido attached to the object of the deceased parent, leaves no accom-modation for personal transformation; in this model the best one can hope for is a return to prebereavement levels of functioning. Some researchers have since criticized the consequent, dominant grief paradigm known as the *breaking bonds hypothesis* (e.g., Wortman & Silver, 1990), while others have conducted qualitative studies to demonstrate that, in contradistinction to conventional thinking, it is normal and healthy for bonds to continue after a loved one dies (Klass, Silverman, & Nickman, 1996). The current study certainly affirms this alternative understanding. Ontologically, when the parent dies, the *relationship to the parent* does not—only the parent's physical manifestation is gone. Insofar as any relationship requires work to maintain it, the participants in this study demonstrated great effort in maintaining the relationship to their deceased parents. That is, in accommodating the loss of a parent, one must *hold on* in addition to *letting go*.

The variety of ways that participants held on to their deceased parents conforms to the registers of experience identified in the Mahayana Buddhist tradition as body, speech, and mind (e.g., Ray, 2000). The *body* dimension is the realm of physicality and action. In this case, the surviving adult son or daughter holds on to physical objects that serve as reminders of the deceased parent, especially when signifying the parent-child relationship. Thus, one participant cherished a crib made by her father for her first-born child whom the father never met. Another held onto a flag from her father's naval ship, the same flag she remembered seeing flying on his ship as a small girl. Following phenomenological historian J. H. van den Berg (1972), we can say that these objects "gather a world," signifying a personal historical reality that the survivor keeps alive. Within the body realm, the adult son or daughter seeks out individuals resembling the parent, as if to secure role models to act as surrogates, or, perhaps, to help them learn how to assume a new station in life. The *speech* realm is reflected in the participants' holding on to the memory of something significant that the parent had said, be it a source of comfort or resentment. The *mind* realm consists of engaging a very active process of imagination with regard to the parent, including the felt experience of the parent's presence. Whether the experience of the parent's presence constitutes more than imagination is a metaphysical question that falls outside the purview of this paper.

Given these ways that middle-aged orphans retain a connection to their deceased parents, let us now examine the psychological functions served by this process. By holding on, middle-aged sons and daughters are provided the psychological and emotional stability they need to undergo changes in personality and cognitive understanding which, ironically, will enable them to further let go in time. For example, holding on permits the survivor to retain a sense of loving connection to the deceased parent and to derive nourishment from that connection. Also, the parent's perceived expectations play a huge role in maintaining sibling relations. Further, the loss of the parent heralds a shift in sense of mortality, and the sense of being "next in line to die," as one participant put it, causing a tremendous sense of loneliness and existential isolation. Actively embracing the lost relationship serves to moderate the intensity of these feelings as one, in time, comes to absorb and be transformed by their impact.

Perhaps the most significant benefit to maintaining this relationship to the deceased parent derives from the way that bereaved middle-aged children use their imaginations to continue learning from the parent. This imaginative engagement takes a number of forms. At one level, surviving adult children perform a life review that enables them to situate the parent's life within a larger context through which they are better able to understand the parent and heal old grievances. They come to forgive their parents for those actions and/or characteristics they had formerly disapproved of or resented. Because the relationship to the parent was such a formative one, the subsequent changes undergone in that relationship are reflected in the adult child's other relationships as well; in cultivating deeper understanding and compassion toward the deceased parent, adult children similarly become more tolerant and accepting of others. In addition, in reviewing the parent's life, bereaved adult children naturally review their own lives, perhaps finding that they regret—with feelings of guilt and/or shame—aspects of how they related to their parent. They come to realize that there were things about the parent they took for granted. By placing the parent's life within a larger perspective, they place their own life there as well, leading to deeper self-understanding and self-forgiveness.

Even in midlife, sons and daughters strongly identify with their parents; the second parent's death in particular threatens that identity. It has been noted previously that in this situation the surviving son or daughter loses the child role (Anderson, 1980; Moss & Moss, 1983-84). The present study revealed that the surviving adult son or daughter gains a new role, that of elder. Making this transition must be gradual, and one function of holding on is to preserve the child role until one has sufficiently gained command of what it is to be an elder. Thus, maintaining a relationship to the deceased parent helps to cushion the impact of the loss as the individual begins to undergo fundamental changes in identity and role. A similar pattern is seen in the early stages of this loss experience. Immediately following their parent's death, surviving adult sons and daughters find themselves busy with tasks and responsibilities which protect them from feeling the full emotional impact of the event until they are psychologically able to absorb it. What might initially appear as denial or unhealthy clinging is perhaps better understood as part of a larger dynamic between the twin processes of holding on and letting go which eases accommodation to the loss and promotes personal transformation.

CROSSING THE GENERATIONAL LINE: RESPONSIBILITY AND COMMITMENT

Holding on to the deceased parent eases the transition into a new level of adulthood brought about by this shift in roles from the child to the elder. In crossing this generational line, the middle-aged son or daughter is also thrust into a confrontation with his or her own finitude (Anderson, 1980). Losing the last buffer between oneself and death challenges one's illusions of immortality, and leads to a confrontation with "the possibility of no more possibilities" (Heidegger, 1962). Analysis of the descriptions offered by the study participants provides a vivid portrait of this process.

Midlife is a time when one must attend to a great many mundane responsibilities. When the parent first starts dying, middle-aged sons and daughters nevertheless feel ambivalent about taking on the project of caring for the parent. Immediately following the parent's death, a new set of responsibilities is born in the form of funeral and estate matters. When these affairs are finally resolved, adult orphans experience a new freedom, but there is a felt sense of a void in their freedom. They begin to feel the full impact of the loss, including profound loneliness and an enhanced sense of personal mortality. In time, however, this process forges a change at the level of Being as a new sense of existential responsibility arises. In this process, the surviving adult orphan becomes more deeply appreciative and motivated to give something back to the world.

Similar to what happens when confronted with being called to care for their dying parent, when called to this more existential responsibility toward others, midlife orphans must grapple with taking it on. They doubt whether they can do it, and yet they persist. They begin to do things for others they have never done before. In making commitments to others, they develop a greater sense of caring, and they find themselves challenged to expand in new ways. These commitments force them to act outside of the rigid patterns to which they have become habituated. In transcending their ego modes in this manner, they develop a deeper awareness of their interconnectedness to others, beginning with family and extending to community and in some cases to a larger spiritual framework. They gain a new sense of identity which is characterized less by an integrated composite of roles and expectations than by a sense of place issuing from the interconnection of caring concerns to which they commit themselves. From this position of greater caring they find themselves becoming more humble, tolerant, generous, understanding, and sensitive to others.

DEVELOPMENTAL PUSH

We can understand the death of the last living parent as providing what Moss and Moss (1989) describe as a "developmental push." In this sense, the changes wrought by midlife orphanhood are along the "normal" developmental trajectory, except that dealing with the last parent's death, and the meanings therein, accelerate the process. As we have discussed, holding on to the parent in a variety of ways, conjoined with a heightened sense of personal mortality, invites a new understanding of oneself and others, and one's place in the world. This new place promotes the transcendence of egoistic concerns, and a caring involvement that enables the resolution of old conflicts and the cultivation of integrity and wisdom. Thus, the psychological dynamics that unfold for the middle-aged individual upon becoming orphaned provide the opportunity to reach new levels of maturity and progress in the direction of full individuation or self-actualization. Under what circumstances an individual realizes this potential is a topic for further study.

References

Anderson, H. (1980). The death of a parent: Its impact on middle-aged sons and daughters. *Pastoral Psychology*, 28(3), 151-167.

Cochran, L., & Claspell, E. (1987). *The meaning of grief: A dramaturgical approach to understanding emotion.* New York: Greenwood Press.

Fischer, W. F. (1974). On the phenomenological mode of researching "being anxious." *Journal of Phenomenological Psychology*, 2, 405-423.

Freud, S. (1957). Mourning and melancholia. In J. Strachey (Ed. and Trans.), *The standard edition of the complete psychological works of Sigmund Freud* (Vol. 14). London: Hogarth.

Giorgi, A. (1975). An application of phenomenological method in psychology. In W. Fischer Giorgi & R. von Eckartsberg (Eds.), *Duquesne studies in phenomenological psychology* (Vol. II). Pittsburgh, PA: Duquesne University Press.

Giorgi, A. P., & Giorgi, B. M. (2003). The descriptive phenomenological method. In P. M. Camic, J. E. Rhodes, & L. Yardley (Eds.), *Qualitative Research in Psychology* (pp. 243-273). Washington, D.C.: American Psychological Association.

Heidegger, M. (1962). *Being and Time.* San Francisco: Harper Collins.

Hogan, N., Morse, J. M., & Tason, M. C. (1996). Toward an experiential theory of bereavement. *Omega*, 33(1), 43-65.

Horowitz, M. J., Krupnick, J., Kaltreider, N., Wilner, N., Leong, A., & Marmar, C. (1981). Initial psychological response to parental death. *Archives of General Psychiatry*, 38, 316-323.

Kessler, B. (1987). Bereavement and personal growth. *Journal of Humanistic Psychology*, 27(2), 228-247.

Klass, D., Silverman, P. R., & Nickman, S. L. (Eds.). (1996). *Continuing Bonds: New Understandings of Grief.* Philadelphia: Taylor & Francis.

Littlewood, J. (1992). *Aspects of grief: Bereavement in adult life.* London: Tavistock/ Routledge.

Neumann, E. (1993). *The origins and history of consciousness.* Princeton, NJ: Bolinger.

Moss, M. S., & Moss, S. Z. (1983-84). The impact of parental death on middle aged children. *Omega*, 14, 65-75.

Moss, M. S., & Moss, S. Z. (1989). The death of a parent. In R. A. Kalish (Ed.). *Midlife loss: Coping strategies* (pp. 89-114). London: Sage Publications.

Owen, G., Fulton, R., & Markusen, E. (1982-83). Death at a distance: A study of family survivors. *Omega*, 13, (3), 191-225.

Ray, R.A. (2000). *Indestructible truth: The living spirituality of Tibetan Buddhism.* Boston & London: Shambhala.

Samuels, A. (Ed.). (1986). *The father: Contemporary Jungian approaches.* New York: New York University Press.

Sanders, C. M. (1979-80). A comparison of adult bereavement in the death of a spouse, child, and parent. *Omega*, 10(4), 303-322.

Scharlach, A. E. (1991). Factors associated with filial grief following the death of an elderly parent. *American Journal of Orthopsychiatry*, 61(2), 307-313.

Scharlach, A. E., & Fredricksen, K. I. (1993). Reactions to the death of a parent during midlife. *Omega*, 27(4), 307-319.

Umberson, D., & Chen, M. D. (1994). Effects of a parent's death on adult children: Relationship salience and reaction to loss. *American Sociological Review*, 59, 152-168.

Wortman, C. B., & Silver, R. C. (1990). Successful master of bereavement and widowhood: A life course perspective. In P. B. Baltes & M. M. Baltes (Eds.), *Successful aging: Perspectives for the behavioral sciences* (pp. 225-265). Cambridge, U.K.: Cambridge University Press.

van den Berg, J. H. (1972). *A different existence.* Pittsburgh, PA: Duquesne University Press.

Wertz, F. J. (1985). Method and findings in a phenomenological psychological study of a complex life-event: Being criminally victimized. In A. Giorgi (Ed.), *Phenomenology and psychological research* (pp. 155-216). Pittsburgh, PA: Duquesne University Press.

Wong, P. T. P. (2004). Editorial: Existential psychology for the 21st century. *International Journal of Existential Psychology and Psychotherapy, 1*, 1-2.

Meaning Making in Illness:
A Potent Human Magic

MAUREEN ANGEN

Abstract

Making sense of a life-threatening illness is a difficult task that is made even more problematic by our societal tendency to blame those who experience illness. Based on multiple conversations with twelve women who felt they were living well after receiving a life-threatening cancer diagnosis, as well as on various first-person accounts of illness, this interpretive work considers how meaning making helps people with cancer establish a renewed sense of well-being. The voices of the women reflect how blame and shame complicated their efforts to grasp the messages illness presented, messages that eventually helped them to transform aspects of their lives in order to live each day more fully. This paper explores how people negotiate this paradoxical pairing of meaning and blame. It considers why we tend to blame the person experiencing illness and what some have done to resist becoming a victim while continuing to search for and find a beneficial sense of meaning in their illness experience.

As human beings we live with the impulse to story our lives into meaning. We give our lives cohesion and direction through our stories, smoothing out the rough and tangled pathways of our attitudes, beliefs, and behaviors. We ease or disturb our minds through the meanings we make of our experiences and the stories we tell others and ourselves. Our narratives are a source of understanding; they have a "moral force," a "healing power," even an "emancipatory thrust" (Sandelowski, 1991, p. 161). "Our narratives are orchestrations of meaning" (Schmookler, 1997, p. 37).

The human drive to make meaning was an important aspect of healing in the illness stories I heard from women who felt they were living well after a life-threatening cancer diagnosis. This drive was complicated by the narratives of illness that surrounded them, the predominant illness narratives of current North American culture, which tend to blame those who become ill for their own misfortune. Yet those who made meaning of their illness preformed a resistance to these dominant narratives that seems essential to their ability to continue to live well.

The material for this chapter comes from "An Interpretive Inquiry into the Experience of Living Well after a Life-threatening Cancer Diagnosis," a dissertation study undertaken to increase our understanding of what it might mean to live well with illness. My desire, as a counsellor in a community cancer care facility, was to open a dialogue around living well during illness. A hermeneutic-phenomenological approach was used to bring into play the myriad of voices/stories of illness and consider them in light of current societal understandings of illness and well-being. The results yielded a collection of paradoxes that people experiencing illness must struggle with. This particular accounting will focus on the meaning/blame paradox as it fits within the cultures of illness and wellness supported by current North American society.

GATHERING THE TEXT

The primary sources of information, the texts that have been most influential in this interpretation, have come from multiple, in-depth conversations with 12 women who felt they were living well after a life-threatening diagnosis, and from numerous autobiographical accounts of the experience of illness. As it turned out, the 12 people who answered the invitation to participate in this project were uniformly female, middle class, and white, with an age range from 30 to 66 years. All were married, except the eldest participant who divorced in her thirties and has since remained single. And all but one of the women have between one and three offspring, many of whom have grown to adulthood and left the family home. These women had each been given a diagnosis of "malignant" cancer: Half had a breast tumor, three had gynecological cancers, one had growths in her bowel, and another had tumors throughout her lymph system. Cancer had metastasized (spread to secondary sites) in more than half of these women, although in three of the women diagnosed with metastases more recent tests had shown no sign of cancer in their bodies at the time of our conversations. Three others had returned to active treatment for a further spread of cancer. One woman died during the research period.

In all our conversations the focus was on the illness experience, the meaning of living well after a life-threatening diagnosis, how well-being is experienced, and what increases or inhibits their sense of wellness. I also had many informal conversations in person, by phone, or through email with several of the women. The taped conversations took place between May 1998 and June 1999; informal conversations are ongoing. Throughout my involvement with this topic I also sought out and read as many first person accounts of illness as I could find. Quotes from these pieces of writing also permeate this account. The conversations and the reading provide horizons of understanding that fuse with the perspectives I have gained through my continued interaction with people who are living with a cancer diagnosis in my work as a counsellor. I have spoken to many individuals, read widely in the literature on illness and well-being, and brought to the endeavor my own understandings and observations. The interpretation of the topic presented here has resulted from a "respiralling" through these various sources and resources of information and understanding available to me.

In my inquiry I heard repeatedly how the illness had been the "breakdown" that provided a clearing in which new life meanings could arise. Illness disrupted one's life story, requiring major rewriting. These women spoke of illness as "a gift" or "a wake-up call." One described cancer as "a wonderful teacher" and claimed that even if some miracle could wipe out the cancer experience she would do it all again to gain the self-knowledge and way of life she had attained. She had no desire to return to the self she was prior to the experience. Many who are inspired to write of their illness experiences also describe the new perspective on life that arose out of their illness, the rearrangement of priorities, and the permission it gave for making meaningful changes in their lives. It seems that illness can provide the crisis that proverbially becomes a dangerous opportunity. The healing that this pursuit of meaning fosters can extend well beyond physical curing to the healing of all of one's interactions with others and the world.

Unfortunately, our society does not easily foster such meaning making efforts during illness; this is the challenge I uncovered as I listened to and read various illness stories. Within the attempt to find a meaningful understanding of the cancer diagnosis, the ill person must be wary of succumbing to numbing levels of guilt and blame that may be heaped upon their efforts. They must disregard or resist the numerous sociocultural messages, the dominant "stories of illness" written largely by our current society.

CULTURES/NARRATIVES OF ILLNESS

Culture, from a postmodern perspective, is constantly constructed by our participation in myriad ongoing discourses or narratives (Anderson, 1995; Kvale, 1995). While "participation" suggests a level of willingness, our individual author-ship or agency is both made possible and constrained by the various societal stories we are caught up in or subjected to (willingly or otherwise). "In the very act of telling a story, the position of the storyteller and the listener, and their place in the social order, is constituted; the story creates and maintains social bonds" (Kvale, 1995, p. 21). The regulation of behavior through the various role definitions and expectations that devolve from different discourses bespeaks the production of power in our society (Foucault, 1988). Narratives or discourses give shape to bodies of knowledge, which in turn give rise to institutions, which in their turn exercise considerable, though often subtle, influence over the embodied lives of those who come into contact with them (Bordo, 1989, 1993b; Butler, 1990, 1993; Grosz, 1994). Some narratives or discourses hold greater sway over others in our society, some provide more opportunity for dialogue and choice than others, and some are ignored or denied a hearing.

Within the culture of health in our society there are numerous competing discourses, narratives, "habits of mind" (Toombs, 1987), or "worlds of meaning" (Kleinman, 1992), that encompass our experiences of illness, disease, wellness, or well-being. Some of these stories wield considerable power over us while others struggle to gain a foothold in our society. Modern biomedicine, for example, having aligned itself with the dominant Western narrative of scientific positivism, has developed vast networks of culturally sanctioned institutions and professional roles. Even so, there is a complex discursive arena in health in which many voices are vying to be heard.

In this century, modern biomedicine has employed scientific technique and technology to alleviate the suffering of illness and to extend life. While there is little question that biomedicine has made great strides, its practitioners tend to overlook or even disparage the human ability to maintain well-being and our capacity for self-healing, relying solely on physiological procedures to dispel disease. Currently though, growing numbers of people, especially those suffering from serious acute and chronic diseases, are searching for ways to take an active role in their own healing processes, recognizing the need to engage their own healing resources.

A Brief History of Western Attitudes to Health

Reaching back to our earliest Western notions I found that health was defined as "the state or condition of being sound or whole" (Payne, 1983, p. 393). The words *healing* and *health* come to us from the Anglo-Saxon root *hale* meaning "making whole or holy" by "restoring integrity and balance" (Weil, 1988, p. 42). Over the past century in Western society though, modern allopathic medicine or biomedicine has dictated the authoritative notion of health. Despite its holistic origins, Western biomedicine seems to have narrowed the perspective on health to a purely mechanistic understanding of the human body. Health, in biomedicine, is defined as the simple absence of physical *disease*; the subjective and social experiences of *illness* are ignored or relegated to other disciplines (Capra, 1982).

Over 50 years ago the World Health Organization realized the restrictive nature of the biomedical conception of health as simply "the absence of disease." They offered the following radical departure from the biomedical understanding: "Health is a state of complete physical, mental, and social well-being and not merely the absence of disease or infirmity" (cited in Dunn, 1961). But it was not until Ivan Illich's (1976) writings that there was any questioning of the dichotomous model of health. He suggested that health is the ability to adapt to, and make meaning of, all aspects of human life—including birth, illness, aging, suffering, and death. He criticized biomedicine for medicalization of such natural aspects of living and disrupting our ability to live well throughout our lives, even during periods of physical duress. Also in reaction to the biomedical model, George Engle (1977) prescribed a shift to what he called the biopsychosocial model of health for use in clinical practice. This model views the individual as a whole system made up of various interacting subsystems embedded in larger family, community, social, and environmental systems. Aaron Antonovsky (1980, 1987), in direct protest of the pathogenic focus of biomedicine, developed what he called a salutogenic model of health encompassing both ease and dis-ease.

The "holistic" and "wellness" models of health that have grown out of such thinking take an openly systemic perspective, focusing on the whole person and person-environment interaction and thereby giving rise to increasingly creative attempts to re-story health experiences. The dichotomous model of wellness versus illness is being reconsidered in many of these new theories. For example, Margaret Newman (1986) developed a notion of health as expanding conscious-ness, in which health and illness are viewed as aspects of "a single process... moving through varying degrees of organization and disorganization, but all as one unitary process" (p. 4). These more complex, transformative approaches to health seem to provide an antidote to the simplistic patho-physiological focus of the prevailing biomedical model, opening up new directions for investigating how one might live well with illness, even though he or she might continue to have some problems.

Biomedicine has yet to take these new models into account. In a 1986 publication of the *International Dictionary of Medicine and Biology* the biomedical conceptualization of health continued to be limited to: "a state of well-being of an organism, or part of one, characterized by normal function and unattended by disease" (cited in Freund & McGuire, 1991, p. 6). Despite the fact that many people are clamoring for an approach to health that focuses more on dignity and caring than on curing and allows them to participate more actively in their own healing, the predominant model for health remains focused on treating the physical aspects of disease (Garrett, 1994).

The scientific worldview adopted by modern biomedicine rooted itself deeply in the soil of Cartesian-Newtonian thought and Newtonian imagery of nature as a giant clockwork. This mechanistic metaphor has had significant ramifications for ill people:

> The patient is the owner of the body-machine which is brought to the physician for repairs. A rational patient adheres to the rules of the sick-role: seeking out medical expertise, giving the body over to be examined and complying with the treatment regimen. When patients deviate at any step in this process they may be judged irrational or responsible for their illness. Even when the norms of illness behavior are strictly followed, if medicine cannot explain or alleviate the illness, the patient may be blamed for its failure. These manoeuvres act to maintain the rationality and coherence of the biomedical world view even while they disqualify the patient's suffering or moral agency. (Kirmayer, 1988, pp. 57-58)

The experiential and existential reality of people as conscious, self-reflective beings situated in a social web is rarely explored, and the bodily manifestation of illness is translated through laboratory findings into a set of quantifiable facts (Berliner & Salmon, 1979; Pelletier, 1992). These "facts" are then statistically compared to the numbers derived from other similarly ill persons in order to construct a diagnosis, a prognosis, and a treatment plan. This scientifically based approach sets the physician up as the authoritative expert, leaving the person who is ill in a passive role, hence the use of words such as "patient" and "invalid" (Hunter, 1991).

Medicine has done little to help us understand what it means to live well in the midst of a serious illness, and less to help us consider how to die with dignity, living well right to the end. In fact, biomedical institutions have segregated us from the ill and dying, resulting in an alienation from human experiences of suffering. We may be one of the first generations of human beings that get through life without ever experiencing the impact of having a relative die at home. This severely limits our ability to accept illness, pain, suffering, and death as part of the human condition. While much has been gained by the scientific approach to health and disease, much has also been concealed.

Holistic health models have attempted to uncover some of the aspects of health lost in the ascendancy of biomedicine, but these models have their drawbacks as well. The focus on individual responsibility has led to viewing those experiencing illness as morally deficient (Newman, 1986). Health is pursued as a lifestyle, as a moral virtue, with the beautiful, youthful, healthy-looking body being the manifest sign of this virtue and therefore, "…illness must be the result of a moral failure or lapse" (Pelletier, p. 28). The idealization of health and youth has fuelled an incredible industry in fitness equipment and centers, as well as cosmetics and cosmetic surgery. Our bodies have become the new temples at which we worship with religious fervor. Wellness-lifestyle models create a new form of "ableism". Those experiencing the disability of illness are positioned as responsible for not caring for themselves sufficiently. Biomedicine carries on as if in a scientifically sanctioned moral vacuum, but wellness models create a new dogmatism, recognizable in the New Age dictum, "You create your own reality."

In all of science there is currently a search going on for more comprehensive models which fit our (relatively new) understanding of the interconnectedness of space and time, mass and energy, mind and body, person and environment, and even consciousness and the universe. In medical science, the application of advanced laboratory science to disease processes is providing increasing evidence of complex, and simultaneous, biochemical interactions occurring throughout the brain and body (Pert, 1991, 1997). Changes in the natural science perspective—from dualisms to continuities, from mechanistic to systemic understandings—are pushing us to understand health in new ways (Kabat-Zinn, 1990).

Medicine, like all of science, is increasingly being located within a nexus of social, cultural, and historical forces (Bernstein, 1985; Kuhn, 1970). The existential fact of embodied experiences of vulnerability and suffering are missing in the biomedical discourse and many theorists are questioning this lack. Writers such as Budd (1992), Kleinman (1992), and Neuhaus (1993) argue that our experiences of ill health could be more promisingly viewed as interpretations, as attempts to ascribe meaning to a set of symptoms. This approach requires that health practitioners listen carefully for ways of approaching illness that fit within the individual's worldview. The ill person's experience, how he/she describes or narrates his/her own engagement with the illness and treatment procedures, becomes equally as important as the biomedical knowledge of the practitioner (Hunter, 1991). This approach has a large popular following judging by the success of such author-practitioners as Bolen (1994), Seigel (1986, 1989, 1993), Northrup (1994), Pearsall (1991), and Weil (1988, 1995), who all advocate getting in touch with the metaphors and meanings presented by the symptoms of an illness. By paying attention to people's stories of illness we have an opportunity to realize the ways in which institutional medicine can support or disrupt the healing needs of people who are experiencing illness.

MAKING SENSE OF ILLNESS

Those who spoke to me of their experiences of living well after a cancer diagnosis, as well as the various first-hand accounts I read, gave evidence of negotiating numerous contradictory pathways on the journey to healing. They gave examples, such as feeling that the life threat of the illness, while incurring physical and psychological limitations and losses, at the same time gave them an unprecedented freedom, a sense of permission to make changes, a release from the banality and grind of everyday life. Paradoxically, they found a more meaningful life in the midst of its threatened loss. Living well with a serious illness, as they described it, requires making sense of the disease, while rejecting any sense of blame. While no two of the illness stories I was exposed to were exactly alike, many described finding an increased significance in living by being present to the fact that one might die sooner rather than later. This recognition of life's preciousness and drive toward making the experience meaningful seems to be a predominant aspect of the phenomenon of living well after a terminal diagnosis.

Finding Meaning

Illness in our society is commonly held to be a negative experience, and yet the women I spoke to often described being blessed by illness in their new-found ability to truly grasp and feel a sense of gratitude for every passing day. Living well after a serious diagnosis involves reframing the experience of illness and reorganizing one's life to make each day more meaningful. The diagnosis of cancer, painful as it was, brought a sudden new awareness of the world and their place in it. In the words of one participant:

> The cancer experience... cancer wasn't the best thing that ever happened to me, but the "cancer experience," the wake-up call.... I'm thankful for that (Jazz1, p.13). One day I looked up at the sky and suddenly felt this immense gratitude.... Suddenly I became aware of the beauty of the sky and the sun. It was always there, but something shifted, that channel opened and since then I really try to be aware of what's happening in my life and be in a thankful mode. (Jazz1, p. 19)

Another woman claimed:

> ...definitely what I have found is that some of the most amazing things in my life, some of the best things in my life, have come through this cancer journey of mine. So that's pretty remarkable. (Beth, p. 6)

Many authors of illness stories, such as Arthur Frank (1991), Kat Duff (1993), and Oliver Sacks (1994), write of their lives being beneficially informed by facing their mortality as well. Audre Lorde (1980), a black feminist activist who had a mastectomy for breast cancer, describes her experience of facing her mortality as follows:

> Living a self-conscious life, under the pressure of time, I work with
> the consciousness of death at my shoulder, not constantly, but often
> enough to leave a mark upon all of my life's decisions and actions.
> And it does not matter whether death comes next week or thirty years
> from now; this consciousness gives my life another breadth. It helps
> me to shape the words I speak, the ways I love, my politic of action,
> the strength of my vision and purpose, the depth of my appreciation
> of living. (Lorde, 1980, p. 16)

Treya Killam Wilber, who died peacefully in her home after living three years with late stage breast cancer, contended that cancer taught her the ongoing lesson of "balancing the will to live with the acceptance of death." She found a place of "passionate equanimity" within herself—a place which allowed her to make the most of however much time she had left (Wilber, 1991).

Illness also grants a certain permission: one is allowed to be more fervently who one is, to do what one really wants to do, with less concern or regard for what others might think. It is as if the societal restrictions which normally keep us from acting too boldly or making radical life changes are suddenly stripped away; living one's life to its fullest and expressing one's innermost desires become much more crucial as the criticisms of others become less inhibiting. Anatole Broyard, a literary critic who wrote throughout his experience of living with and dying from prostate cancer claimed:

> A critical illness is like a great permission, an authorization or
> absolving. It is all right for a threatened man to be romantic, even
> crazy, if he feels like it. All your life you think you have to hold back
> your craziness, but when you're sick you can let it out in all its garish
> colors. (1992, p. 23)

There is a sense in which living well requires that each of us do what we need to do for ourselves, not in a selfish way, but in an authentic way which does not concern itself with the external judgments of "proper" behavior.

The occasion of "breakdown" that illness provides becomes in this way a "clearing" (Dreyfus, 1991; Heidegger, 1962); it creates a space in which one can live with exuberance and freedom we generally deny ourselves, with room for dancing out all the many colours and feelings of our life, and time in which to recollect our unique abilities and sense of purpose. Many religious and mystic writers have suggested that living well requires a life informed by the constant awareness of death. Buddhist practitioners engage in meditations visualizing their own death in order to become mindful of the ephemeral quality of all living things, to develop compassion for the fears we all harbour—fears which keep us from acknowledging pain, suffering, and death as inevitable aspects of life. Jean Vanier (1999) says that those who come to face their own fears and vulnerabilities

> begin to realize that to become fully human is not a question of following what everyone else does, of conforming to social norms, or of being admired and honored in a hierarchical society; it is to become free to be more fully oneself, to follow one's deepest conscience, to seek truth, and to love people as they are. (p. 95)

Perhaps living well requires that each of us face up to our mortality, to our vulnerability and fears, regardless of whether we have a life-threatening diagnosis.

Avoiding Blame

We live in a society that collectively assumes that each person is a rational agent acting on his or her own behalf. "Our commitment to rational mastery means that we would like to believe that if we do everything right, that is act sensibly, we will not get sick" (Kirmayer, 1988, p. 62). As a result, most of us tend to blame those who get sick for their own misfortune (like women are often blamed for being raped or AIDS sufferers for their disease) assuming that they must have done something wrong. Remaining secure in the knowledge that we have acted more sensibly and therefore will not get sick, we allow ourselves to retain our illusion of rational control. This way of thinking protects us from the need to face our own fears of illness and death. We can continue to assume that we are doing everything right and therefore have no need to worry that we might someday find ourselves in the same position. By blaming, we avoid the very conversations which might transform our understandings of illness.

Guilt and shame, from the perspective of those living with a serious illness—questions such as "Why me?" and "What did I do to deserve this?"—seem only to get in the way of well-being, while blaming allows the undiagnosed to distance themselves from those who are ill. Possibly the only good answer to the question "Why me?" is "Why not me?" Kat Duff, who suffers from chronic fatigue syndrome suggests that, for her, the only answer to the suffering and injustices of illness is to "come to see the universality of [the illness] experience" and, in doing so, allowing the thread of one's own life to be "woven back into the web of our world" (Duff, 1993, p. 132). Viewing her illness as something that is integral to the human experience, something that can happen to anyone at any time, is a form of resistance to the culturally held notion of blame. This resistance is often enacted by those who are living well with illness. Dwelling on the reasons for one's own possible guilt seems to decreases one's sense of well-being.

Sharon Batt (1994) struggled with this notion of blaming as she engaged with her experience of breast cancer. She wrote:

> I was offended by the underlying implication... that some personal failing of my character had caused me to get cancer and that—if I really wanted to live—I would quickly perform the necessary major surgery on my life, if not my basic essence. The prospect was exhausting, even demoralizing. (p. 144)

Yet she, like many others, was unwilling to reject the idea that there might be a connection between the way she lived her life and the cancer. She describes herself as yearning for an answer to the question her diagnosis posed to her. "Something had caused me to get cancer; understanding it might help me survive" (p. 144). Paradoxically, resisting the culture of guilt and blame does not equate to a negation of all sense of responsibility to the illness.

This is a quandary that I heard voiced repeatedly. People's stories of living well with a life-threatening diagnosis were rife with the need to consider the meaning of their illness and at the same time expiate themselves from any sense of guilt or shame for having become ill in the first place—a difficult process of negotiation when one is surrounded by those who, often with little awareness, impart blame. One participant, in a forthright manner, placed blame in its place very bluntly saying: "Ya, and these babies... babies get cancer you know.... Nobody can be blamed for getting their own cancer" (Linda, p. 17).

Yet, even as they avoid the sticky path of blaming themselves, they are quite willing to look for the significance of the illness in their own life pattern. It seems as if accepting serious illness as a meaningless event, as something inconsequential to be borne stoically and as quickly as possible left behind, is not a pathway towards living well with illness. One participant described it this way: "I really felt this was a wake-up call and I've been trying to listen to what the experience wanted to teach me" (Jazz1, p. 6). Another echoed this sentiment:

> Part of what I was trying to do was get reoriented, as well as dig back into who I was as a person that might've... precipitated the fact that cancer cells in my body could've taken hold....Ya, that made good sense to me and I had said right from the beginning, my words were, "This is a wake-up call" and I didn't know what I was saying about it being a wake-up call until I started to delve in, I just knew it was. (Lynn, p. 11)

Having an intuitive sense that she may have created the conditions for cancer to establish itself in her body, she has tried to understand herself better by delving into her past and seeing how it contracts her present ways of being.

Problematically, many of the early, popular, self-help books on illness promote the sentiment that the growing acceptance of the body-mind link can be directly translated into the New Age dictum "you create your own reality" (Wilber, 1991). The Simonton's (1978) approach to visualization, Louise Hay's (1995) positive attitude philosophy, and Bernie Siegel's (1986, 1989, 1993) early works on exceptional cancer patients, have all been accused of making promises that can turn into a serious pitfalls for the unwary (Batt, 1994; Handler, 1996; Lerner, 1994). The New Age "logic" of karmic lessons to be learned interferes with a person's ability to see that: "While we can control *how we respond* [italics added] to what happens to us, we can't control everything that happens to us" (Wilber, 1991, p. 220).

Numerous recent authors have tried to mitigate the damage that such guilt-inducing approaches can do in the lives of people who are already suffering (Lerner, 1994; LeShan, 1990). While many of the people I had contact with used body-mind techniques, such as meditation, yoga, deep relaxation, and visualization, or simply improved their self-care through exercise, diet, and getting sufficient rest, none ascribed to a sense of conscious control over having caused, or being capable of curing their illness. Illness presented them with an opportunity to find deeper meaning in life and their goal is to find ways of making whatever time remains to them a richer, more fulfilling experience.

HEALING BEYOND CURING

This interplay between meaning and blame represents a delicate balancing act. Living well with illness requires taking up an active, responsible role by acknowledging that there is some meaning in the symptoms of the dis-ease one is experiencing, using that meaning as the impetus for making changes in one's life, while, at the same time, retaining a sense of not being responsible for having caused the illness. Perhaps the difference is between being "responsible to" (as in able to respond) and "responsible for" (as in blameworthy). This might seem a minor distinction, but it appears to be significant for the cultivation of well-being during illness.

Arthur Frank (1997a) calls the need to make sense of being sick the "potential consciousness of illness" (p. 136). He suggests that this drive to find meaning in illness should not be dismissed as unproductive, magical, or superstitious thinking. For him it is a "uniquely human capacity to grasp suffering as a moral opening, an occasion for witness and change"—it is a "potent human magic" which allows people to make the best of the difficult times illness presents (Frank, 1997a, p. 143). Without this "potent human magic," despair, depression, and hopelessness can never be far away.

In *The Alchemy of Illness*, Kat Duff (1993) suggests "...we would lose ourselves altogether if it were not for our stubborn, irrepressible symptoms, calling us, requiring us to recollect ourselves and reorient ourselves to life" (p. 33). She worries that biomedicine, or as she calls it,

> Cosmopolitan medicine banishes that knowledge by insisting that suffering is without meaning, and unnecessary, because pain can be technically eliminated. Symptoms are divorced from the person who has them and the situations that surround them, secularized as mechanical mishaps, and so stripped of their stories, the spiritual ramifications and missing pieces of history that make meaning. (pp. 45-46)

The interruption of illness provides an opening that our self-reflective nature can use as an opportunity to reconnect with self and renegotiate one's way in the world.

My interpretation of these narratives of living well with illness shows their capacity to expand upon the prevailing discourses of illness in our society. These stories make a moral claim on those of us whose professional efforts put us in relationship with people experiencing illness (Frank, 1997; Walker, 1998). As practitioners perhaps we could tune our ears to hear more of the possibilities for transformation and growth in the stories ill people tell.

The understandings, which have unfolded throughout the body of this text, hopefully serve to deepen your awareness of the possibilities in this approach to illness. I have tried to uncover the ongoing process of negotiation and renegotiation that occurs as people struggle to find well-being within illness. I am not prepared to argue that everyone who would live well after a life-threatening diagnosis must find meaning in the ways suggested here. What I do want to argue is that through careful attention to people's stories of well-being within illness, we are called into a new conversation about health and what it means to live well.

Einstein is credited with having suggested that the biggest question that human beings have to answer for themselves is whether the universe is a friendly place. Somehow, despite all the suffering of their illness experience, people who are living well have gained a sense that the universe is a friendly place, that our experiences of living and dying make some kind of sense within a grander scheme of things. Perhaps the sacrifices of illness convey to us a deeper understanding of the sacredness, the wholeness, of all life—restoring us to a greater sense of integrity and balance, as in "health" or *hale* (Latin for whole, holy).

References

Achterberg, J. (1985) *Imagery in healing*. Boston: New Science Library.

Anderson, W. T. (Ed.). (1995). *The truth about the truth: De-confusing and re-constructing the postmodern world*. New York: Tarcher/Putnam.

Barasch, M. I. (1993). *The healing path: A soul approach to illness*. New York: Putnam Press.

Batt, S. (1994). *Patient no more: The politics of breast cancer*. Charlottetown, PE: Gynergy Books.

Bordo, S. (1989). The body and the reproduction of femininity: A feminist appropriation of Foucault. In A. Jagger & S. Bordo (Eds.), *Gender/body/knowledge: Feminist reconstructions of being and knowing* (pp. 13-33). New Brunswick, NJ: Rutgers University Press.

Frank, A. (1991). *At the will of the body: Reflections on illness*. Boston: Houghton Mifflin.

Frank, A. W. (1997). Illness as a moral occasion: Restoring agency to ill people. *Health, 1(2)*, 131-148.

Hay, L. (1995). *Life: Reflections on your journey*. Carson, CA: Hay House.

Heidegger, M. (1962). *Being and time*. New York: Harper.

Hunter (1991). *Doctors' stories: The narrative structure of medical knowledge*. Princeton, MA: Princeton University Press.

Kirmayer, L. J. (1988). Mind and body as metaphors: Hidden values in biomedicine. In M. Lock & D. Gordon (Eds.), *Biomedicine examined* (pp. 57-93). Boston: Kluwer Academic Publishers.

LeShan, L. (1990). *Cancer as a turning point*. New York: Plume Printing.

Lorde, A. (1980). *The cancer journals*. San Francisco, CA: Aunt Lute Books.

Pearsall, P. (1991). *Making Miracles*. New York: Prentice Hall Press.

Pert, C. (1997). *Molecules of emotion*. New York: Schribner.

Remen, R. N. (1996). *Kitchen table wisdom: Stories that heal*. New York: Riverhead Books.

Schmookler, A. B. (1997). *Living posthumously: Confronting the loss of vital powers*. New York: Henry Holt.

Simonton, O. C., & Mathews-Simonton, S. (1978). *Getting well again*. New York: Tarcher.

Toombs, K. S. (1987). The meaning of illness: A phenomenological approach to the patient-physician relationship. *The Journal of Medicine and Philosophy, 12*, 219-240.

Vanier, J. (1999) *Becoming human*. Toronto, ON: House of Anansi Press.

Wilber, K. (1991). *Grace and grit*. Boston: Shambhala.

Author Note

I wish to thank the Social Science and Humanities Research Council of Canada, the Killam Foundation at the University of Calgary and the Canadian Institutes of Health Research for support during various aspects of bringing this study to print. I am also indebted to Dr. Sharon Robertson and Dr. Jim Field for their mentoring and seeing me through the dissertation process.

Posttraumatic Growth:
Finding Meaning through Trauma

PATRICIA FRAZIER
AMY CONLON
TY TASHIRO,
SARAH SASS

Abstract

A growing body of research suggests that many victims of traumatic events, in addition to experiencing symptoms of posttraumatic stress, report positive changes in their lives as a result of the trauma (e.g., Tedeschi & Calhoun, 1995). These changes include realizing how strong they are, growing closer to friends and family, and appreciating life more. Posttraumatic growth relates to the general topic of "meaning" in two ways. First, finding positive aspects of a traumatic event can be a way of finding meaning in the event. Second, traumatic events can lead to a greater sense of meaning in life, as a result of rebuilding schemas that were shattered by the traumatic event. This paper addresses three questions: (a) What is the prevalence of posttraumatic growth at various points posttrauma? (b) How is growth related to more commonly recognized symptoms of posttraumatic distress? and (c) What factors are related to growth following a traumatic event?

PREVALENCE OF POSTTRAUMATIC GROWTH

In terms of prevalence, posttraumatic growth is fairly common. Although there is variability across studies, in most studies, about 50-60% of the sample reports some positive change as a result of various traumas. The four most common broad areas of growth are positive changes in self, relationships, life philosophy, and empathy (Tedeschi & Calhoun, 1995).

Even though growth following trauma does seem to be fairly common, various limitations of the research make it difficult to estimate its actual prevalence. First, in many studies, posttraumatic growth has not been assessed systematically. For example, some prevalence rates are based on the number of people who spontaneously reported some type of positive change to the researcher who actually was studying the *negative* effects of trauma. Other studies have used open-ended questions to assess the effects of trauma, only some of which directly ask about positive changes. A second limitation is that research has tended to focus on certain types of traumatic events, particularly illness. However, other types of trauma may result in different types or amounts of positive changes. For example, unlike illness, a sexual assault involves the intentional infliction of harm and therefore may be less likely to lead to positive changes. Finally, most studies have been cross-sectional and have assessed positive changes months or years after the trauma. This fits with the general assumption that growth is the result of a long recovery process (e.g., Calhoun & Tedeschi, 1998). However, since change generally is not assessed in the early posttrauma period, this assumption has not been tested adequately.

In an effort to address some of these limitations, we assessed positive change more systematically and in survivors of an event that is not often studied—namely, sexual assault. We also collected data longitudinally in one sample so that we could assess the prevalence of positive change at different points in the posttrauma recovery process, including soon after the assault.

POSITIVE CHANGE AND DISTRESS

While it is encouraging that traumatic events can have positive effects, it is important to know how these self-reported positive changes relate to more traditional measures of posttraumatic distress. For example, people who are able to find some positive aspect of the trauma might report less distress. On the other hand, because more severe events tend to lead to more positive change, growth may be *positively* related to distress. Finally, reports of growth and distress may be unrelated (see Park, 1998, for a review). Research to date on the relations between positive changes and distress is somewhat equivocal. Although there is some support for each of these hypotheses, most studies find that positive change is related to less distress.

Research on the relations between positive change and distress also has limitations. Some of these were mentioned before, such as the lack of systematic measurement and the fact that most studies have been conducted months or years posttrauma. This second limitation is particularly important because it means that we have little information regarding whether reports of positive change are more adaptive at certain points than at others. For example, early reports of change may reflect denial, whereas reports of growth reported years after the trauma may reflect actual life changes. We also know very little about whether certain types of positive changes are more or less associated with psychological distress. Information on which kinds of changes are most adaptive (or harmful) seems particularly important in terms of identifying possible areas for therapeutic intervention.

To address these questions, we assessed the relations between reports of positive change and standard distress measures at various points post-rape. We also assessed the relations between specific types of positive changes and distress measures.

CORRELATES OF POSITIVE CHANGE

The final question concerns identifying factors related to reporting positive change. We focus here on two broad areas: coping strategies and perceived control. In regard to coping, quite a lot of research supports a link between approach and avoidance coping strategies and traditional distress measures. Generally, approach-coping strategies, in which individuals attempt to work through and deal with the traumatic event, are associated with fewer symptoms while avoidance strategies are associated with more symptoms. There is far less research exploring the relationship between coping strategies and posttraumatic growth, although it seems likely that the strategies people use to cope with trauma would be associated with the extent to which they report posttraumatic growth. Specifically, the ability to perceive positive change seems to require that trauma survivors acknowledge and deal with the trauma. Thus, use of approach-coping strategies should be associated with more positive change whereas avoidance strategies should be associated with fewer positive changes. Another coping-related variable that has been found to be related to posttraumatic growth is religiosity (Calhoun, Cann, Tedeschi, & McMillan, 2000). This makes sense in that religious beliefs are likely to facilitate the meaning-making process.

In regard to perceived control, it is important to distinguish between various types of control: perceived control over the past, perceived control over the present recovery process, and perceived control over the future. We examined perceived control because finding benefits or positive change has been conceptualized as a form of secondary control, or a way of trying to gain control over an uncontrollable situation (Affleck, Tennen, & Gershman, 1985). Little research has examined the relations between these aspects of control and growth; what does exist has yielded inconsistent results.

In summary, the three goals of our research were to assess the prevalence of posttraumatic growth at various points of posttrauma, the relations between growth and commonly recognized symptoms of posttraumatic distress, and the correlates of self-reported growth among two samples of sexual assault survivors.

METHOD
Participants

One group of participants was 174 female sexual assault survivors who were contacted through the Sexual Assault Resource Service (SARS) which is an agency that works with several hospitals in Minneapolis, MN, to perform evidentiary exams and provide counseling for survivors who report to the emergency room (ER) following a sexual assault (ER sample). SARS clients who chose to participate in our study completed questionnaires at four points post-assault: two-weeks, and two, six, and twelve months. We received approximately 90 completed questionnaires at each time period. Most of the participants were Caucasian and their average age was 28 years.

The second sample (community sample) was sexual assault survivors identified via a random phone interview regarding trauma experiences and post-traumatic stress disorder (PTSD). Briefly, women who were willing to participate in a follow-up study after the phone interview were mailed questionnaires. We received 135 completed questionnaires from women who had experienced a sexual assault at some point in their life. The average time since the assault was 16 years. Most of the respondents were Caucasian, and had an average age of 39.

Measures

Positive change. To identify the specific aspects of life that had changed as a result of the assault, participants completed a 14-item life change measure. Items were developed based on open-ended responses of sexual assault survivors obtained in an earlier study and the broader literature on posttraumatic growth. The items reflected the four life domains mentioned earlier: changes in self (e.g., ability to be assertive), relationships (e.g., relationships with friends and family), spirituality or life philosophy (e.g., appreciation of life), and empathy (e.g., concern for others in similar situations). Items were rated on a 5-point scale with 1 indicating that area of life had gotten "much worse" as a result of the assault,

3 indicating no change, and 5 indicating that it had gotten "much better." To determine the total number of positive changes reported, we added the number of items rated as either a 4 or a 5. For the correlational analyses, we created a scale out of the 14 items, with higher scores reflecting more overall positive change.

Distress. We combined scores on the depression, hostility, and anxiety subscales of the Brief Symptom Inventory (Derogatis, 1977) to create an overall index of distress.

Coping. Five 9-item subscales of the Coping Strategies Inventory (Tobin, Holroyd, Reynolds, & Wigal, 1989) were used to assess the strategies participants used to deal with the assault. We combined the cognitive restructuring and expressing emotions subscales into an approach coping scale and the social withdrawal, problem avoidance, and wishful thinking subscales into an avoidant coping scale. The degree to which participants used religious coping was assessed with a 10-item measure developed from other religious coping scales.

Control. Past control was assessed via 25 items assessing the extent to which survivors blamed the assault on themselves (both their behavior and character; 10 items) or external factors (society, the rapist, or chance; 15 items). Present control was assessed via a 5-item measure of control over the recovery process. Future control was assessed via a 5-item measure of the likelihood of future assaults.

RESULTS
Prevalence of Positive Change

We first report the mean number of positive changes reported by the ER sample at each of the four assessments and by the community sample, which was assessed an average of 16 years post-assault. Interestingly, participants were able to report areas of positive change quite soon after the assault—at the two week assessment an average of slightly over four areas of positive change were identified. The most common positive changes at two weeks post-assault were concern for others in similar situations (80%), greater appreciation of life (46%), and positive changes in family relationships (46%). With time, participants reported more positive changes, with the biggest increase occurring between two weeks and two months post-assault. By the two-month assessment, the average number of positive changes reported stabilized at about six. The most common positive changes at 12 months post-assault were concern for others in similar situations (76%), greater appreciation of life (58%), and being more assertive (48%). In the community sample, the average number of positive changes reported was almost seven. The most common changes in this sample were concern for others (79%), increased assertiveness (63%), and ability to recognize strengths (63%).

Positive Change and Distress

Across all four time periods in the ER sample, and in the community sample, individuals who reported more positive changes in their lives as a result of the assault also reported less distress (i.e., less depression, anxiety, and hostility). Interestingly, the relations between positive change and distress were very similar over time, from 2 weeks (r = -.52, p<.001) to an average of 16 years post-rape (r = -.49, p<.001). This suggests that even early reports of change may be adaptive. In terms of specific types of change, positive changes in self and spirituality/life philosophy tended to be more strongly related to lower distress levels than were changes in relationships or empathy.

Correlates of Positive Change

To examine correlates of positive change in the ER sample, we calculated correlations between the positive change measure and the four coping and the seven control measures across the four time periods and averaged them. Correlations also were calculated with the community sample data. In regard to coping, approach coping was strongly related to greater reports of positive change in the ER sample (mean r = .61, p<.001). On the other hand, individuals who engaged in more avoidant coping tended to report fewer positive changes (mean r = -.25, p<.05). Religious coping was also fairly strongly related to positive change (mean r = .44, p<.001). Similar correlations were found in the community sample between positive change and approach (r = .24, p<.01), avoidant (r = -.32, p<.001), and religious (r = .35, p<.001) coping.

In regard to past control, self-blame was negatively related to positive change in both samples (r's= -.20 and -.19, p's<.05, in the ER and community samples, respectively), whereas blaming external factors generally was not related to post-traumatic growth (r's = .04 and -.03 in the ER and community samples, respectively). Thus, focusing on the past, on why the rape occurred, does not appear to facilitate the growth process. On the other hand, present control, or control over the recovery process, was strongly related to posttraumatic growth (r's = .63 and .47, p's< .001, in the ER and community samples, respectively). In fact, it had the highest correlations with growth of any of the variables examined. Control over the recovery process involves statements such as "I can get over this if I work at it" and "I know what I must do to help myself recover." Finally, perceived control over future assaults was somewhat related to growth (r = .21, p<.05, and r = .29, p<.001, in the ER and community samples, respectively) but not as strongly as control over the recovery process.

DISCUSSION

To summarize, our data suggest that growth is common among sexual assault survivors, just as it is in survivors of other types of traumatic events. Across two very different samples of sexual assault survivors, the most common positive changes are increased empathy for others; changes in self, such as increased assertiveness; and changes in spirituality or life philosophy, such as greater appreciation of life. These are similar to the changes reported by survivors of other traumatic events (Tedeschi & Calhoun, 1995).

Many survivors report at least some positive life changes even as soon as two weeks post-assault, which is contrary to the notion that positive change necessarily results from a long recovery process. This suggests that theoretical models need to focus on the antecedents and consequences of abrupt as well as gradual change. In terms of the process of change over time, the number of self-reported positive changes increases over time, with the biggest period of change between two weeks and two months post-assault (see Frazier, Conlon, & Glaser, 2001).

In regard to the second research question, survivors who report more positive changes, particularly in themselves and their life philosophy, also report less distress. This is true even at two weeks post-assault, suggesting that early positive change does not reflect denial.

In terms of the factors that are associated with greater posttraumatic growth, both approach and religious coping are associated with reporting more positive changes following a sexual assault. Thus, it appears that individuals who report positive change are, indeed, dealing with, rather than denying, the trauma. In terms of perceived control, control over the present recovery process is most strongly related to reports of growth. Thus, control is important but it seems most adaptive to focus on what you can control now rather than focusing on past control and why the assault happened.

In regard to clinical implications, it is important for clinicians to be aware of the growing literature on posttraumatic growth and to use this knowledge in their work. From a clinical standpoint, an exclusive focus on the negative effects of trauma may influence how therapists approach clients and how clients see themselves, leading both to ignore the positive changes that may result from traumatic life events. We need to widen our focus so that both the positive and negative changes accruing from trauma are addressed in research and practice.

A second counseling implication concerns the timing of interventions. Specifically, our data suggest that the period between two weeks and two months post-assault is the time of greatest flux in self-reported positive life changes. According to crisis theory, people are especially receptive to outside influence in times of flux, making this early posttraumatic period a good time to intervene.

References

Affleck, G., Tennen, H., & Gershman, K. (1985). Cognitive adaptations to high-risk infants: The search for mastery, meaning, and protection from future harm. *American Journal of Mental Deficiency, 89,* 653-656.

Calhoun, L., Cann, A., Tedeschi, R., & McMillan, J. (2000). A correlational test of the relationship between posttraumatic growth, religion, and cognitive processing. *Journal of Traumatic Stress, 13,* 521-527.

Calhoun, L., & Tedeschi, R. (1998). Posttraumatic growth: Future directions. In R. Tedeschi, C. Park, & L. Calhoun (Eds.), *Posttraumatic growth: Positive changes in the aftermath of crisis* (pp. 215-238). Mahwah, NJ: Erlbaum.

Derogatis, L. (1977). *Manual for the SCL-90.* Baltimore: Johns Hopkins School of Medicine.

Foa, E., & Rothbaum, B. (1998). *Treating the trauma of rape: Cognitive-behavioral therapy for PTSD.* New York: Guilford.

Frazier, P., Conlon, A., & Glaser, T. (2001). Positive and negative life changes following sexual assault. *Journal of Consulting and Clinical Psychology, 69,* 1048-1055.

Park, C. (1998). Implications of posttraumatic growth for individuals. In R. Tedeschi, C. Park, & L. Calhoun (Eds.), *Posttraumatic growth: Positive changes in the aftermath of crisis* (pp. 153-178). Mahwah, NJ: Erlbaum.

Tedeschi, R., & Calhoun, L. (1995). *Trauma and transformation: Growing in the aftermath of suffering.* Thousand Oaks, CA: Sage.

Tobin, D. L., Holroyd, K. A., Reynolds, R. V., & Wigal, J. K. (1989). The hierarchical factor structure of the Coping Strategies Inventory. *Cognitive Therapy and Research, 13,* 343-361.

Influences of Global Meaning on Appraising and Coping with a Stressful Encounter

CRYSTAL L. PARK

Transactional models of coping have highlighted the importance of appraisal processes in coping with stressful encounters; these appraisals involve the meaning people assign to the stressor at hand. However, the roles that global meaning (such as an individual's life purposes and goals) play in determining these situational meanings have rarely been addressed. This paper has three goals: (a) to present a model of the ways that global meaning is brought to bear in the process of appraising and coping with stress, (b) to present data that illustrate the influence of global meanings on situational appraisals, and (c) to draw some conclusions about the role of global meaning in the process of coping with stress.

The transactional stress and coping model proposes that adaptation to a stressor is influenced by the coping processes in which people engage following that stressor (Lazarus & Folkman, 1984). This model focuses on cognitive appraisals of the situation and the coping strategies that follow from this appraisal. Cognitive appraisals involve assessing the meaning of an event by determining the extent to which the event is threatening, controllable, and predictable, and then deciding what can be done. These appraisals, in turn, influence the coping efforts put forth by the individual. Coping is typically divided into the categories of problem-focused coping strategies (attempting to directly change the problem) and emotion-focused coping strategies (attempting to regulate the distress) (Lazarus & Folkman, 1984; Aldwin, 2007).

A MEANING-MAKING COPING MODEL

Because so much of the coping needed to deal with major life events, especially losses, involves intrapsychic processes or *meaning making*, some theorists have argued that the transactional stress and coping model is of limited usefulness in studying adjustment to these kinds of events (e.g., Mikulincer & Florian, 1996). Park and Folkman (1997) drew upon the work of numerous theorists, including Greenberg (1995), Horowitz (1991), Rothbaum, Weisz, and Snyder (1982), and Taylor (1983), to develop a meaning-making model of coping. This model suggests that events cause distress by violating people's basic goals and their assumptions about the world. In order to decrease their distress, people must adjust their views of the

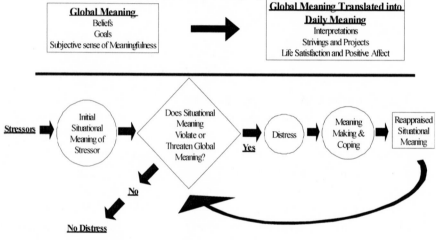

event or revise their goals and assumptions about the world to accommodate the new information (Park, 2005a; Parkes, 1993). This model is depicted in Figure 1.

Figure 1. Model of global meaning and meaning making.

According to this model, when individuals encounter potentially stressful events, they appraise the meaning of the event (i.e., "What has happened?") and then determine the extent to which this appraised meaning is discrepant with their global meaning system. Global meaning systems are the internal cognitive structures that orient and guide people, consisting of individuals' fundamental ways of construing reality and structuring the goals that orient and motivate them throughout life (i.e., their global beliefs and goals) (see Silberman, 2005; Park & Folkman, 1997). The level of distress caused by events is determined by the level of this discrepancy. Depending on the circumstances surrounding the stressful event or trauma, individuals' beliefs can be shattered and their goals rendered unattainable. For example, a robbery might violate one's beliefs about the fairness or justness of the world or his or her sense of controllability and invulnerability, but an accident resulting in an injury will not only violate one's beliefs but also one's goals of being a healthy, intact person. The distress caused by the event is therefore determined by the extent to which its appraised meaning violates the individual's beliefs (e.g., fairness, justice, benevolence) and goals (e.g., the extent to which the event is not what the person wants to have had happened; the extent to which other goals are now appraised as being less attainable).

This model posits that this discrepancy between appraised and global meaning is a highly uncomfortable state, involving a sense of loss of control, predictability, or comprehensibility of the world. In order to recover, the discrepancy between the appraised meaning of the event and the beliefs and goals that have been disrupted by it, must be reduced (Park, 2005b; see Park & Folkman, 1997, for a review). The processes through which people reduce this discrepancy involve changing the appraised meaning of the situation, changing their global beliefs and goals, or both, to achieve integration of the appraised meaning of the event into their global meaning system (Parkes, 1993; Klinger, 1998). This meaning-making coping is considered necessary when dealing with loss because the situation is not changeable or reparable; only through cognitive adaptation can individuals transform the meaning of the stressful experience. Meaning-making coping is characterized by attempting to see the event in a better light (e.g., Pearlin, 1991) and by cognitively "working through" the event by repeatedly thinking about the event and its implications (McIntosh, Silver, & Wortman, 1993).

THE INFLUENCES OF GLOBAL MEANING IN A COPING TRANSACTION

Accumulating research suggests that aspects of global meaning can have profound influences on the coping in which individuals engage following a stressful event. For example, research on one aspect of global meaning—religiousness—indicates that global meaning can play a strong and pervasive role in appraisal and coping processes; people higher in religiousness may appraise at least some situations as less stressful and more controllable, and use more religious coping than those who are less religious (see Pargament, 1997, for a review). However, few studies have taken a broader approach to examine multiple dimensions of global meaning and their relationships with appraisal and coping processes, especially across a period of time. Such research provides an opportunity to examine the influences of global meaning on the unfolding processes of meaning making, and was the explicit goal of the present study.

In the present study, five dimensions of global meaning were assessed in an attempt to broadly capture its important aspects. These dimensions included beliefs in self-controllability of events that occur, in randomness in the way that events occur, and in luck. Also included was a measure of life meaningfulness, the degree to which life makes sense and the demands of life are perceived as being worth responding to. Finally, intrinsic religiousness, the extent to which religion is held as the respondent's master motive, was assessed; intrinsic religiousness includes elements of both belief and motivation. To assess coping processes, three types of appraisals were assessed, challenge (the extent to which the event is manageable and positive outcomes are possible), threat (the extent to which the event is perceived to likely do harm), and controllability (the extent to which one has the ability to control the outcome of the event). Coping was conceptualized broadly as the responses that one might deliberately make to deal with the problem, including problem-focused coping activities, emotion-focused coping activities, and meaning-focused coping activities.

METHOD
Participants

Participants were 131 college students (100 women, 31 men, mean age = 19.2 years) at a midwestern American university.

Procedures

Participants were drawn from the Psychology Department participant pool. They completed packets of questionnaires in a small group setting (Time 1) and, one month later, returned to complete a second packet of questionnaires (Time 2). At Time 1, participants completed measures of global meaning and appraisal and coping; at Time 2, they completed only measures of appraisals and coping. They received research credit for their participation.

Measures_

Global Meaning Measures. A number of measures were used to assess dimensions of global meaning, broadly defined, including beliefs (worldviews, religiousness) and general purposefulness or meaning in life. Worldviews were measured with three subscales from the World Assumptions Scale (WAS; Janoff-Bulman, 1989): self-controllability, randomness, and luck, each of which is assessed by four items. Previous research using the WAS indicates that it possesses reasonably good psychometric properties (Janoff-Bulman, 1989; Schwartzberg & Janoff-Bulman, 1991). Religiousness was measured using the intrinsic scale of the Age-Universal Intrinsic/Extrinsic Scale-Revised (Gorsuch & McPherson, 1989). Participants rated each of seven items on a scale from 0 (strongly disagree) to 4 (strongly agree). Meaningfulness of life was assessed with the meaningfulness scale of the Sense of Coherence Scale (Antonovsky, 1987), consisting of 9 items, with each item having a seven point scale with appropriate anchors on each end. (For this item, anchors were "totally without meaning or purpose" and "full of meaning and purpose").

Measures of Coping Processes. At Time 1, participants were asked to list the most stressful event that they had experienced in the past three months. They were then asked to complete coping process measures (appraisals and coping) regarding this event. At Time 2, participants were asked to again complete the coping measures in reference to the event that they had identified at Time 1. Appraisals were assessed with three subscales from the Stress Appraisal Measure (SAM; Peacock & Wong, 1990) assessing perceptions of self-controllability, threat and challenge with regard to the identified stressful event. For each item, participants rated their perceptions of the situation on a scale ranging from 1 (not at all) to 5 (a great amount). Coping was assessed with the COPE (Carver, Scheier, & Weintraub, 1989), a widely-used instrument with good psychometric properties. The COPE consists of 60 items; participants were asked the extent to which they used each of the items to deal with the identified stressor on a scale from "not at all" (1) to "a lot" (4). The 60 items form 15 subscales.

RESULTS
Relationships among Aspects of Global Meaning

To examine how the five dimensions of global meaning were related to one another, bivariate correlations were conducted, and results of which are presented in Table 1. Interestingly, luck and meaningfulness of life were the most highly interrelated dimensions of global meaning, and luck was also related positively to belief in self-control. Meaningfulness of life was also positively related to belief in self-control. Intrinsic religiousness was not related to meaningfulness of life, self-control, or luck, but was negatively related to luck. None of the interrelationships were particularly strong, which indicates that the dimensions are relatively independent aspects of global meaning.

Table 1
Relationships among dimensions of global meaning

	Belief in Randomness	Belief in Self-Control	Intrinsic Religiousness	Meaningfulness of Life
Belief in Luck	-.16	.28**	.11	.53***
Belief in Randomness	--	-.08	-.27**	-.21*
Belief in Self-control		--	.11	.39***
Intrinsic Religiousness			--	.09

$p < .10$ * $p < .05$ ** $p < .01$ *** $p < .001$

CROSS-SECTIONAL RELATIONS BETWEEN DIMENSIONS OF GLOBAL MEANING AND COPING PROCESS VARIABLES

To examine relationships between global meaning and coping process variables at Time 1, a series of bivariate correlations were conducted between the five dimensions of global meaning and the appraisal and coping variables. Results are presented in Table 2. It is important to note that large numbers of correlations are presented without adjusting significance levels, which may result in some relationships appearing to be significant but which, in fact, are due to chance. Because this study is exploratory and these findings are presented primarily to suggest directions for future research, the correlations are presented for the reader to consider.

Beliefs in luck and self-control, intrinsic religiousness, and meaningfulness of life were all related positively to appraisals of challenge and controllability. Religiousness and meaningfulness in life were also negatively related to appraisals of threat. A belief in randomness was only negatively related to appraisals of challenge. Meaningfulness of life appeared to be related to the most adaptive appraisals.

Belief in randomness was only related to a few coping strategies, most of which are considered maladaptive (e.g., behavioral disengagement, denial). Belief in luck was also only minimally related to coping activities. Beliefs in self-control and meaningfulness in life had similar patterns of relationships with coping activities, although meaningfulness in life was related more strongly to coping activities, and this pattern of relationships indicated that meaningfulness in life was related to coping that is typically regarded as adaptive, including the use of more social support and active coping, and less disengagement and denial. The coping strategies considered most closely related to meaning making, acceptance and positive reappraisal, were related to belief in self-control, meaningfulness of life, and, less strongly, intrinsic religiousness.

Table 2
Cross-sectional relations of global meaning dimensions with appraisals and coping

	Belief in Randomness	Belief in Luck	Belief in Self-Control	Intrinsic Religiousness	Meaningfulness of Life
Appraisals					
Challenge	-.19*	.18*	.27**	.23*	.35***
Threat	.09	-.08	-.09	-.18*	-.24**
Controllability	-.06	.31**	.41**	.31***	.46***
Coping					
Acceptance	.11	.10	.27**	.06	.17*
Active coping	-.12	.03	.24**	.05	.17*
Behavioral Disengagement	.25**	-.22*	-.04	-.03	-.25**
Positive Reinterpretation	-.12	.09	.37**	.19*	.32**
Planning	-.06				
Alcohol/Drug Use	.06	.10	.05	-.08	.00
Denial	.19*	-.09	-.05	.03	-.29**
Humor	.23**	-.04	.06	.02	-.02
Restraint	-.03	-.11	-.08	.10	-.11
Suppression Of Competing Activities	-.01	.04	-.01	.11	-.01
Social Emotional Support	.06	.13	.21*	.11	.27**
Social Instru-mental Support	.13	.14	.11	.01	.17*
Venting	.07	-.05	.06	-.08	.06
Religious Coping	-.25**	.07	.10	.72***	.18*
Mental Disengagement	.10	-.01	.13	.01	-.13

$^f p < .10$ $^* p < .05$ $^{**} p < .01$ $^{***} p < .001$

LONGITUDINAL RELATIONS BETWEEN DIMENSIONS OF GLOBAL MEANING AND COPING PROCESS VARIABLES

To examine relationships of global meaning and coping process variables longitudinally, a series of bivariate correlations were conducted between the five dimensions of global meaning assessed at Time 1 and the Time 2 appraisal and coping variables. Results are presented in Table 3. The longitudinal correlations are much weaker, but the global meaning variables did appear to influence the appraisals and coping activities one month later. Meaningfulness in life, belief in self-control, and (marginally) belief in luck were related to appraised controllability of the stressor. Beliefs in randomness and luck were related to only a few of the coping activities, some of which had not been present at Time 1 (e.g., relations between belief in randomness and substance use to cope and seeking social emotional support). Belief in self-control was related to the meaning-making coping strategies of positive reappraisal and (marginally) acceptance. Both belief in self-control and meaningfulness in life were related to active coping and planning. Religiousness was related (marginally) to positive reinterpretation and strongly to religious coping.

Table 3
Longitudinal relations between dimensions of global meaning and appraisals
and coping

	Belief in Randomness	Belief in Luck	Belief in Self-Control	Intrinsic Religiousness	Meaningfulness of Life
Appraisals					
Challenge	.04	.03	.08	.06	.14
Threat	.09	.03	-.14	-.07	-.04
Controllability	-.04	.14 ^{f}	.19*	.05	.31***
Coping					
Acceptance	.10	-.01	.17 ^{f}	.12	.10
Active coping	.11	-.02	.25**	-.01	.29**
Behavioral Disengagement	.03	-.14 ^{f}	-.18 ^{f}	-.14 ^{f}	-.27
Positive Reinterpretation	-.04	.06	.25**	.17 ^{f}	.12
Planning	.11	.16 ^{f}	.22*	.04	.28**
Alcohol/Drug Use	.25**	-.08	-.11	.17 ^{f}	-.16 ^{f}
Denial	.01	-.08	-.10	.06	-.16 ^{f}
Humor	.12	.07	-.07	-.05	-.13
Restraint	.10	-.13	.03	-.09	-.12
Suppression Of Competing Activities	-.00	.08	.14 ^{f}	-.02	.05
Social Emotional Support	.25**	.02	.14 ^{f}	-.01	.11
Social Instru-mental Support	.10	-.05	-.04	.01	.07
Venting	.19*	.01	.07	.09	.03
Religious Coping	-.13	.10	.16 ^{f}	.64***	.18*
Mental Disengagement	.13	-.01	-.04	.08	.18*

$^f p < .10$ $^* p < .05$ $^{**} p < .01$ $^{***} p < .001$

DISCUSSION

Results of this study suggest that dimensions of global meaning exert fairly strong influences on coping processes and that the patterns of influence differ among different dimensions of global meaning. In general, it appears that certain dimensions of global meaning, such as belief in randomness, are related to less adaptive coping, while others, such as meaningfulness in life, are related to more adaptive coping.

The correlational analyses were exploratory, and the results raise many more questions than they answer in terms of mechanisms of effect. The patterns of relationships between dimensions of global meaning with appraisals and coping strategies examined cross-sectionally and longitudinally also differed. For example, cross-sectionally, meaningfulness in life and belief in self-control were related to adaptive appraisals and coping strategies, including meaning-making coping, but these relationships weakened or disappeared by Time 2. It may be that those higher in meaningfulness in life and belief in self-control have resolved their distress over the event and are less in need of meaning making.

There were a number of limitations to the study. For example, the measures of global meaning used were those developed by others for various purposes and may not be the best measures of global meaning. There may also be other critical dimensions of global meaning that were not assessed in this study. Correlational analysis and the use of only two time points limited the informativeness of the study regarding the mechanisms of effect as these processes unfolded over time. Future research should be conducted employing longitudinal designs to examine dimensions of meaning and their influences in the processes of coping with stressors and making meaning from difficult life events.

References

Aldwin, C. M. (2007). *Stress, coping, and development* (2nd ed.). New York: Guilford.

Antonovsky, A. (1987). *Unraveling the mystery of health: How people manage stress and stay well.* San Francisco: Jossey-Bass.

Carver, C. S., Scheier, M. G., & Weintraub, J. G. (1989). Assessing coping strategies: A theoretically-based approach. *Journal of Personality and Social Psychology, 56,* 267-283.

Gorsuch, R. L., & McPherson, S. E. (1989). Intrinsic/Extrinsic measurement: I/E-Revised and single item scales. *Journal for the Scientific Study of Religion, 28,* 348-354.

Greenberg, M. A. (1995). Cognitive processing of traumas: The role of intrusive thoughts and reappraisals. *Journal of Applied Social Psychology, 25,* 1262-1296.

Horowitz, M. (1991). Person schemas. In M. Horowitz (Ed.), *Person schemas and maladaptive interpersonal patterns* (pp. 13-31). Chicago: University of Chicago Press.

Janoff-Bulman, R. (1989). Assumptive worlds and the stress of traumatic events: Applications of the schema construct. *Social Cognition, 7,* 113-136.

Klinger, E. (1998). The search for meaning in evolutionary perspective and its clinical implications. In P. T. P. Wong & P. S. Fry (Eds.), *The human quest for meaning* (pp. 27-50). Mahwah, NJ: Erlbaum.

Lazarus, R. S., & Folkman, S. (1984). *Stress, appraisal, and coping.* New York: Springer.

McIntosh, D. N., Silver, R. C., & Wortman, C. B. (1993). Religion's role in adjustment to a negative life event: Coping with the loss of a child. *Journal of Personality and Social Psychology, 65,* 812-821.

Mikulincer, M., & Florian, V. (1996). Coping and adaptation to trauma and loss. In M. Zeidner & N. S. Endler (Eds.), *Handbook of coping: Theory, research, applications* (pp. 554-572). New York: Wiley.

Pargament, K. I. (1997). *The psychology of religion and coping.* New York: Guilford.

Park, C. L. (2005a). Religion and meaning. In R. F. Paloutzian & C. L. Park (Eds.), *Handbook of the psychology of religion and spirituality* (pp. 295-314). New York: Guilford.

Park, C. L. (2005b). Religion as a meaning-making framework in coping with life stress. *Journal of Social Issues, 61,* 707-729.

Park, C. L., & Folkman, S. (1997). Meaning in the context of stress and coping. *General Review of Psychology, 1,* 115-144.

Parkes, C. M. (1993). Bereavement as a psychosocial transition: Processes of adaptation to change. In M. S. Stroebe, W. Stroebe, & R. O. Hansson (Eds.), *Handbook of Bereavement: Theory, research, and intervention* (pp. 91-101). New York: Cambridge University Press.

Peacock, E., & Wong, P. (1990). The stress appraisal measure (SAM): A multidimensional approach to cognitive appraisal. *Stress Medicine, 6,* 227-236.

Pearlin, L. I. (1991). The study of coping: An overview of problems and directions. In J. Eckenrode (Ed.), *The social context of coping* (pp. 261-276). New York: Plenum.

Rothbaum, F., Weisz, J. R., & Snyder, S. S. (1982). Changing the world and changing the self: A two-process model of perceived control. *Journal of Personality and Social Psychology, 42,* 5-37.

Schwartzberg, S. S., & Janoff-Bulman, R. (1991). Grief and the search for meaning: Exploring the assumptive worlds of bereaved college students. *Journal of Social and Clinical Psychology, 10,* 270-288.

Silberman, I. (2005). Religion as a meaning system: Implications for the new millennium. *Journal of Social Issues, 61,* 641-663.

Taylor, S. E. (1983). Adjustment to threatening events: A theory of cognitive adaptation. *American Psychologist, 38,* 1161-1173.

Meaning in Life and Resilience to Suicidal Thoughts Among Older Adults

MARNIN J. HEISEL
GORDON L. FLETT

Abstract

We examined the associations among protective factors, risk factors, and suicide ideation in older adults. A heterogeneous sample of 107 older adults completed the Geriatric Suicide Ideation Scale (GSIS; Heisel & Flett, 2006), a multidimensional self-report measure of late-life suicide ideation, and measures of psychological resiliency (recognition of meaning and purpose in life, and life satisfaction) and risk factors (depression, hopelessness, and physical health complaints). The findings supported predicted associations between suicide ideation and the protective and risk factors, and suggested the role of existential and spiritual factors in promoting psychological resiliency and in protecting against suicidal thoughts among seniors. These findings have implications for prevention and intervention practices with despairing and potentially suicidal older adults.

Adults 65 years and older have high rates of suicide worldwide (Bertolote, 2001) and employ highly lethal means of self-harm (Krug, Dahlberg, Mercy, Zwi, & Lozano, 2002). Shifting population demographics necessitate improved understanding of suicide risk detection and prevention strategies. Suicide prevention is predicated upon accurate assessment of risk and protective factors; to date, research on protective factors has been overshadowed by a focus on suicide risk among seniors (Heisel, 2006), despite increased attention to psychological resiliency in the suicide literature more generally (Heikkinen, Aro, & Lönnqvist, 1993; Heisel & Flett, 2004; Kay & Francis, 2006; Lubell & Vetter, 2006). In the present study, we examined the associations among a set of protective factors, risk factors, and suicide ideation among older adults, replicating a methodology employed in our research with an adult psychiatric sample (Heisel & Flett, 2004), to inform theory, research, and practice with suicidal seniors.

Shneidman (1996) theorized that suicide risk is driven by psychache, a condition defined by intolerable psychological pain. Research findings have indicated robust associations between late-life suicide ideation and indices of intense psychological pain: depression, hopelessness, loneliness and poor perceived social support, and experienced or anticipated health problems (Awata et al., 2005; Bartels et al., 2002; Cook, Pearson, Thompson, Black, & Rabins, 2002; Friedman, Heisel, & Delavan, 2005; Uncapher, Gallagher-Thompson, Osgood, & Bongar, 1998; Vanderhorst & McLaren, 2005). A majority of depressed and/or hopeless older adults do not engage in suicidal behavior, however, suggesting that it is a combination of suicide risk factors and an absence of key protective factors that instigate suicidal thoughts and behavior.

Linehan and colleagues (1983) have demonstrated that adaptive cognitions regarding reasons for living can quell suicidal thoughts. Frankl (1971, 1984, 1988) theorized that a lack of recognition of meaning in life could lead to the experience of spiritual emptiness, termed the "existential vacuum," which, if left unresolved, might engender despair and suicidality. Empirical support exists for Frankl's theory. Perceived meaninglessness has been associated with stress, despair, depression, and pathological responses to aging, loss, and terminal illness (Krause, 2004; Pintos, 1988; Prager, Bar-Tur, & Abramowici, 1997; Reker, 1997; Reker & Wong, 1988; Ulmer, Range, & Smith, 1991). Moore's (1997) phenomenological study of meaning in life among suicidal older adults identified a broad association of alienation with perceived meaninglessness, with underlying themes of psychache, social isolation ("nobody cares"), and powerlessness. Recognition of meaning in later life has, conversely, been associated positively with creativity, psychological well-being, and an orientation towards others (Fry, 2000, 2001; Hickson & Housley, 1997; Prager, 1996; Zika & Chamberlain, 1992). Weisman (1991) posited that life's main tasks consist of (a) searching for meaning, (b) maintaining morale, and (c) negotiating with mortality (Weisman, 1991, p. 195). Moody (1991) stated that the experience of aging can help underscore the meanings inherent in one's life, supporting research that has demonstrated a greater recognition of meaning in life by seniors in comparison with younger adult populations (Ebersole &

DePaola, 1989; Van Ranst & Marcoen, 1997). Clinical findings have demonstrated the effectiveness of existential psychotherapy, reminiscence, and life review in fomenting meaning recognition among seniors (Brown & Romanchuk, 1994; Farran, 1997; Kotarba, 1983; Saul, 1993; Silver, 1995). We thus hypothesized that perception of meaning in life may be a critical factor in promoting resiliency and in mitigating thoughts of suicide among seniors.

In our previous research we administered measures of suicide ideation, and of risk (depression, social hopelessness, and neuroticism) and protective factors (purpose in life and satisfaction with life) to 49 patients of a tertiary care psychiatric hospital (M = 37.5 years of age; SD = 8.2), a majority of whom had a mood and/ or personality disorder (Heisel & Flett, 2004). We found that suicide ideation was associated positively with depression (r= .75, $p < .001$), social hopelessness (r = .77, $p < .001$), and neuroticism (r = .47, $p < .001$), and negatively with purpose in life (r = -.69, $p < .001$) and life satisfaction (r = -.33, $p < .05$). A hierarchical multiple regression analysis with suicide ideation as outcome found that addition of the protective factors substantially improved the proportion of variance accounted for by the risk factors alone. We further detected a significant interaction of depression and purpose in life on suicide ideation, as those with high depression and high purpose in life reported significantly less suicide ideation than equally depressed participants reporting less life purpose.

A similar methodology was used in the present study, in which we examined the associations between suicide ideation and a set of protective factors and risk factors potentially associated with late-life suicide ideation. It was hypothesized that late-life suicide ideation would be associated negatively with perceived meaning and purpose in life, and satisfaction with life, and positively with depression, global and social hopelessness, and perceived health problems. We further hypothesized that the protective factors might explain significant additional variance in suicide ideation scores, after accounting for the risk factors, replicating our findings with an adult clinical sample (Heisel & Flett, 2004). Finally, we hypothesized a significant interaction of depression and perceived meaning in life on suicide ideation, anticipating that those high in depression and meaning in life would endorse less suicide ideation than would equally depressed individuals perceiving less meaning in life.

METHOD
Participants

The present sample included 107 seniors (76% female; M = 81.5 years of age, SD = 7.7, Range: 67 to 98 years), living independently or in care-providing facilities. Voluntary participants were recruited from community centers or community-based senior's programmes (n = 10), retirement residences (n = 9), nursing residences (n = 45), general hospital wards (n = 25), and from psychogeriatric practices or psychogeriatric hospital wards (n = 18). Recruitment procedures and methods are described more fully elsewhere (Heisel & Flett, 2006).

PROCEDURE

Participants completed the Geriatric Suicide Ideation Scale (GSIS; Heisel & Flett, 2006), a reliable and valid multidimensional, 31-item, 5-point Likert-scored measure of Suicide Ideation, Death Ideation, Loss of Personal and Social Worth, and Perceived Meaning in Life developed among seniors. Participants additionally completed self-report measures assessing purpose in life (PIL; the 9-item purpose in life subscale of Ryff's (1989) multidimensional measure of psychological well-being), an item assessing meaning in life (MIL; derived from the Geriatric Suicide Ideation Scale; "I feel that my life is meaningful"), satisfaction with life (Satisfaction With Life Scale or SWLS; Diener, Emmons, Larsen, & Griffin, 1985), depression (Geriatric Depression Scale or GDS; Yesavage et al., 1983), global hopelessness (Beck Hopelessness Scale or BHS; Beck, Weissman, Lester, & Trexler, 1974; scored on a 1-5 point Likert scale as in Heisel, Flett, & Hewitt, 2003), an interpersonal form of hopelessness (Social Hopelessness Questionnaire or SHQ; Flett, Hewitt, Heisel, Davidson, & Gayle, 2006), and an item assessing self-reported severity of physical health problems (scored 1-7). Participants with severe visual or motor limitations were administered the measures verbally by the first author. Participants were fully debriefed upon completion of the study, and were referred for appropriate care, if deemed necessary.

RESULTS

Descriptive statistics and zero-order correlation coefficients between the GSIS and measures of protective factors and risk factors are presented in Table 1. All analyses with the GSIS excluded its MIL item. Hierarchical multiple regression analysis findings are presented in Table 2. A test of the potential interaction effect of depression and meaning in life on suicide ideation is presented in Table 3 and in Figure 1.

Table 1
Correlational Matrix for Suicide Ideation, Resilience, and Risk Factors

	2	3	4	5	6	7	8	M	SD	β
1. GSIS-MIL	-.62**	-.57**	-.54**	-.54**	.77**	.70**	.54**	57.21	16.28	.93
2. MIL		.45**	.39**	.30**	-.46**	-.53**	-.29**	3.92	.81	--
3. PIL			.36**	.12	-.61**	-.68**	-.55**	36.04	6.42	.65
4. SWLS				.22*	-.55**	-.48**	-.46**	23.97	6.82	.83
5. Health Ratings					-.38**	-.30**	-.18†	5.08	1.42	--
6. GDS						.71**	.56**	9.20	6.28	.88
7. BHS							.70**	48.00	9.87	.82
8. SHQ								51.96	11.75	.86

Note. $*p<0.05$ $**p<0.01$ $†p<0.10$ $N=102$

GSIS-MIL = Geriatric Suicide Ideation Scale total scores minus the GSIS meaning in life item; MIL = GSIS Meaning in Life item; PIL = Purpose in Life subscale of the Multidimensional Psychological Well-Being Scale; SWLS = Satisfaction with Life Scale; Health Ratings = Self-Reported Physical Health Ratings (scored in the direction of wellness); GDS = Geriatric Depression Scale; BHS = Beck Hopelessness Scale; SHQ = Social Hopelessness Questionnaire.

Table 2
Summary of a Hierarchical Multiple Regression Analysis of Risk and
Protective Factors on Suicide Ideation (GSIS-MIL)

	Variable	B	SE B	β	t	p
Step 1	(Intercept)	44.88	17.59	---	2.55	.013
	Sex	.15	3.94	.00	.04	.969
	Age	.13	.22	.07	.59	.559
Step 2	(Intercept)	43.25	11.68	---	3.71	.000
	Sex	-.31	2.39	-.01	-.13	.898
	Age	-.10	.14	-.06	-.75	.454
	Health Rating	- 2.43	.77	-.23	-3.17	.002
	GDS	.99	.24	.42	4.19	.000
	BHS	.52	.15	.36	3.46	.001
Step 3	(Intercept)	77.24	18.45	---	4.19	.003
	Sex	.24	2.33	.01	.10	.920
	Age	-.09	.14	-.05	-.67	.503
	Health Rating	- 2.36	.74	-.22	-3.17	.002
	GDS	.88	.24	.37	3.64	.001
	BHS	.31	.17	.21	1.85	.068
	MIL	-3.59	1.53	-.18	-2.34	.022
	PIL	-.16	.22	-.07	-.73	.467
	SWLS	-.18	.17	-.08	-1.09	.280

Note. $R^2 = .00$, $F_{(2,78)} = .17$, $p=.84$ for step 1; $R^2 = .66$, $\Delta R^2 = .65$, F-change$_{(3,75)} = 47.61$, $p<0.0001$ for step 2; $R^2 = .69$, $\Delta R^2 = .04$, F-change$_{(3,72)} = 2.83$, $p<.05$ for step 3. $N = 85$. GSIS-MIL = Geriatric Suicide Ideation Scale total scores minus the GSIS meaning in life item; MIL = GSIS Meaning in Life item; PIL = Purpose in Life subscale of the Multidimensional Psychological Well-Being Scale; SWLS = Satisfaction with Life Scale; Health Ratings = Self-Reported Physical Health Ratings (scored in the direction of wellness); GDS = Geriatric Depression Scale; BHS = Beck Hopelessness Scale.

Table 3
Summary of a Hierarchical Multiple Regression Analysis Predicting Suicide Ideation (GSIS-MIL) with Participant Sex, Age, Meaning In Life, and Depression Scores, and the Interaction of Meaning in Life and Depression

	Variable	B	SE B	β	t	p
Step 1	(Intercept)	61.83	12.58	--	4.92	<.001
	Sex	.54	2.26	.01	.24	.81
	Age	.07	.13	.03	.53	.60
	GDS	1.65	.17	.63	9.72	<.001
	MIL	- 6.39	1.30	-.32	-4.91	<.001
Step 2	(Intercept)	54.40	13.22	--	4.12	
	Sex	.35	2.25	.01	.16	.88
	Age	.10	.13	.05	.83	.41
	GDS	1.61	.17	.62	9.55	<.001
	MIL	- 5.38	1.42	-.27	-3.78	<.001
	MILXGDS	- .27	.16	-.11	-1.69	<.05a

Note. ª This analysis is one-tailed. R^2=.69, $F_{(4, 94)}$=53.00, p<.0001 for step 1; R^2=.70, ΔR^2=.01, F-change$_{(1, 93)}$=2.84, p<0.05, one-tailed for step 2. GSIS-MIL = Geriatric Suicide Ideation Scale total scores minus the GSIS meaning in life item; GDS = Geriatric Depression Scale; MIL = GSIS meaning in life item; MILxGDS = Centered interaction of MIL and GDS; N = 99.

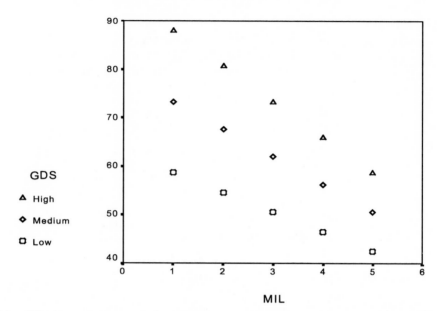

Note. GSIS-MIL = Geriatric Suicide Ideation Scale total scores minus the GSIS meaning in life item; MIL = GSIS meaning in life item; GDS = Scores on the Geriatric Depression Scale lying at the sample mean (GDS = 9.2), one standard deviation above the mean (GDS = 15.5), and one standard deviation below the mean (GDS = 2.9).

Figure 1. Interaction of Meaning in Life and Depression on Suicide

The results demonstrated acceptable approximations of univariate and multivariate normality for the measures of protective factors and risk factors (Tabachnick & Fidell, 1996). Sample statistics (see Table 1) revealed relatively low severity suicide ideation on the GSIS (M = 57.21, SD = 16.28), moderate to high purpose in life (PIL; M = 36.04, SD = 6.42) and satisfaction with life (SWLS; M = 23.97 SD = 6.82), and low to moderate depression and hopelessness on the GDS (M = 9.20, SD = 6.28), the BHS (M = 48.00, SD = 9.87), and the SHQ (M = 51.96, SD = 11.75).

As predicted, the correlational findings indicated significant negative associations between suicide ideation and the protective factors (recognition of meaning and purpose in life, and satisfaction with life), and positive associations with the risk factors (depression, global and social hopelessness, and physical health ratings) (see Table 1). The protective factors were significantly intercorrelated with one another. The risk factors were significantly intercorrelated with one another for the most part, as there was only a trend towards an association between perceived health ratings and social hopelessness ($p < 0.10$). The protective factors and risk factors were largely inversely correlated; for instance, higher meaning in life, purpose in life, and life satisfaction were associated with lower depression and hopelessness. Greater meaning in life and life satisfaction were associated with better health ratings; purpose in life was not associated with this variable, suggesting differential patterns of correlations between meaning and purpose in life with measures of health and impairment. We next computed a pair of exploratory hierarchical multiple regression analyses predicting suicide ideation separately with the protective factors and risk factors (available upon request). We included participant age, sex, meaning in life, purpose in life, and satisfaction with life scores in the first analysis, and age, sex, depression, global hopelessness, social hopelessness, and perceived health ratings in the second, employing backwards elimination, in order to produce parsimonious models of protective and risk factors associated with late-life suicide ideation. Perceived meaning in life, purpose in life, and satisfaction with life entered the trimmed protective factor model, and accounted for 48% of the variance in suicide ideation scores. Physical health ratings, depression, and global hopelessness remained in the trimmed risk factor model, together accounting for 69% of the variance in suicide ideation scores.

We next entered participant age, sex, and the remaining risk and protective factors into a hierarchical multiple regression analysis, investigating whether the protective factors contributed significant incremental variance in suicide ideation scores above and beyond that contributed by the risk factors (see Table 2). This regression analysis was statistically significant (R^2 =.69, ΔR^2 = .04, $F(3, 72)$ = 2.83, $p < .05$), suggesting value in attending to both resilience and pathology when investigating late-life suicide ideation. A trimmed final model using backwards elimination (not shown) indicated that meaning in life (β = -3.95, $SE\,\beta$ = 1.49), physical health ratings (β = -2.30, $SE\,\beta$ = .72), depression (β = .99, $SE\,\beta$ = .22), and global hopelessness (β = .35, $SE\,\beta$ = .14) all significantly contributed to a predictive model of late-life suicide ideation (R^2 =.68, $F(4, 81)$ = 41.14, $p < .001$).

We finally conducted a hierarchical multiple regression analysis testing our hypothesized interaction of depression and meaning in life on suicide ideation (see Table 3 and Figure 1). Participant age, sex, meaning in life, and depression scores were entered on step 1, and the centered interaction of meaning in life and depression on step 2. The results indicated a significant interaction effect of meaning in life and depression on suicide ideation, above and beyond the unique main effects of those variables. Meaning in life appears to protect against suicide ideation at high, medium, and low levels of depression, as those endorsing high meaning recognition reported less suicide ideation than those with lower levels of meaning recognition.

DISCUSSION

The present study examined the associations between late-life suicide ideation and a set of potential resilience and risk factors in order to inform theory, research, and treatment with at-risk older adults. We found support for hypothesized negative associations between suicide ideation and recognition of meaning in life, purpose in life, and satisfaction with life, and for hypothesized positive associations between suicide ideation and depression, global and social forms of hopelessness, and perceived physical health problems. These findings accord with previous research demonstrating close links between depression, hopelessness, physical complaints, and late-life suicide ideation in seniors (Bartels et al., 2002; Friedman et al., 2005; Pearson & Brown, 2000; Uncapher et al., 1998), and additionally suggest the need to attend to the role of key salutary factors in mitigating suicide risk among older adults.

The present findings broadly support Frankl's (1971, 1984, 1988) contention that recognition of sources of meaning in life, irrespective of one's age and health, helps protect against loneliness, hopelessness, despair, dissatisfaction with life, and suicidal contemplations. The results further replicate our previous findings with an adult clinical sample (Heisel & Flett, 2004), suggesting that meaning and purpose in life contribute to suicide resiliency among disparate populations at elevated suicide risk. Although significantly intercorrelated, meaning and purpose in life are somewhat distinct constructs that might differentially protect against suicide ideation in different populations. Purpose in life scores were significantly negatively associated with suicide ideation in the present analyses, but did not enter the final trimmed model of risk and protective factors. Purpose in life was additionally not associated with perceived health problems, but health problems were associated significantly with perceived meaninglessness. Inspection of the PIL items revealed an element of future orientation that may be less relevant to meaning recognition among seniors. As one reaches one's senior years, the temporal focus of meaning recognition may turn from future possibilities to past accomplishments (Frankl, 1988; Lukas, 1986, 1991), corresponding to successful resolution of "ego integrity," Erikson's (1963) final stage of psychosocial development.

Findings of a strong negative correlation between meaning in life and social hopelessness lend support for Moore's (1997) framework linking perceived meaninglessness with social isolation and alienation among suicidal older adults. These data suggest the importance of perceived social support and of social integration in protecting against late-life suicide (Duberstein et al., 2004), and suggest a role for interpersonally oriented forms of psychotherapy in helping to reduce late-life suicide risk (Bruce et al., 2004).

The present findings further indicated a significant interaction of recognition of meaning in life and depression on suicide ideation, similar to our previous clinical research findings (Heisel & Flett, 2004). These findings support Frankl's (1984) contention that recognizing meaning in suffering can preserve a wish to live. Findings also support research demonstrating that seniors can develop and maintain meaning in life and profound existential awareness (Petrie & Brook, 1992; Pintos, 1988; Reker, 1997).

Overall, the present study suggests that attending to both suicide resiliency and risk may benefit theory and clinical practice with at-risk older adults. The present findings are limited by a single-item measure of meaning in life, a cross-sectional methodology, and a largely culturally homogeneous sample. Despite its limitations, the present study reflects efforts to investigate psychological resiliency to late-life suicide ideation, exploring the protective role of key existential variables. Clinical implications include the importance of assessing for resiliency to suicide when assessing late-life suicide risk, and the potential value in drawing on seniors' stores of life experience and potentially burgeoning existential awareness (Lukas, 1986; Weisman, 1991) when working to effect psychological change, to enhance health and well-being, and ultimately to prevent suicide.

References

Awata, S., Seiki, T., Koizumi, Y., Sato, S., Hozawa, A., Omori, K., et al. (2005). Factors associated with suicidal ideation in an elderly urban Japanese population: A community-based, cross-sectional study. *Psychiatry & Clinical Neurosciences, 59*(3), 327-336.

Bartels, S. J., Coakley, E., Oxman, T. E., Constantino, G., Oslin, D., Chen, H., et al. (2002). Suicidal and death ideation in older primary care patients with depression, anxiety, and at-risk alcohol use. *The American Journal of Geriatric Psychiatry, 10*(4), 417-427.

Beck, A. T., Weissman, A., Lester, D., & Trexler, L. (1974). The measurement of pessimism: The hopelessness scale. *Journal of Consulting and Clinical Psychology, 42*, 861-865.

Bertolote, J. M. (2001). Suicide in the world: An epidemiological overview 1959-2000. In D. Wasserman (Ed.), *Suicide: An unnecessary death* (pp. 3-10). London: Martin Dunitz.

Brown, J. A., & Romanchuk, B. J. (1994). Existential social work practice with the aged: Theory and practice. *Journal of Gerontological Social Work, 23*(1/2), 49-65.

Bruce, M. L., Ten Have, T. R., Reynolds III, C. F., Katz, I. I., Schulberg, H. C., Mulsant, B. H., et al. (2004). Reducing suicidal ideation and depressive symptoms in depressed older primary care patients: A randomized controlled trial. *JAMA, 291*(9), 1081-1091.

Cook, J. M., Pearson, J. L., Thompson, R., Black, B. S., & Rabins, P. V. (2002). Suicidality in older African Americans: Findings from the EPOCH study. *The American Journal of Geriatric Psychiatry, 10*(4), 437-446.

Diener, E., Emmons, R., Larsen, R., & Griffin, S. (1985). The Satisfaction with Life Scale. *Journal of Personality Assessment, 49*, 71-75.

Duberstein, P. R, Conwell, Y., Conner, K. R., Eberly, S., Evinger, J. S., & Caine, E. D. (2004). Poor social integration and suicide: fact or artifact? A case control study. *Psychological Medicine, 37*, 1331-1337.

Ebersole, P., & DePaola, S. (1989). Meaning in life depth in the active married elderly. *The Journal of Psychology, 123*(2), 171-178.

Erikson, E. H. (1963). *Childhood and society* (2nd ed.). New York: Norton.

Farran, C. J. (1997). Theoretical perspectives concerning positive aspects of caring for elderly persons with dementia: Stress/adaptation and existentialism. *The Gerontologist, 37*(2), 250-256.

Flett, G. L., Hewitt, P. L., Heisel, M. J., Davidson, L. A., & Gayle, B. (2006). *The Social Hopelessness Questionnaire: Development of a domain-specific measure.* Manuscript submitted for publication.

Frankl, V. E. (1971). *The doctor and the soul: From psychotherapy to logotherapy* (R. & C. Winston, Trans.). New York: Bantam.

Frankl, V. E. (1984). *Man's search for meaning.* New York: Simon & Schuster.

Frankl, V. E. (1988). *The will to meaning: Foundations and applications of Logotherapy.* New York: Penguin.

Friedman, B., Heisel, M. J., & Delavan, R. L. (2005). Psychometric properties of the 15-item Geriatric Depression Scale in functionally impaired, cognitively intact, community-dwelling elderly primary care patients. *Journal of the American Geriatrics Society, 53*(9), 1570-1576.

Fry, P. S. (2000). Religious involvement, spirituality and personal meaning for life: Existential predictors of psychological wellbeing in community-residing and institutional care elders. *Aging & Mental Health, 4*(4), 375-387.

Fry, P. S. (2001). The unique contribution of key existential factors to the prediction of psychological well-being of older adults following spousal loss. *The Gerontologist, 41*(1), 69-81.

Heikkinen, M., Aro, H., & Lönnqvist, J. (1993). Life events and social support in suicide. *Suicide and Life-Threatening Behavior, 23*(4), 343-358.

Heisel, M. J. (2006). Suicide and its prevention among older adults. *Canadian Journal of Psychiatry, 51*(3), 143-154.

Heisel, M. J., & Flett, G. L. (2006). The development and initial validation of the Geriatric Suicide Ideation Scale (GSIS). *The American Journal of Geriatric Psychiatry, 14*, 742-751.

Heisel, M. J., & Flett, G. L. (2004). Purpose in life, satisfaction with life and suicide ideation in a clinical sample. *Journal of Psychopathology and Behavioral Assessment, 26*(2), 127-135.

Heisel, M. J., Flett, G. L, & Hewitt, P. L. (2003). Social hopelessness and college student suicide ideation. *Archives of Suicide Research, 7*(3), 221-235.

Hickson, J., & Housley, W. (1997). Creativity in later life. *Educational Gerontology, 23,* 539-547.

Kay, W. K., & Francis, L. J. (2006). Suicidal ideation among young people in the U.K.: Churchgoing as an inhibitory influence? *Mental Health, Religion & Culture, 9*(2), 127-140.

Kotarba, J. A. (1983). Perceptions of death, belief systems and the process of coping with chronic pain. *Social Science and Medicine, 17*(10), 681-689.

Krause, N. (2004). Stressors arising in highly valued roles, meaning in life, and the physical health status of older adults. *Journals of Gerontology Series B: Psychological Sciences & Social Sciences, 59*(5), S287-S297.

Krug, E. G., Dahlberg, L. L., Mercy, J. A., Zwi, A. B., & Lozano, R. (Eds.) (2002). *World report on violence and health.* Geneva, Switzerland: World Health Organization.

Linehan, M. M., Goodstein, J. L., Nielsen, S. L., & Chiles, J. A. (1983). Reasons for staying alive when you are thinking of killing yourself: The reasons for living inventory. *Journal of Consulting and Clinical Psychology, 51,* 276-286.

Lubell, K. M., & Vetter, J. B. (2006). Suicide and youth violence prevention: The promise of an integrated approach. *Aggression and Violent Behavior, 11*(2), 167-175.

Lukas, E. (1986). *Meaning in suffering: Comfort in crisis through logotherapy* (J. B. Fabry, Trans.). Berkeley, CA: Institute of Logotherapy Press.

Lukas, E. (1991). *Psychological ministry.* (W. Schulte, Trans., corrected by R. Sonner & T. Pritchard). Original published as *Psychologische Seelsorge*, Verlag Herder, Germany, 1985.

Moody, H. R. (1991). "Rational suicide" on grounds of old age? *Journal of Geriatric Psychiatry, 24*(2), 261-276.

Moore, S. L. (1997). A phenomenological study of meaning in life in suicidal older adults. *Archives of Psychiatric Nursing, 11*(1), 29-36.

Pearson, J. L., & Brown, G. K. (2000). Suicide prevention in late life: Directions for science and practice. *Clinical Psychology Review, 20*(6), 685-705.

Petrie, K., & Brook, R. (1992). Sense of coherence, self-esteem, depression and hopelessness as correlates of reattempting suicide. *British Journal of Clinical Psychology, 31,* 293-300.

Pintos, C. C. G. (1988). Depression and the will to meaning: A comparison of the GDS and PIL in an Argentine population. *Clinical Gerontologist, 7*(3/4), 3-9.

Prager, E. (1996). Exploring personal meaning in an age-differentiated Australian sample: Another look at the Sources of Meaning Profile (SOMP). *Journal of Aging Studies, 10*(2), 117-136.

Prager, E., Bar-Tur, L., & Abramowici, I. (1997). The sources of meaning profile (SOMP) with aged subjects exhibiting depressive symptomatology. *Clinical Gerontologist, 17*(3), 25-39.

Reker, G. T. (1997). Personal meaning, optimism, and choice: Existential predictors of depression in community and institutional elderly. *The Gerontologist, 37*(6), 709-716.

Reker, G. T., & Wong, P. T. P. (1988). Aging as an individual process: Toward a theory of personal meaning. In J. E. Birren & V. L. Bengtson (Eds.), *Emergent theories of aging* (pp. 214-246). New York: Springer.

Ryff, C. D. (1989). Happiness is everything, or is it? Explorations on the meaning of psychological well-being. *Journal of Personality and Social Psychology, 57*(6), 1069-1081.

Saul, S. (1993). Meaningful life activities for elderly residents of residential health care facilities. *Loss, Grief and Care, 6*(4), 7986.

Shneidman, E. S. (1996). *The suicidal mind.* New York: Oxford University Press.

Silver, M. H. (1995). Memories and meaning: Life review in old age. *Journal of Geriatric Psychiatry, 28*(1), 5773.

Tabachnick, B. G., & Fidell, L. S. (1996). *Using multivariate statistics* (3rd ed.). New York: HarperCollins.

Ulmer, A., Range, L. M., & Smith, P. C. (1991). Purpose in life: A moderator of recovery from bereavement. *Omega, 23*(4), 279-289.

Uncapher, H., Gallagher-Thompson, D., Osgood, N. J., & Bongar, B. (1998). Hopelessness and suicidal ideation in older adults. *The Gerontologist, 38*(1), 62-70.

Van Ranst, N., & Marcoen, A. (1997). Meaning in life of young and elderly adults: An examination of the factorial validity and invariance of the life regard index. *Personality and Individual Differences, 22*(6), 877-884.

Vanderhorst, R. K., & McLaren, S. (2005). Social relationships as predictors of depression and suicidal ideation in older adults. *Aging & Mental Health, 9*(6), 517-525.

Weisman, A. D. (1991). Vulnerability and suicidality in the aged. *Journal of Geriatric Psychiatry, 24*(2), 191-201.

Yesavage, J. A., Brink, T. L., Rose, T. L., Lum, O., Huang, V., Adey, M., et al. (1983). Development and validation of a geriatric depression screening scale: A preliminary report. *Journal of Psychiatric Research, 17*(1), 37-49.

Zika, S., & Chamberlain, K. (1992). On the relation between meaning in life and psychological well-being. *British Journal of Psychology, 83,* 133-145.

Author's Note

This study was part of Dr. Heisel's doctoral dissertation conducted at York University under Dr. Flett's supervision, and written while Dr. Heisel was the

Stephen Godfrey Fellow in Suicide Studies in the Department of Psychiatry, University of Toronto. Thank you to Drs. Kenneth Shulman, Robert van Reekum, and Marcus Feak for their assistance in GSIS item development, and to Dr. Heisel's on-site supervisors: Drs. Gary Challis, Howard Dombrower, Corinne Fischer, Alastair Flint, Rosemary Meier, Ivan Silver, David Streiner, Gary Teare, Fran Kleiner, M.S.W., and Earl Smith, M.S.W. We appreciate the helpful comments and suggestions of Dr. Heisel's Doctoral Dissertation committee: Drs. Paul Kohn, Clarry Lay, Toyomasa Fusé, Joseph Levy, and Michael Kral. Thank you to the study participants and to the Research Ethics Boards and staff of the Ahavath Achim Retirement Home, Bathurst Jewish Centre, Baycrest Centre for Geriatric Care, Bernard Betel Centre for Creative Living, Brookside Retirement Residence, Cheltenham Nursing Home, Extendicare sites, Harold & Grace Baker Centre, Hilltop Retirement Residence, King Garden Retirement Centre, Lansing Retirement Residence, Markham-Stouffville Hospital, Meals on Wheels, Mount Sinai Hospital, North York Seniors Walkers, Providence Centre, St. Michael's Hospital, Strathaven Retirement Residence, Sunnybrook and Women's Health Sciences Centre, Toronto General Hospital, University Health Network, University of Toronto, Whitby Mental Health Centre, York University, and the YMCA for their assistance in conducting this study.

This research was funded by a Social Sciences and Humanities Research Council of Canada (SSHRC) Doctoral Fellowship to Dr. Heisel, and by a grant from the SSHRC awarded to Dr. Flett. Dr. Heisel currently holds a Young Investigator award from the American Foundation for Suicide Prevention. Dr. Flett holds a Canada Research Chair in Personality and Health.

Finding Meaning in Chronic Pain: The Dynamics of Acceptance

EARL D. BLAND
DOUGLAS D. HENNING

Abstract

Those who treat individuals with chronic pain are aware of the pervasive and often devastating effect this pain can have on individual lives including shaking the very foundations of a person's being. Crises of meaning (defined by the authors as questions involving *why* and *how*) are frequent for people with chronic pain as they try to make sense of their lives in the face of significant challenges to functional abilities and comfort. Along with physical impairment, chronic pain engenders a host of emotional, cognitive, spiritual, relational, and socioeconomic problems. While these difficulties seem insurmountable, perhaps the greatest challenge underlying these struggles is construing a new or modified worldview that includes the inescapability of pain. Reorienting one's expectations, self-perception, and future possibilities is often a slow and arduous journey. This paper proposes that acceptance is a dynamic *process catalyst* whereby people with chronic pain incorporate new meanings of self, others, and the world. Not only does acceptance promote positive adjustment and well-being, it stimulates hope, optimism, and self-efficacy in spite of troublesome realities.

Pain is a ubiquitous human phenomenon. Current estimations place the number of Americans suffering from chronic pain resulting in partial or total disability at about 50 million. Estimates of physician appointments involving Americans seeking assistance for acute or chronic pain may run to 100 million visits annually (Eimer & Freeman, 1998). The negative economic impact of chronic and acute pain syndromes is significant, in the United States (AMA, 1995; Eimer & Freeman, 1998; Garofalo & Polatin, 1999) and internationally (Linton, 1998). Additionally, chronic pain affects worker productivity (Feuerstein, Huang, & Pransky, 1999; Fishbain, Cutler, Rosomoff, Khalil, & Steele-Rosomoff, 1997; Helliwell, Mumford, Smeathers, & Wright, 1992), family relationships (Kerns & Payne, 1996), and overall psychological and social well-being (Eimer & Freeman, 1998; Gatchel & Turk, 1999). Philosopher and theologian C. S. Lewis (1962) observed "creatures cause pain by being born, and live by inflicting pain, and in pain they mostly die" (p. 14).

Regardless of the source, pain is a phenomenon that impacts the entire person. Biopsychosocial approaches to treating medical and psychological problems have clearly demonstrated that rigid dualistic perception of a mind-body split is misguided and insufficient in our understanding of humans (Turk & Flor, 1999). Both medicine and psychology have embraced the notion that physical pain (or other medical pathology) can have devastating psychosocial consequences (Eimer & Freeman, 1998). Merskey & Bogduk (1994) recognized this systemic attribute of pain in their broadly accepted definition: "Pain is an unpleasant sensory and emotional experience associated with actual or potential tissue damage, or described in terms of such damage" (p. 210).

As an extension of the biopsychosocial view of pain, this paper will address how two processes, meaning making and acceptance, interact in the process of pain management. There is extensive literature documenting the positive impact psychosocial interventions have on managing chronic pain conditions, but much of it has focused on specific cognitive and behavioral interventions (Eimer & Freeman, 1998; Fordyce, 1976, 1988; Gatchel & Turk, 1996; Gatchel & Turk, 1999). Managing pain behaviors, addressing emotional sequelae such as depression and anxiety, increasing positive coping, and applying the positive benefits of biofeedback, relaxation, and hypnosis have all demonstrated promise. In contrast, direct deliberation of meaning and acceptance has been explored on a much more limited basis (McCracken, 1998; McCracken, Spertus, Janeck, Sinclair & Wetzel, 1999; Morris, 1999). We believe that meaning making, especially the process of acceptance, is a crucial aspect of active pain management. However, meaning is seldom addressed specifically, or recognized at all. It is our goal to highlight the function of acceptance as it relates to finding positive meaning for those who deal with chronic pain. First, the biopsychosocial perspective of pain management will be outlined followed by the role that meaning making plays in coping with pain. Finally, the process of acceptance and how it acts as a catalyst to healthy meanings will be discussed.

THE BIOPSYCHOSOCIAL CONTEXT

The average individual tends to hold to the traditional *biomedical model* of disease—if someone is ill or in pain there must be an observable biological condition causing the disease or discomfort. A related expectation is that, once the particular condition has been treated, provided the necessary tincture-of-time for healing has been allowed, the symptoms of disease/discomfort will abate. Thus, a linear singular cause and cure are assumed. A corollary involves the process of diagnosis to include labelling and treatment planning. Although diagnostic labelling has obvious merit, much debate has centered on problems associated with the process since the middle part of the twentieth century (Fordyce, 1976; Szasz, 1997).

Fordyce (1976), in his work with chronic pain patients, has stressed the power of the diagnosis as well as the patient's subjective experience in shaping and maintaining the symptomatic behavior in chronic conditions. Over the last 30 years a social-learning model of the role symptoms play in chronic conditions has gained increasing support in the field of behavioral pain management. This model allows for a variety of causal, contributing, and correlated factors that form a cluster of chronic symptoms, including social and psychological events, as well as biological origins. Specifically, this has lead to a *biopsychosocial* model of chronic pain. Each area impacts, to a lesser or greater degree, the maintenance, exaggeration, and/or alleviation of the symptoms; therefore, different interventions are needed for *pain* and *suffering*. Suffering is

> an affective or emotional response in the central nervous system, triggered by nociception[1] *or* other aversive events, such as loss of a loved one, fear, or threat. Further, suffering is observed only in the indirect sense of the person engaging in some behavior [avoiding specific activities that makes the pain worse] that is attributed to suffering. (p. 278)

Thus experiences such as physical discomfort, functional limitations, and social impairment serve to validate the presence of pain and disease (i.e., give *meaning* to the experience of pain). Therefore, a major focus of treatment involves the role suffering/illness plays in the individual's daily life.

In acute conditions, pain and suffering often go together and may even be adaptive, with suffering allowing for adequate healing to take place. However, in chronic conditions pain becomes a more enduring part of the individual's life. If treatment can reduce the degree of *suffering*, even though the intensity of the pain may remain the same, the amount of distress one experiences can be decreased significantly, thereby, increasing the degree of functionality. In other words, "Special efforts [are] made to help patients recognize that *hurt and harm are not the same.* That one hurts on moving does not necessarily *mean* (author's italics) that healing has not occurred or that residual injury is present" (Fordyce, 1988, p. 282). These models set the stage for discussing the role that meaning plays in chronic pain conditions. For instance, the degree of suffering one experiences is often one way of validating the extent of the injury, or as a way to give meaning and significance to injury and loss.

PAIN AND CRISIS OF MEANING

When life situations fail to match the ideal or expected experience, emotional pain and distress are often the result. The amount of distress experienced is frequently in direct proportion to the degree of difference between the actual and ideal. Some theorists attribute significant responsibility for emotional pain/ discomfort to the amount of incongruence between these two perspectives—who one thinks he or she is, versus who one believes he or she should be (Frankl, 1984; Rogers, 1942). In fact, Rogers' primary goal of counseling is to assist the individual in reconciling the incongruent relationship between perceived and ideal self (Corey, 1996). Similarly, Frankl's existential crisis, being unable to exist in the moment [with who one is at that moment] must be resolved in order to experience self-acceptance.

To some degree this incongruence seems to be a universal experience among individuals with chronic pain, and, particularly in Western cultures, is often secondary to the expectation that all illness/pain can and should be fixed. Thus, less than complete amelioration of pain is viewed as failure. So when an individual finds him- or herself in this condition that does not fit with his or her self-expectation—severe pain and disability—a crisis is experienced.

This crisis, relative to meaning and chronic pain, is often magnified when the facing of one's unfixable illness, or coming to grips with one's own mortality, occurs at a particularly young age—out of the expected developmental sequence. For example, it may be hard enough for individuals in the young-old age range, 60 to 75, to adjust to the normal aging processes, such as having difficulty moving from a sitting to a standing position because of stiff joints, mild arthritis, and relatively normal levels of pain. It is quite another thing for someone at the age of 30 to experience profound difficulty moving about. The increased difficulty in coping is in large part due to the fact that the conditions are occurring earlier than expected; the conditions have occurred out of developmental sequence.

In summary, for individuals seen in behavioral pain management clinics there is a strong likelihood that in addition to pain, they are experiencing various levels of emotional discomfort—depression, anxiety, and a sense of hopelessness. This emotional pain is often related, at least in part, to a crisis of meaning. Thus, the humanistic and existential perspectives as mentioned above (Corey, 1996) are quite helpful in assisting individuals learn how to cope with, and view themselves as whole and complete individuals apart from, pain that has become a central part of their life.

ACCEPTANCE

The exercise of finding and generating meaning appears to be a fundamental aspect of human existence. We give rise to meanings spontaneously. When events make sense we are often unaware of the meaning-making process. A person who complains of acute pain just after a bad motor vehicle accident does not spark curiosity about meanings. We expect the accident victim to be suffering. However, as mentioned earlier, when the pain appears without the benefit of trauma or corroborating medical diagnosis, when the source is a mystery or the pain persists long after a normative healing cycle, the ability to form adequate meanings becomes elusive.

It is at this point of meaning crisis that the process of acceptance becomes critical to those who suffer from persistent pain conditions. Acceptance, a common but difficult word to define, can often evoke a plurality of emotional responses depending on the situation or event that is in need of being accepted. Acceptance of a gift can generate excitement or joy, while trying to accept that a loved one has died may breed resistance, sadness, anger, or fear. There is a difference between accepting positive circumstance or events and accepting that which is seen as negative or unwanted.

Hayes (1994) defines acceptance as "experiencing events fully and without defense, as they are and not as they say they are" (p. 30). Hayes believes that context is vital to understanding the nature and process of acceptance. While energy is often spent changing the *content* of people's problems (e.g., altering thoughts, feelings, behaviors, attitudes, or memories), Hayes believes that changing the context of psychological problems is equally important. He sees acceptance as a strategy that complements manipulation and coping. Hayes speaks to the interaction of meaning and acceptance:

> The meaning of psychological events is found in the relationship
> between those events and their psychological context… psychological
> events in another context are no longer "the same psychological
> events…." By establishing a posture of psychological acceptance,
> events that formerly were taken to be inherently problematic become
> instead opportunities for growth, interest, or understanding. (p. 13)

Recently, researchers have investigated acceptance as it specifically relates to chronic pain (Geiser, 1992; Large & Strong, 1997; McCracken, 1998; McCracken et al., 1999). McCracken et al. (1999) has attempted to operationally define acceptance as "acknowledging one's pain, giving up unproductive attempts to control pain, acting as if the pain does not necessarily imply disability, and being able to commit one's efforts toward living a satisfying life despite [the] pain" (p. 284). This definition speaks not only to the cognitive events but the whole of psychosocial operations. In addition, McCracken's definition involves action, which, according to Dougher (1994) is important when understanding the process of acceptance. Dougher believes that "acceptance is something one does" (p. 37). Other components of acceptance include abandoning of avoidance, taking in an event, and letting go of dysfunctional efforts to change (Hayes, Strosahl, & Wilson, 1999). Hayes et al. (1999) goes on to propose that acceptance is an active process where one acknowledges feelings, thoughts, and memories without getting trapped in negative verbalizations or interpretations of these psychological events.

Acceptance is a complex multilayered phenomenon best understood as an evolving process that leads to new meaning. The following are three components of the acceptance process: control, emotional regulation, and cognitive behavioral structuring. After a brief description of each we will discuss the integration of meaning making as it relates to acceptance.

CONTROL

People who live with chronic pain often experience their most profound sense of distress in the area of perceived personal control. Several studies have demonstrated that a person's perceived ability to control their pain contributes to the degree of positive or negative psychological consequences secondary to pain (Jensen, Romano, Turner, & Karoly, 1991; Rudy, Kerns, & Turk, 1988; Turk, Okifuji, & Scharff, 1995). The typical misperception is that anything short of complete amelioration or escape from symptoms is seen as a lack of control. The inability to escape the noxious stimuli of pain particularly after countless physician visits, surgical procedures, and medication trials leaves one in a perplexing state of hopelessness and helplessness.

Depression, anxiety, anger, helplessness, and hopelessness accompany the pain because one cannot escape the torment. In addition, when pain is inescapable, definitions of self must be reworked to incorporate that which is not desired and frequently loathed. Not only is the pain a threat to the biological integrity of the self, but all other definitions of self (e.g., social, psychological, spiritual) demand revision. Persistent pain frequently means uncontrolled bodily sensations, disrupted social contacts, economic uncertainty, and alterations in one's worldview.

Command of one's life becomes increasingly tenuous as the person with persistent pain scrambles to accommodate the stress of instability. This accommodation can be an extremely difficult and emotionally wrenching process marked by continual efforts to reinstate the desired "normal" way of life.

Hayes (1994) believes that attempting to change situations that are inherently unchangeable is [obviously] pointless and acceptance is the only reasonable course of action. Therefore, since it is true that some pain is intractable or that the side effects of achieving the absence of pain are unacceptable (e.g., total anesthesia), then it appears acceptance is part of a rational approach. Persons with persistent pain must move to a definition of self and a worldview that incorporates new limitations on their ability to directly control the self and environment. In addition, these patients may need to progress from a dominant context of control/escape, to a context of acceptance where at a minimum, the person is able to operate effectively within their limitations, learning to control their reaction to the pain.

EMOTIONAL REGULATION

In concert with decreased sense of control from chronic pain conditions is the emotional upheaval influencing much of a pain patient's world. Although there are many different emotions generated by persistent pain, it appears that depression, anxiety, and anger (or derivatives such sadness, grief, fear, frustration, irritability, etc.) are the most significant ones.[2] Banks and Kerns (1996) have hypothesized that high rates of depression in people with chronic pain can be explained by looking not only at the symptom of pain, but also at the level of impairment and disability, the level of secondary losses (e.g., economic, social, work, leisure, self-esteem), and the general hassles involved in working with the medical system as additional stressors for the person with chronic pain.

Along with the source of the negative emotions, the importance of the emotional environment or context in which the chronic pain resides must be considered (Eccleston & Crombez, 1999). The presence of positive or negative emotional contexts may impact the attentional demand pain has for a given individual. The person who experiences chronic pain in the midst of a relatively unencumbered low stress environment will probably face different hurdles than the person whose chronic pain is one more stressor in the midst of a life situation full of distressing events.

Thus, if one is to move to a point of acceptance and positive meaning with regards to persistent pain, negative emotional states will have to be addressed. This is especially true for those emotions associated closely to definitions of self. "How can I be worthwhile if I don't work?" "No one wants to be around a person who is always in pain." "Why isn't healing occurring?" "Is God punishing me?" These and similar questions are laden with negative emotions, such as sadness, anxiety, depression, rejection, and frustration. The process of acceptance requires that one acknowledges his/her feelings without spiraling into negative interpretations or meanings. Additionally, through acceptance and the discovery of new meanings, one must address the cognitive structures that help maintain negative emotions regarding current life circumstances.

COGNITIVE BEHAVIORAL STRUCTURING

The cognitive aspects of chronic pain are based on the idea that sensory data, including pain, is cognitively mediated as it enters into conscious awareness (Eimer & Freeman, 1998; Fordyce, 1976, 1988; Gatchel & Turk, 1996, 1999). This cognitive processing of pain leads to any number of interpretations, meanings, beliefs, attitudes, and emotional sequelae and is significantly influenced by pre-existing cognitive structures or schema, such as current and historical context, intensity and novelty of pain, prior experiences, and learning (Chapman, Nakamura, & Flores, 1999; Eccleston & Crombez, 1999).

The meaning attributed within the context of acute pain (e.g., pain as danger, warning, or threat) is essentially an overlearned cognitive process that impacts the context of chronic pain structures of self-perception, self-identity, and emotional regulation. Chapman et al. (1999) believe this meaning-making process is inherently a construction, which can be seen in the different stories and perceptions held by people who deal with persistent pain. Each story, while similar, carries its own unique flavor that can change dramatically depending on the current experience of pain within the psychosocial context. Meaning making is a dynamic phenomenon that allows the individual to construct and reconstruct the subjective experience.

This constructivist perspective is useful because it helps inform our discussion in two important areas: cognitive distortions and the cognitive aspect of acceptance. First, persistent pain can produce multiple cognitive distortions (Jensen, Romano, Turner, Good, & Wald, 1999; Shutty, Degood, & Tuttle, 1990; Stroud, Thorn, Jensen & Boothby, 2000; Sullivan, Stanish, Waite, Sullivan, & Tripp, 1999). Pain and its related emotions contribute to distortions of self, others, past events, and the future. Concepts such as catastrophizing, over-generalization, learned helplessness, and other errors in thinking, are helpful in understanding the thought life of pain patients. Changing these destructive patterns of thinking is believed to be a crucial component of healthy coping and therefore a focus of psychological treatment. Inherent in this change process is the restructuring of relational connections that lead to meanings. If one is to see the self and pain more productively, he or she must accept and alter his or her perception of pain.

Therefore, acceptance becomes a dynamic process catalyst, helping the person to move away from negative interpretations of self, others, and the future, towards perceptions that have benign or positive meaning. As persons with persistent pain increase their degree of acceptance, they often diffuse the power cognitive distortions and negative beliefs have had, and begin to consider alternative meanings of their current condition. For example, as the patient with persistent pain begins the process of acceptance, he or she moves from negative self-statements such as "I am useless because of my pain" to statements that allow for a new meaning of self to germinate: "What can I do despite my pain?" Because persistent pain conditions frequently interrupt many facets of life, acceptance of this interruption diffuses the need to escape from the inescapable and to explore new alternative meanings and options regarding self-identity, relationships with others, and future prospects. If new meanings are the end goal, acceptance is the impetus that allows and encourages these new meanings to develop.

The concept of acceptance also helps to clarify how a person changes his/her actions, decreasing the function of pain behaviors. Pain behaviors are actions that communicate disability and discomfort (e.g., wincing, limping, decreased activity) and have been shown to play a significant role in reducing an individual's level of functioning and exacerbating the pain condition (Fordyce, 1976). In chronic pain conditions, where pain is inescapable and the warning function of pain has lost much of its relevance, new meanings must be developed that allow one to function as optimally as possible. Acceptance that one must tolerate a certain degree of pain during life activities reduces the anxiety surrounding pain and increases functioning. Although chronic pain patients may need to operate within certain behavioral parameters (e.g., allowing for more time to complete tasks, taking rest breaks, judicious use of short acting pain medication), they are still able to participate in life. Acceptance allows pain patients to find positive meaning in their actions as they move from focusing on limitations to embracing what is possible.

MEANING AND ACCEPTANCE

If, as proposed, acceptance of persistent pain is not a passive or singular event but a complex endeavor involving emotional, cognitive, and behavioral reorganizations it stands to reason that meaning making is a corollary developmental occurrence. The new meanings of self, others, past events, and future include new self-definitions, which involve perceived gender roles, life roles, capabilities, social connections, and spirituality. Acceptance and the development of more workable meanings act synergistically to move the individual towards greater functioning and health.

Hayes (1994) beckoned a rethinking of the contexts of change. The acceptance schema allows persons with chronic pain and those involved in their care to balance efforts at alleviating pain by realistically exploring what degree of discomfort and pain will not be ameliorated. When biomedical efforts to stop pain are unsuccessful, patients must be delivered from the dizzying exploration for "the cure" involving endless referrals, medication trials, and surgical procedures. These patients should not be left with simplistic and linear conclusions that there is nothing more to be done; they will just have to live with it. Using our best efforts at reducing pain and providing clear strategies that encourage acceptance of the remaining discomfort will stimulate patients to find new meanings and a new worldview that allows persistent pain to be part of a healthy productive life.

References

American Medical Association (1995). Pain. In T. C. Doege & T. P. Houston (Eds.), *Guides to the evaluation of permanent impairment* (4th ed.). Chicago: Author.

Banks, S. M., & Kerns, R. D. (1996) Explaining high rates of depression in chronic pain: A diathesis-stress framework. *Psychological Bulletin, 119,* 95-110.

Chapman, C. R., Nakamura, Y, & Flores, L. Y. (1999). Chronic pain and consciousness: A constructivist perspective. In R. J. Gatchel & D. C. Turk (Eds.), *Psychosocial factors in pain: Critical perspectives* (pp. 35-55). New York: Guilford Press.

Corey, G. (1996). *Theory and practice of counseling and psychotherapy* (5th ed.). Brooks/ Cole Publishing Co.

Dougher, M. J. (1994). The act of acceptance. In S. C. Hayes, N. S. Jacobson, V. M. Follette, & M. J. Dougher (Eds.), *Acceptance and change: Content and context in psychotherapy* (pp. 37-45). Reno, NV: Context Press.

Eccleston, C., & Crombez, G. (1999). Pain demands attention: A cognitive-affective model of the interruptive function of pain. *Psychological Bulletin, 125,* 356-366.

Eimer, B. N., & Freeman, A. (1998). *Pain management psychotherapy: A practical guide.* New York: John Wiley & Sons.

Feuerstein, M., Huang, G. D., & Pransky, G. (1999). Work style and work-related upper extremity disorders. In R. J. Gatchel & D. C. Turk (Eds.), *Psychosocial factors in pain: Critical perspectives* (pp. 175-192). New York: Guilford.

Fishbain, D. A., Cutler, R. B., Rosomoff, H. L., Khalil, T., & Steele-Rosomoff, R. (1997). Impact of chronic pain patients' job perception variables on actual return to work. *The Clinical Journal of Pain, 13,* 197-206.

Fordyce, W. E. (1988). Pain and suffering: A reappraisal. *American Psychologist, 43*(4), 276-283.

Fordyce, W. E. (1976). *Behavioral methods for chronic pain and illness.* St. Louis, MO: C.V. Mosby.

Frankl, V. (1984). *Man's search for meaning* (Rev. ed.). New York: Washington Square Press, Pocket Books.

Garofalo, J. P., & Polatin, P. (1999). Low back pain: An epidemic in industrialized countries. In R. J. Gatchel & D. C. Turk (Eds.), *Psychosocial factors in pain: Critical perspectives* (pp. 164-174). New York: Guilford.

Gatchel, R. J., & Turk, D. C. (Eds.). (1996). *Psychological approaches to pain management: A practitioner's handbook.* New York: Guilford

Gatchel, R. J., & Turk, D. C. (Eds.). (1999). *Psychosocial factors in pain: Critical perspectives.* New York: Guilford Press.

Geiser, D. S. (1992). *A comparison of acceptance-focused and control-focused psychological treatments in a chronic pain treatment center.* Unpublished doctoral dissertation, University of Nevada, Reno.

Hayes, S. C. (1994). Content, context, and the types of psychological acceptance. In S. C. Hayes, N. S. Jacobson, V. M. Follette, & M. J. Dougher (Eds.), *Acceptance and change: Content and context in psychotherapy* (pp. 13-32). Reno, NV: Context Press.

Hayes, S. C., Stosahl, K. D, & Wilson, K. G. (1999). *Acceptance and commitment therapy: An experiential approach to behavior change.* New York: Guilford.

Helliwell, P. S., Mumford, D. B., Smeathers, J. E., & Wright, V. (1992). Work related upper limb disorder: The relationship between pain, cumulative load, disability, and psychological factors. *Annals of the Rheumatic Diseases, 51,* 1325-1329.

Jensen, M. P., Turner, J. A., Romano, J. M., & Karoly, P. (1991). Coping with chronic pain: A critical review of the literature. *Pain, 47,* 249-483.

Jensen, M. P., Romano, J. M., Turner, J. A., Good, A. B., & Wald, L. H. (1999). Patient beliefs predict patient functioning: Further support for a cognitive-behavioral model of chronic pain. *Pain, 81,* 95-104.

Kerns, R. D., & Payne, A. (1996). Treating families of chronic pain patients. In R. J. Gatchel & D. C. Turk (Eds.), *Psychological approaches to pain management: A practitioner's handbook* (pp. 283-304). New York: Guilford

Large, R., & Strong, J. (1997). The personal constructs of coping with chronic low back pain: Is coping a necessary evil? *Pain, 73,* 245-252.

Lewis, C. S. (1962). *The problem of pain.* New York: MacMillan Publishing Company.

Linton, S. J. (1998). The socioeconomic impact of chronic back pain: Is anyone benefitting? *Pain, 75,* 163-168.

McCracken, L. M. (1998). Learning to live with pain: Acceptance of pain predicts adjustment in persons with chronic pain. *Pain, 74,* 21-27.

McCracken, L. M., Spertus, I. L., Janeck, A. S., Sinclair, D., & Wetzel, F. T. (1999). Behavioral dimensions of adjustment in persons with chronic pain: Pain-related anxiety and acceptance. *Pain, 80,* 283-289.

Merskey, H., & Bogduk, N. (Eds.). (1994). *Classification of chronic pain: Descriptions of chronic pain syndromes and definitions of pain terms* (2nd ed., p. 210). Seattle, WA: IASP Press.

Morris, D. B. (1999). Sociocultural and religious meanings of pain. In R. J. Gatchel & D. C. Turk (Eds.), *Psychosocial factors in pain: Critical perspectives* (pp. 118-131). New York: Guilford

Rogers, C. (1942). *Counseling and psychotherapy.* Cambridge, MA: The Riverside Press.

Rudy, T. E., Kerns, R. D., & Turk, D. C. (1988). Chronic pain and depression: Toward a cognitive-behavioral mediation model. *Pain, 35,* 129-140.

Shutty, M. S., DeGood, D. E., & Tuttle, D. H. (1990). Chronic pain patients' beliefs about their pain and treatment outcomes. *Archives of Physical Medicine & Rehabilitation, 71,* 128-132.

Sullivan, J. L., Stanish, W., Waite, H., Sullivan, M., & Tripp, D. A. (1998). Catastrophizing, pain, and disability in patients with soft tissue injuries. *Pain, 77,* 253-260.

Stroud, M. W., Thorn, B. E., Jensen, M. P., & Boothby, J. L. (2000). The relation between pain beliefs, negative thoughts, and psychosocial functioning in chronic pain patients. *Pain, 84,* 347-352.

Szasz, T. S. (1997). *The Manufacture of Madness: A Comparative Study of the Inquisition and the Mental Health Movement* (Reprint ed.). New York: Syracuse University Press. (Original work published 1970)

Turk, D. C., Okifugi, A., & Scharff, L. (1995). Chronic pain and depression: Role of perceived impact and perceived control in different age cohorts. *Pain, 61,* 93-101.

Turk, D. C. (1996). Biopsychosocial perspective on chronic pain. In R. J. Catchel & D. C. Turk (Eds.), *Psychological Approaches to Pain Management: A practitioner's Handbook* (pp. 3-32). New York: Guilford Press.

Turk, D. C., & Flor, H. (1999). Chronic pain: A biobehavioral perspective. In R. J Gatchel & D. C. Turk (Eds.), *Psychosocial factors in pain: Critical perspectives* (pp. 18-34). New York: Guilford Press.

Endnotes

1. *Nociception*—a mechanical, thermal, or chemical energy impinging on specialized nerve endings that in turn activate [specific] … fibers thus initiating a signal to the central nervous system that aversive events are occurring.

2. For a review of negative emotions and pain see Robinson & Riley, 1999.

PART THREE

SUFFERING, DEATH, & GRIEVING

Spirituality and Pain: Finding Purpose, Meaning, and Hope in the Midst of Suffering

HAROLD G. KOENIG

[Keynote address delivered at the 4th International Meaning Conference.]

I am going to be talking about spirituality and pain as the focus of my presentation: A bit on pain, about suffering as a gift, the role in which spiritual transformation can help people cope with pain, and how religion influences coping. I will also review some of the research on religion and coping with illness, and then look at some spiritual approaches to pain with regard to application. Pain has multiple components or expressions. There is physical pain—the kind of pain that people have that is caused by disease or illness (e.g., arthritis). I experience chronic pain. I have for about 30 years and it is pain that is related to inflammation of the joints and the tendons. Then there is emotional pain—the pain that people experience because they feel bad emotionally. They feel depressed or anxious. Depression is probably one of the strongest forms of emotional pain where people feel so desperately in pain that they would rather kill themselves than be alive. Then there is spiritual pain—pain that derives from existential kinds of feelings like, "Why am I here?" "Why did God allow such and such to happen?" These are the kinds of spiritual struggles that we experience. Then there is the experience of all of these interacting together. Physical pain causes emotional pain because people become depressed over their physical pain and then they wonder, "Why is it that they have been picked to experience pain in life?"

NOW WHAT ABOUT SUFFERING AS A GIFT?

You know, pain is the gift that nobody wants. I think there is a book by that title, *The Gift That Nobody Wants*, and yet pain can do a lot for us. Medical societal views toward suffering and pain are: Avoid it at all cost. There is no real value or worth seen in pain or suffering other than to get rid of it. There are some risks involved in pain and also some benefits that we will take a look at. Pain can be destructive. I see a lot of patients with chronic pain, young and old, as part of my clinical practice. And it can be destructive, even in very devoutly spiritual people. If living day in and day out with pain rivets your attention to it and causes you not to be able to pray or read scriptures, it can be destructive. It makes you irritable so you are short with your family and loved ones. It can destroy people. Pain can lead to addiction as people try to struggle with relieving it, wanting to have just a little bit of comfort and not having pain in their life. That is one of the gifts of pain—being without pain is a wonderful thing. But many of us who do not have that pain, do not really realize how wonderful it is to lie in bed at night and not have any pain. So people get addicted because they take medicines to give them those short periods of relief.

Pain can be isolating because it affects your functioning and you do not feel like socializing with people. You want to just be alone and not have any more stimulation at all and it affects your socialization and you start to feel isolated and lonely. Pain can cause anger and frustration. After a while, day in and day out with pain and suffering, it is frustrating and it pushes people to become angry. I have a patient who is a very devout man in his thirties suffering from chronic pain and there is nothing he can do to get away from it and he is so angry. Pain can make life burdensome for both oneself and other people trying to care for somebody in chronic pain. Many of you may know what I am talking about—you may have a loved one that you are trying to help. Pain makes people irritable. It is hard for them to express appreciation. People begin to feel that they are not only a burden to others but they are a burden to themselves, and of course that is part of the driving thing that causes people to become depressed. Pain can lead to depression, loss of hope, and suicide. These results manifest regularly in older people with chronic medical illness and chronic disability and a lot of times we do not even hear about it. People end up just not complying with their medications or taking a little bit too much of a medication, and people are reported as dying from natural causes.

What about the benefits of pain? Well, when you are in pain you are unlikely to be able to feel that pain has any value at all. All you want to be is without the pain. However, pain does provide a person with an understanding that others who are not in pain do not have: a depth of understanding and appreciation for what others who are going through pain are really going through. It is one of those things that you just cannot really appreciate unless you have been through it. It provides insight. Hopefully, it provides compassion. If it is not too destructive, pain can provide compassion for others, although compassion usually is not there when the person is having pain. It usually comes afterwards. And, of course, it can cause spiritual transformation. Pain can cause people to become more intimate with God. It can draw them to God as they seek Him in their striving for relief. Pain can also drive them away from God because they are angry and so they direct that anger at the One who ultimately is responsible for their pain. So it can go either way.

WHAT ABOUT TRANSFORMING PAIN THROUGH FAITH?

All religions of the world address the problem of pain and suffering; it is one thing religions have in common. In Christianity, faith can transform pain. Having faith, believing in God, and having a religious worldview can help people see their pain as having a sense of purpose or contributing to some kind of good. When they can get to that point, that purpose lightens the burden of their pain. When they can see that pain has some kind of meaning behind it, the burden of pain is lessened. Faith also enables the use of the pain to help others and that is perhaps the greatest benefit of pain. It can motivate us to try to help others with similar circumstances. Humans in general have a deep need to help others; when they are no longer able to do so because of disease or disability, they find that depression can begin very quickly. There is a deep human need to contribute to others' lives and to feel useful, especially for those people who feel that they have been a burden on others. Pain enables one to help others who likewise suffer from pain. It is the best certification you can have in reaching out to, supporting, and spending time with others one can have. There is no way you can be trained in school to really to have the same thing you get from having pain. A sense of participating in Christ's redemptive suffering can be spiritually transformative. This view comes primarily from the Catholic tradition. In the Protestant tradition, people believe that Christ did it all—there is nothing left to do. However, pain somehow allows us to participate in that redemptive suffering that Christ went through, which has saved all of humanity.

GENERATING STRENGTHS FROM OTHERS' WORK

People in pain can contribute to the work of others. This idea is actually from a book by Mother Teresa called *The Joy of Loving*. In Minneapolis, a woman in a wheelchair suffering from continuous convulsions from cerebral palsy asked me what people like her could do for others. I told her, "You can do the most. You can do more than any of us because your suffering is united with the suffering with Christ on the cross and it brings strength to us all." There is tremendous strength that is growing in the world through this continuous sharing, praying together, suffering together, and working together. It is almost based on the principle of justice—justice that the suffering of pain contributes something. There are sick and crippled people who cannot do anything to share in the work. So they adopt a sister or a brother who then involves the sick co-worker fully in whatever he or she does. The two become like one person and they call each other their second half. Mother Teresa writes, "I have a second half in Belgium. Each time I have something special to do it is she behind me that gives me all the strength and courage to do it." If you have a ministry and you have someone else who is deeply suffering or disabled who is praying for you, it may help. I have experienced that strength myself when I know people are praying for me, when I may be very tired or want to give up or feel that this is just not worth it. So I think we are linked in that way or can link with those who suffer.

HOW DOES RELIGION INFLUENCE COPING?

Religion provides a positive worldview, a worldview that sees this beautiful universe, created by a Creator with whom we can communicate, talk to, relate to, pray to, and influence. What a wonderful worldview it is where the creator cares for us and, in the Christian worldview, cares enough to have become a human and to have fully experienced the pain and suffering that humans go through. What a beautiful worldview it is, where people with pain can identify with that worldview as opposed to the scientific worldview which sees the world as basically random, that humans are simply organisms that have evolved from lower organisms into some higher form of organisms, and that we are really not very significant at all in this vast universe. There is really no purpose or meaning to the individual life. But in the religious worldview there is purpose and meaning. Every person is important; every person has a calling, whether they recognize it or not. Every person's life is meaningful, so much so that there is a scripture verse that talks about the shepherd leaving the entire flock for the one sheep that wanders off. I do not know if you have seen the movie with George Burns, in which he is God and the devil, entitled, *Oh God! You Devil*. In that movie I was struck by the fact that God and the devil are sitting at a table and there is this one person whom God wants to be able to have, who really is in Satan's clutches. So God bets all of humanity for that one person's life and I think that is what is so significant with the religious worldview—meaning and purpose in life.

PSYCHOLOGICAL INTEGRATION

When bad things happen—when you have a bad diagnosis or you are suffering with pain or you have a traumatic event, lose a loved one, or even you know a disaster might occur to you or you might have a major loss, you need to be able to psychologically integrate that event into your worldview before you can move on. Even religious worldviews that may seem pretty destructive, for example, fundamentalist religious worldviews that emphasize the role of the devil and sin and hell and you might think there is not much positive emotion, when bad things happen, many people in those groups feel that it was caused by their sin and that by confessing their sin they can prevent it from occurring again. And you know it is a worldview that gives them a sense of meaning and purpose, explains the event, and gives them control over the event.

There was a major disaster that occurred in some small islands out on the South Pacific and, at one point, there were psychologists that went and were counseling the people. They became very upset by the local religious community who were attributing the disaster to God's wrath over the attention paid to the pearl industry around the island and the fact that people were spending time on Sundays working in the pearl industry. They said that the people needed to repent and if they did so, things would become better. There was a lot of conflict between the psychologists and the religious people. I do not think the psychologists realized the role that the religious beliefs of that population was playing in psychologically integrating that disastrous event and giving them control over that event.

Again, religion provides a sense of hope that there is always something good that can come out of it, that God can either relieve people's pain or can give them the strength to cope with the pain or can give the pain meaning, so there is that hope. When hope goes, people do not last very long. Hope is a real motivating force for just about everything, including compliance with treatments and people have to be able to see into the future that there is some way out of the situation in which they find themselves. If they cannot see that, they will not last very long. Of course, that is what happens when people commit suicide: hope is gone.

PERSONAL EMPOWERMENT

If we can talk to the creator, it gives us power in a situation that we may otherwise feel powerless. When in sickness or chronic pain where you are dependent upon the doctors or the nurses, you can lie there and just be at the mercy of the treatments, or you can pray and you can influence your situation through that mechanism. The later is empowering. It gives the person a sense of control over the situation even though it is an indirect form of control through God.

ROLE MODELS FOR SUFFERING THAT HELP PEOPLE TO ACCEPT THEIR PAIN

The book of Job is my favorite book in the Bible. It is one of the oldest books and one that really provides a wonderful illustration of somebody coping with pain: losing all of his family and children. Imagine if you lost your children suddenly.

What would happen if you lost your job—your work to which you have devoted your life. It happened to Job. All of his sheep and goats were suddenly all gone. What then would happen if you became depressed and sad over all of that had happened to you and you then had that emotional pain to bear? It happened to Job. What if you then became sick with painful boils over your body? It happened to Job and Job responded like we would all respond: He became angry and asked, "Why me, God?"

As counsellors, we can learn from how Job's friends helped him. At first they were doing very well. They sat with him for seven days and said not a single word. Then, of course, they started to try to fix the problem for Job and tried to explain the problem. That is when things did not work out so well. In fact, Job even had to pray for his counsellors before God would forgive them for that kind of advice that they gave. Those of us in the health care professions are trained to fix things and offer advice, not to listen. But Job was angry and he asked God why and God answered him. I think his answer really helps people with chronic pain. He said, "Job, did you create the fishes in the sea? Did you create the sun and the moon, the whole universe? Do you know the past, eternal past, and do you know the future, eternal future? No you don't. But I do, I know all these things. You see only a very tiny slice of reality. There's a lot more going on here than you are seeing right now. I know this; trust in me; trust in me." And then ultimately Job had a good outcome. He is a wonderful role model.

GUIDANCE FOR DECISION MAKING THAT REDUCES STRESS

People experiencing pain and suffering a lot of times will turn to alcohol or drugs and become addicted. Religion helps them to make better decisions that reduce stress over the long term and provide answers to ultimate questions like, "Why me?" It provides support—both human support and support from the divine. Especially important is the fact that support is not lost with severe illness and disability. The philosophers, the atheistic and agnostic philosophers, did well as long as they were healthy and independent and young. But when they got into their old age and when they became sick with illness and disease, all of that philosophy did not help them much. They became very empty in those days when, as we say in the United States, "the rubber met the road."

How common is religion in coping? What are some consequences of religious coping? And what about religion and coping with pain specifically? There is a little study we did at Duke Hospital, a very simple study. We gave a consecutive series of patients in medicine, neurology, and cardiology, a scale from 0 to 10 and we said: "To what extent do you use religion to help you to cope?" All patients were over the age of 60 and, yes, this was in the Bible belt. However, 40 percent of this random sample indicated 10 on that 0 to 10 scale. Another 50 percent indicated between 5 and 9.9 on that scale so that in the end only about 1 in 10 indicated less than 5 on that 0 to 10 scale. So older adults, at least in Duke Hospital, rely upon their faith to help them to cope.

This happens not just in Duke Hospital. There have been studies in arthritis patients in California, diabetes patients in New York, kidney disease patients in Washington, cancer patients all over the country, heart disease patients, heart transplant patients, lung disease patients, lung transplant patients, and HIV and AIDS patients out of Miami and Los Angeles. There have been studies of individuals with cystic fibrosis (younger people as well as older), sickle cell disease, amyotrophic lateral sclerosis, Lou Gehrig's disease, chronic pain, and adolescents who were severely ill. Well over 80 studies have documented high rates of religious coping in these conditions, largely in the United States.

Remember that little scale from 0 to 10? Well, we divided the scores into low, moderate, high, and very high quartiles and then looked at the percent of the patients with various levels of depression. You can see those in the very high, the highest quartile of religious coping have about half the rate of depression compared to those in the lowest quartile. This is nearly a thousand consecutively admitted patients to the neurology and medicine services at Duke Hospital. We are now looking at depressed medically ill patients. We identify them as depressed. We do a diagnostic evaluation and then we track them over time and we see what happens to their depression; how quickly they go into remission. These are not psychiatric patients but medical patients. We divided what is called intrinsic religiosity, which is another measure of religiousness and tracked those with low, medium, and high. We divide the score in thirds and look at their recovery rates from depression. This is the probability of non-remission. They are all enrolled at time zero with depression and then they recover at varying rates. Those with high religiosity are recovering at every time point faster than those with low religiosity. This is statistically significant and independent of other predictors of depression. So now we have a model to try to understand how religion or spirituality affects mental health in severe illness. Certainly there are genetic and biological factors deriving personality, depression, anxiety. There are developmental factors, whether or not we were loved as children or whether or not our parents were available to us, that sense of development, that sense of our basic needs being met at critical times in our development, all influencing our vulnerability to depression and psychological pain later in life. Then there is religion that influences and provides training and ultimately influences decision making in adulthood. Religion influences the likelihood of experiencing stressful life events based on decision making as well as coping with those stressful life events that occur and cannot be avoided. It then mobilizes these coping behaviors. But religion also influences future goals, prior experiences, and, of course, mobilizes coping resources such as the support of the faith community, all influencing these various outcomes.

RELIGION AND COPING WITH PAIN

There is an older study of 71 patients with advanced cancer from regional cancer centers in Vermont. Ninety-two percent believed in God, 83 percent believed in a personal God, 80 percent believed that prayer was helpful, two-thirds felt close to God and about half indicated the church was very important. All of these religious measures were correlated with greater well-being and lower pain level.

There is a prospective study of 74 patients with persistent low back pain for six months or more. A "prayer or hoping" subscale of this coping strategies questionnaire was the third most commonly used coping strategy out of the six strategies studied. The praying subscale was significantly and positively related to average pain at baseline. This is understandable; people who are in more pain are more likely to pray, because pain is a driving force that causes people to pray. So it was positively correlated cross-sectionally but increased use of prayer or hoping strategies over time was significantly related to decreases in pain intensity over time. It is very important to look at these relationships prospectively, not just cross-sectionally, because pain is driving prayer. This is Kabat-Zinn's work in terms of mindfulness meditation on self-regulation. It is one of the few clinical trials that has looked at the effects of meditation on pain relief. In fact, they were able to show statistically significant reductions in pain, mood disturbances, etc.

There is a study coming out of Duke (Keefe, et al) which looks at rheumatoid arthritis patients. Thirty-five patients with RA were asked to keep a structured daily diary for 30 consecutive days, to assess spiritual experiences, religious and spiritual coping with pain, salience of religion in coping, as well as religious coping efficacy. What they found was that those who reported more frequent daily spiritual experiences had a higher level of positive mood, lower levels of negative mood, and higher levels of social support. No relationship, however, was found with pain levels. So, you know, sometimes it takes awhile for these things to work but in terms of mood and attitude, those who are more religiously involved and having spiritual experiences regularly are certainly coping better.

Here is a little story about a patient out of an article in *JAMA* published July 24, 2002. This was a patient of one of the editors at *JAMA* who also happened to be a professor of medicine at Harvard. This patient impressed the doctor so much that they decided to publish an article on it in *JAMA*. It is probably the longest article on religion and coping with illness that has ever been published in a journal such as *JAMA, New England [Journal of Medicine]* or *Lancet*. The lady was older, had multiple serious medical problems resulting in chronic, progressive, unrelenting pain. She had conditions like diabetes and peripheral neuropathy and painful neuropathy in her extremities caused by the effects of the blood sugar. She had widespread rheumatoid arthritis and osteoarthritis. Her spinal column was developing bone spurs that were digging into her spinal cord, causing loss of feeling and strength in her legs and feet. In fact, she had what is called neuropathic pain—where the pain is coming from changes in the nervous system and is not responsive to narcotic analgesics. So she can take as much Dilaudid or Demerol as she wants but she remains in pain as long as she is conscious. Alternative medical treatments have not been effective. They tried healing touch, massage, acupuncture, and all sorts of alternative strategies; none were effective. She has limited material resources. She lives alone and does not have much support, but despite all of this she is doing well psychologically. She is positive, hopeful, and optimistic. And this is what impressed the medical doctor who is not particularly interested in religion but sees this patient in his office every couple of weeks and cannot do anything for her but sit there with her and just listen. She tells the doctor that she is positive and hopeful. She is functioning completely independently with no assistance and, in fact, he even finds her sometimes being wheeled around in the hospital, praying with patients, and encouraging other patients with conditions like chronic pain. She says that religion is how she does it. Exactly how does she cope with pain? These are her words taken out of the *Journal of the American Medical Association*:

> I don't dwell on the pain. Some people are sick and have pain and it
> gets the best of them—not me. I pray a lot. I believe in God and I
> give my whole heart, body and soul over to him. Sometimes I pray
> and I'm in deep serious prayer and all of a sudden my pain gets easy,
> it slackens up and I drop off to sleep and wake up and I can do things
> for myself. So prayer helps me a lot. I give God my heart and soul,
> you don't have to worry about nothing. He leads you and directs you;
> He takes care of you. I believe in that; that is my belief.

Now let us dissect this just for a moment and see how it works for her. "I don't dwell on the pain." Now when people have pain, one thing it does is rivet their attention to the pain and the more they pay attention to pain, the larger it gets. So she is not dwelling on it; she is able to distract herself by praying. So praying helps to get her mind off the pain and gets her focused upon something greater than just herself. And it is not just the praying—she emphasizes the fact that "I believe in God," and not just a simple assent to believe, but a wholehearted commitment to God. So when she is praying she is not talking to a stranger; she has a relationship with God. God and she have been communicating for some time. She is not just praying to relieve her pain. This is part of an ongoing relationship with the Divine that is going both ways and is involving her wholeheartedly—her whole life is turned over to her God.

She goes on to say, "Now sometimes I pray and I'm in deep serious prayer and all of a sudden my pain gets easy." The relaxation response Herbert Benson talks about, that in deep meditation the body relaxes and people go into this deep state of meditation. That, I think, is exactly what is happening here. She is becoming relaxed and then she can drop off to sleep, her muscles relax, she wakes up and she can do things after getting a little bit of sleep here. "So prayer helps me a lot," she says. But then she goes back to this statement: "I give God my heart and soul." Again, she is back to this wholehearted turning her life over to God. "And you don't have to worry about nothing." So she is not worrying about her pain, she is not worrying about when it is going to come back or whether it is ever going to go away. She feels taken care of and supported.

So that gives you a sense of how this particular patient dealt with the pain. I will summarize: How do you deal with pain? Well, work on your attitude. Develop a spiritual attitude toward pain. Submit, as this woman did, to your understanding of God or a higher power. Submit completely, accept the pain for now. That does not mean you should not do everything possible to relieve the pain, but with whatever pain that is left after you have done everything possible to relieve it, there is a certain amount of acceptance that needs to be done. Realize that—and this is very, very important—realize that joy, fulfillment, and meaning are still possible whether you are in pain or not. They are not irrevocably linked with your pain. If you are having pain you can experience those emotions. You can because of a spiritual attitude. Recognize your pain as a special calling, a special calling for you to reach out to others in pain and help those people because you know what they are going through. Get involved in a faith community. That faith community needs you if you have chronic pain. They need you. You are not necessarily going there just to be supported by them; they need you among them so that they have an opportunity to minister to the suffering among them. Seek inspiration, look for role models in Scripture, pray for relief. I pray for relief. When I am sleeping at night and my hip and back are bothering me, I pray that God will take that pain. And you know, sometimes God does—that pain goes away and it is wonderful. Pray also for God's will to be done because God may be using the pain in your life. Pray for the ability to cope with the pain, even if it does not go away. Finally, pray for others and help them with their pain.

Suffering—an Existential Challenge: Understanding, Dealing, and Coping with Suffering from an Existential-Analytic Perspective

ALFRIED LÄNGLE

Abstract

The paper begins with a description of an existential-anthropological classification of different types of suffering. These classifications are then deepened through an elaboration of the essence of suffering. The structure of existence derived from the *existential analytic model* is used to elucidate this essential understanding of suffering. The existential analytic model is used to describe both the content of suffering and the impaired structures of existence. From this perspective, a model of coping with, and treatment of, suffering is developed. The paper closes with some logotherapeutic remarks on possible meanings of suffering.

People suffer in numerous ways. They either suffer silently, or express their pain through complaining, crying, hoping, self-sacrifice, or rebellious behavior. People suffer for countless reasons. Suffering is manifold in both form and content. It may be helpful, therefore, to provide an overview of suffering and to categorize the reasons for suffering. We will then look at suffering from an existential point of view and suggest specific activities we feel are necessary in order to cope with suffering.

FORMS OF SUFFERING—AN EXISTENTIAL-ANTHROPOLOGICAL CLASSIFICATION

The various domains in which we may suffer can be structured according to the three anthropological dimensions that Frankl (e.g., 1967, pp. 136ff.) has described. We can complement Frankl's three "classical" dimensions (somatic, psychological, and spiritual/personal) with a fourth "dynamic" one. This dimension

223

emerges when we consider the dialogical reality of the person with the world, what we call the "existential dimension" (Längle, 1999):

- Physical suffering is pain: injuries, illnesses, functional disorders, such as problems with sleep or migraines. Just think of how much suffering can be caused by a simple toothache!

- Psychological suffering is experienced by the loss of something valuable or dear: feelings, such as anxiety, heaviness and strain, the absence of emotion, emptiness, and psychological pain or injury.

- Suffering has an underlying pattern: an experience of self-alienation, of not being oneself. This particular form or type of suffering is attributed to a loss of something that is essential for a person to experience a fulfilled existence. Feelings attributed to these experiences include: insecurity, breach of trust, despair, absence of relationship, injustice, remorse, or guilt.

- Existential suffering evokes feelings of futility, meaninglessness. This form of suffering emerges from a lack of orientation with a larger context, in which we can understand our life and our activities, our success or senseless fate.

All possible forms of suffering from our perspective can be attributed to one of these four categories, or a combination of any of them.

The quality or degree to which a person suffers depends on personality factors and maturity. Let us look at these qualitative differences in the following two examples:

Example 1

I recently met a young active man of 34 years who was at the beginning of a successful career in his firm. We met at a moment in his life when he was not well. He was anxiously awaiting a diagnosis for the cause of his walking difficulties: Was it a simple infection or was it indeed this incurable disease leading gradually to paralysis—multiple sclerosis (MS)? It soon turned out that it was indeed MS. He was so shocked by this diagnosis that he could not work for the next two months. This neurological disease and his difficulty in walking were very real, but this young man suffered most of all from the blow of fate, which he experienced as annihilating. The man experienced persistent and painful questions: "How do I continue? What is to become of my situation, what am I to expect?"

What would become of this man and his life? This diagnosis surely meant an earlier death, years in a wheelchair, dwindling capacities, and increasing dependence. Would he be able to withstand that? Could he accept this fate? What was there left to do in a life marked by illness? What would one live for? Was this a life worth living?

The man's immediate and personal experience with this diagnosis leads to his questioning the perception of his disease by others: How would he respond to other people's questions? Would he be able to accept their pity and superficial comments that were meant to console him? Would he want to meet them at all in his changed state? This man was not looking for the essence of his disease. Life had not become hopeless for him, for he knew that he could live out of his personal depth. But he did not feel strong enough to accept this disease and how his life had changed at this particular point. What does it take to live with such a disease? He had never thought about this question, not even hypothetically. The very real implications of this question had now come to him with a vengeance: he could not even walk anymore! He did not feel strong enough at present to meet other people. He had to come to terms with his reactions, feelings, and changed relationships. He had to recover from this shock and to clarify his position in the world for himself—before that, nothing else was possible. He was personally devastated and overcome by his suffering. He experienced trembling, crying, and insecurity. He retreated and did not want to be asked about his disease and his state of being. He was afraid of losing face, crying, and being submerged by the pain of this incomprehensible fate.

Example 2

A few weeks ago I visited with a 70-year-old patient. He had been hospitalized for the 15th time within the past year. Metastases were in his liver, lungs, bones, and back. Because of insufferable pain, one metastasis had now been surgically removed from his sacral canal.

This patient was asleep when I arrived. He had not closed his eyes all night long because of the pain that persisted in spite of the operation. Some time after he awoke I asked how he felt about his life. This man had always been an avid tennis player and was now obliged to stay in bed. His answer was sober and in keeping with his whole attitude towards life. He stated:

> I cannot change it. This is how it is. Of course, I would love to play tennis, and it is not easy to give that up. But I have always been a realist, and now I see this realistically as well. I will never be able to play again.

I was curious about the clear answer he gave me. Is he covering up and hiding his suffering? I therefore asked him more directly whether not being able to play again was not in fact terribly sad and how he could cope with that? My patient replied, "Well, this is the way it is. I am trying to cope the best I can. But this is the way it is now." How much pain had this man already suffered and how much more was in store for him? I did not know, but now I understood his words. I could feel that his strength as a person and his capacity to endure were rooted in this strict matter-of-fact attitude he had adopted throughout his life.

If we look at the fate of these two people we may ask ourselves: Who is suffering more? Knowing of course that it is difficult to compare the subjective expressions and experiences of suffering, we may nonetheless ask ourselves: Who seems to be suffering more? The man who is near death and in terrible pain or the younger patient, with Multiple Sclerosis, who does not have any physical pain and has many years ahead of him? For the young man, it seems his fate is much harder to carry. From such observations, which you may have occasionally made yourself, we would ask the following question: What is suffering?

THE ESSENCE OF SUFFERING

It might seem almost childlike to ask: Why do we actually suffer? But let us expand on this question. What is it that constitutes suffering? What do we suffer from in suffering? Do we suffer because we do not comprehend a particular sensation? Is it a conscious or an unconscious feeling of meaninglessness that turns an experience into one of suffering? Or is suffering merely the sensation of something negative, disagreeable, troubling, or painful that has either a physical or psychological origin? Indeed, as a preliminary observation we can say that suffering is felt when we undergo an emotional experience of this sort. Suffering is not necessarily an encompassing experience of meaninglessness. One thing can be said with certainty: Suffering is linked to emotions. Even mental suffering goes along with unpleasant feelings. A preliminary explanation of suffering would be the "sensation of disagreeable feelings" that arise in connection with the above-mentioned categories of physical pain, troubling loss of something dear, painful self-alienation, or meaninglessness.

But does this preliminary description stand up to closer examination? Is the disagreeable feeling really the decisive criterion of suffering, the effective agent that turns a specific experience into suffering instead of joy or delight? Disagreeable feelings are not always equal in their meaning and effect on our lives since they are subjectively understood and integrated in a variety of ways. An effort, a trouble, or an exertion may cost a lot of energy or cause unpleasant feelings, but if we know that these feelings serve a purpose or have meaning, then what constitutes suffering is blurred. Even if writing an article means painful renunciation of more pleasant activities and many hours of work at night, this activity will not necessarily be conceived of as suffering. This is precluded by the simple fact that the activity was undertaken voluntarily (cf. Frankl's concept of the "will to meaning", 1967, pp. 5-13; 1976). In general, we might suggest that the sting of suffering is broken if the unpleasant situation is freely chosen. This is akin to one of Camus' statements when he calls Sisyphus a *happy* man. Sisyphus must roll a stone to the top of a mountain with enormous effort only to see that his effort is always in vain because the stone will not stay at the top. Camus (1955) makes Sisyphus proudly defy the punishment the gods intend for him by doing his work *voluntarily*. Thus the work acquires meaning by resisting absurdity and meaninglessness. Are the pains of labour, for example, soon forgotten in the wake of joyous feelings for a newborn child?

The feelings of the two patients described above are extremely strong but there is an enormous difference in the degree of their suffering. Whereas one patient is full of anxiety and on the brink of despair, the other copes with his suffering with what seems to be a sense of calm and equanimity.

A closer examination reveals that suffering is not completely identical to experiencing painful feelings. Suffering can be seen as a *spiritual perception of a content* based on the specific feelings of pain. These feelings cause suffering only when they are perceived as destructive. We can therefore define suffering from an existential point of view as "the felt destruction of something dear and/or vital." Or stated briefly, suffering is a feeling of loss or impairment to one's existence. This is the central understanding of suffering from an existential-analytical point of view. The perception and feeling of destruction is commonly experienced with suffering. What is decisive for the experience of suffering is the subjective feeling of destruction of something vitally important, the sensation of something being torn apart or annihilated, a sensation that one's existential foundations are being split. What is decisive are the subsequent emotions elicited by this perception.

THE ENDANGERED ELEMENTS OF LIFE

What is destroyed in the experience of suffering? What is this destruction related to? What are the elements that we may regard as life preserving or life supporting? Existential analysis has developed a comprehensive theory of *existential fundamental motivations* to address these questions (cf. Längle, 1992, 2003). From an existential-analytic perspective, an experience is experienced as suffering if it threatens *fundamental structures of existence*. These fundamental structures relate to the four fundamental realities of human existence: (a) the world and its conditions, (b) one's life and its force, (c) one's identity and relationship to others, and (d) the demands of the situation and the horizon of our lives.

What effect does the impairment of these foundations have when they are subjectively felt and lead to the experience of suffering? The impairment of the first fundamental condition leads to the feeling of not being able to be here at all, and to a feeling of being unable to overcome new conditions. This feeling undermines any integrating activity. The ability to integrate new conditions leads to an acceptance of the present reality. Without this ability, increased insecurity and anxiety are the results. Suffering in this dimension consists of an inability to accept what is here.

An impairment of the second fundamental condition engenders subjective feelings of dislike, a preference for not relating anymore, of not wishing to act, not wanting or being able to enjoy, not being moved or internally turned in the direction of experiencing or acting, and not experiencing anything as worthwhile. This hinders the integrating activity of turning to whatever is dear or precious in one's life. This leads to a loss of vitality and will increase feelings of being troubled, torn, guilty, worried, or sorrowful, all of which may eventually lead to depression. Suffering in this dimension means a loss of vitality, of enjoyment, a loss of something dear, and the feeling of not being able to live under these conditions.

The subjectively felt impairment of the third fundamental condition is tied to the feeling of not knowing oneself anymore, to the feelings of self-alienation and, as a consequence, of not being able to engage with others or encounter others. The ability to integrate both one's own inner dialogue and a dialogue with others is blocked. This leads to an inner emptiness, to self-alienation, with its specific absence of emotion. A person may feel inconsolable, accompanied by a loss of self that can further escalate into histrionic and personality disorders. A loss of self in this dimension involves a feeling that one lacks authenticity, self-esteem, and appreciation or produces feelings of alienation and loneliness.

If the fourth fundamental condition for a fulfilling existence is impaired, a person is unable to respond to the world, to be engaged, to participate in a larger context. The future is not worth envisioning; there is no possible meaning that could provide an orientation to a person's life and render it worth living. The predominant feeling is one of futility, that nothing positive will come in the future and that one's achievements are in fact worthless. These feelings block any possibility of integration and identification with the actual situation (commitment). The result is a pervasive feeling of emptiness and meaninglessness, an experience of "existential vacuum" (Frankl, 1963, pp. 167–171; 1973, pp. 51ff.) and, finally, despair. There can be tendencies toward suicide or actual suicide attempts. Suffering in this dimension consists of a feeling of loss as far as a future or a larger context is concerned, a context that might otherwise provide orientation and point to a positive development.

The question of meaning arises when one's orientation towards the future is in doubt. Although a worthwhile and meaningful future is much harder to discern when one experiences suffering, it is not completely impossible. Meaning can still be found. Meaning, for example, can be derived when a person is physically suffering or endures a night full of pain, as in the case of the 70-year-old patient. Meaning can be found in the hope and faith for a reunion with one's daughter before dying or in a final reunion with a loved one as in the case of the man who lost his daughter in a car accident (see below). In this case, spiritual or religious faith is of particular value because it may provide meaning beyond all situational demands. Faith may open horizons in the most difficult situations of life and allow for a deeper understanding of what is happening. On the other hand, and this must be considered, faith may be misplaced and used to camouflage the situation, to neglect the truth, to avoid the disagreeable facts, or to avoid suffering altogether. To avoid the process of authentic suffering, when it occurs, is in fact a loss. To suffer authentically is necessary. It helps to integrate and overcome psychological and spiritual loss.

These fundamental dimensions form four layers, each an integration of the other. At the same time, each layer has its own distinct element, but requires the integration of each preceding dimension. For example, "to be oneself" in the third dimension is not contained in the first and second dimensions. For its full realization, however, it is necessary to comfortably be in the world (first layer) and to have a satisfying emotional life (second layer). This includes a good relation with oneself, with one's own feelings, and with others. Therefore, in each case of suffering where there is a corresponding problem with meaning, we must ask whether the feelings of meaninglessness are due to a blockage in: (a) not being able to (loss of capacities), (b) not wanting to, a dislike (loss of vitality and inner strength), or (c) a lack of connection, relation, and dialogue with one's self.

If a person cannot endure her suffering because she does not have enough strength, she will be unable to recognize any meaning in a situation since she is unable to envisage any future for herself. The inability to recognize or discover meaning may be the case even when a person has faith and hope or imbues a situation with religious meaning. The problem of meaninglessness in suffering must be diagnosed more precisely. Meaninglessness is connected foremost with a blockage in one of the preceding fundamental conditions for a fulfilled existence. Therapy must focus on this blockage, otherwise the problem of meaninglessness may obscure the underlying problem. An example of this kind of blockage will be illustrated in the next case study.

ANALYSIS OF A FEELING OF MEANINGLESSNESS

A mother and father lose their daughter in a car accident on an icy road on the day of her 21st birthday. They have a son who is two years younger. The daughter worked in the family's firm. Her father had hoped, if not considered, his daughter to be the future of this firm. She was gentle and always ready to help, courteous, adroit, and popular with everyone. The parents were looking forward to having her close by and had prepared for this. They had anticipated a family with grandchildren who would be living in the neighborhood. This terrible loss had annihilated the parents' hopes and devastated their lives. While the mother slowly overcame her paralysing sorrow after nine months, the father remained in a state of passive resignation. For the father, all meaning was lost. Why should he go on working or living since there was no future worth striving for? His faith, his family, his wife, his relatively young age (he had just entered his fifties), his work, the clients, his favourite pastimes, and his inner life meant little to him. The loss of his daughter simply hurt too much.

In conditions such as these, where we see a person with a rich life who is nonetheless both disinterested and disengaged, it points to one of the first three fundamental conditions not being fulfilled. In this case, the father could not accept the loss of this dear and central value in his life. Without that personal acceptance, he could not get over the loss. As a consequence, the father had become depressed and did not allow for the grieving process. Although his level of activity was still sufficient to enable him to continue working, his defensive attitude made him unwilling to take medication or seek help in order to work through his loss. He held onto his depression because he felt that this was his only means to keep in touch with his daughter. His depression allowed him to maintain an illusory hope of not having to let go of his daughter completely. In this case, all the other fundamental conditions had been impaired as well.

The man experienced a feeling of not being able to bear these conditions. This had led to a fear of being annihilated and, as a consequence, an attitude of massive defense. His relationship to life was disturbed and this was the central subject of his suffering: the loss of this love and the incalculable value of the relationship. The father's subsequent loss of vitality had led to depression. As the third fundamental condition became impaired, a piece of his identity had come apart: Who was he now, having lost his daughter? Was he still the same person after the loss of this dear treasure with whom he had identified? With a blockage as severe as this, it is not surprising that he could not envisage a future any more and perceived everything as meaningless. With the loss of his child, his connection to the future had been cut off.

Holding onto the question of meaning provided this father with a certain degree of protection. It protected him against having to accept the situation and it provided him with a reason to hold onto his despair. His logic concluded that it was reasonable not to accept something that would render one's own life senseless. At the same time, however—and this seems particularly important to me—by refusing to accept a situation we make it possible to keep the destructive event at a distance, to push it away, in fact. Attention that is focused solely on the meaninglessness of one's suffering and the meaninglessness of one's future is a consequence of being unable to come to terms with the reality of the situation. If a person focuses on the meaninglessness of life generally, a person extricates himself or herself from fault or responsibility if life does not go on. This is akin to heaping a sulky reproach upon life: If life is an insoluble dilemma then it is impossible to engage oneself in life. The conditions of life are considered too difficult and therefore unacceptable.

Rather than dealing with the suffering and trying to come to terms with it, a passive attitude is being reinforced and one waits for an answer to the *ontological meaning* of the suffering. The question would be: What is the meaning of this suffering, what good can come of this suffering? Such questions, in fact, cannot be answered. The question itself belongs to the realm of faith or philosophy and not to the realm of pure reason. Individuals who hold on to the question of ontological meaning may in fact reinforce a defensive attitude and create a distance to the problem because they are not striving or finding the ability to accept what has happened.

THE LOST EXISTENTIAL ABILITIES IN SUFFERING—THE STRUCTURE OF SUFFERING

In the above example, I elaborated on how the existential-analytic model describes what we suffer from when we suffer. We can link the characteristics of suffering and its elements with distinct approaches necessary for gradually coping with suffering. For each of the fundamental structures of existence there is a specific activity that is blocked by the suffering:

- The suffering may have its root in the fact that one's being in the world is threatened. The consequence of this is an inability to accept the facts. Such suffering can be accompanied by fear. Emphasis must be placed on re-establishing the ability to cope under the new conditions that a person is facing, such as with paralysis or cancer.
- Suffering may have its root in the fact that one's enjoyment of life, or vitality, is impaired. The consequence of this impairment is a lack of motivation to turn to what makes life dear and precious, an unwillingness to feel emotions because they are too painful. This unwillingness easily gives rise to depression. Coping involves a re-establishment of life under the new conditions, such as after the death of a loved one.
- Furthermore, suffering may be caused by a loss of self-esteem or shame. The consequence is an unwillingness to be seen, a tendency to hide and to feel that one is unable to be the person he or she is. Suffering at this

level produces hysterical developments. Coping strategies aim to recapture an authentic sense of being, to restructure and/or to build up one's personality, e.g., after experiencing rape, shame or guilt.

- Finally, suffering can be caused by a loss of context that would give meaning to one's actions and one's life. Generally, development or change is seen as worthless because it is perceived as leading nowhere. The consequence is a renunciation of adjustment to the actual situation, a renunciation of adjustment to what is waiting, or a renunciation of what is calling for a commitment. Suicide and addiction can easily result. Coping strategies are linked to re-establishing a relationship with the future and to bringing about a focus or orientation that is directed towards a larger, more encompassing and even metaphysical sphere.

HOW CAN WE SUFFER?—A STEP-BY-STEP MODEL OF COPING

Coping with suffering is a process. The existential-analytic model provides practical steps that can be applied to this process. These steps deal with all different forms of suffering, which is often composed of several dimensions.

If the inability to be under the changed conditions is the cause of suffering, the structures of one's existence should be worked on in order to re-establish an ability to be. It is helpful to begin by focusing on the ability to endure and to accept suffering in order to integrate it into one's life. A fulfilled existence is constructed on the basis of engagement with reality. Feeling "courage to be" and being able to confront reality is fundamental for existence.

Enduring pain, hurt, and problems is the most basic human ability. To endure suffering is important even if the cause of suffering, fortunately, may often be altered or even eliminated. When suffering imposes itself, it has to be taken into account. The present moment of suffering has to be accepted. In order to do so, we have to ask ourselves whether we have the strength and sufficient support to bear it. To bear one's suffering means accepting it as part of one's existence. To bear the moment means withstanding the emotion through its duration, "en-during" it. This demands considerable psychological energy and the willingness to face this disagreeable emotion. One has to be sure that one can survive this suffering, that there is enough space and support to endure the suffering. Only then can suffering be accepted as a given of human existence, a given that can be endured. We can ask ourselves practical questions such as:

- Am I able to stand this problem at all? How long? A day? An hour? Indefinitely?

- Am I willing to try? Or does everything in me cry out against that?

- Does this suffering leave me with the space to be?

If the suffering is caused by impairment in one's joy of life, the approach is to restore motivation and a *relation to life* through various small steps and personal decision making. This requires turning toward the source of suffering, toward whatever has been lost. By entering into a relationship with it, by approaching it honestly and by giving oneself time or space, grieving can arise naturally. Through grieving we are touched by life itself. By turning toward our loss, we feel our pain intensely. This moves us inwardly, makes us cry and invites us to draw empathically towards ourselves. In order to do this we need relationship and closeness. These are contingent upon our experiences of relationship and closeness in the past and/or through the attention and closeness of other people during the painful situation. We can ask ourselves concrete questions such as:

- Which feelings are caused by this suffering? Does it hurt very much?
- Can I sustain these feelings? Do I want to deal with them? Can I allow these feelings, can I live with them, because they belong to me? Can I endure the link these feelings have with the loss I have gone through?
- Can I recognize and appreciate how these feelings bring me in touch with myself and strengthen my relation to myself?

If the suffering is due to a loss of identity and of being oneself and self-alienation, the focus must be on what we regard as right and suitable for ourselves, on what is authentic and ethically responsible. This theme is the foundation of personhood, which has been impaired either through events or our own behavior. This foundation of personhood requires encounter with other persons. Through encounter, a person finds himself or herself. Through encounter a person sees, feels, and grasps his/her essence. This leads to processes of repentance, of pardon, and of reconciliation. Through repentance a person encounters himself or herself. There is a reconnection with one's true essence through an analysis, often with pain and shame, of what one has done wrong and what has led to the losing of oneself. In the process of mourning, the presence and sympathy of others are helpful. In these cases, respectful face-to-face encounter and the establishment of appropriate distance are asked for. Practical questions can be asked, such as:

- What is my opinion about what has happened to me or about what I have done?
- Can I stand by this opinion, can I stand up to my behavior, to my decisions? Do I respect myself or do I feel shame?
- Am I really myself, am I authentic? Can I appreciate myself?

If suffering is caused by the loss of an orientation towards the future, an orientation that has context and meaning into which one can integrate one's actions and life in a constructive way, then the focus must be on an openness to the demands and opportunities of the given situation, and the larger contexts in which the client finds himself or herself. This requires adjustment, harmonization, and a dialogical way of dealing with the circumstances. By adjusting to the circumstances on the basis of one's ability, motivation, and inner consent, it will be possible for a person to become committed to the situation.

The act of committing or responding to the situation itself enables a person to find an activity that opens the door to creative and meaningful possibilities and actions. These in turn open the door to the future. To realistically see, to take in, to assess, and to adjust to the demands of the situation leads to existential meaning. The ability to see, to feel, or to believe in a wider context provides a window to the ontological meaning (Längle, 1994a) and in turn, the threshold of faith.

From this perspective, the question of meaning is placed in a dialogical relation with the ability to accept, to relate, and to be oneself. If these "personal conditions" are in place, a person will be more open to the meaning of the situation and better able to respond, to cope, and to act. If the situation can be seen, felt, or understood within a larger context and a possible meaning for the suffering emerges, a person will be better able to accept the suffering and to face it without losing a sense of self.

ABOUT THE MEANING OF SUFFERING

Frankl (1963) pointed out that suffering cannot be directly experienced as meaning. If we understand meaning as something worthwhile and precious, then suffering clearly runs contrary to this definition of meaning. To suffer suggests an experience or experiences of loss, destruction, and/or pain. Suffering is therefore experienced as meaningless (this does not exclude that suffering may be considered ontologically necessary or meaningful in the larger context of faith or a particular ideology).

By activating the potential of the inner person, Frankl described a "turn" in the experience of suffering. Even if suffering itself is meaningless, there may be a possible meaning in the way we suffer. The meaning of suffering can therefore lie in the way we deal with it. But it can also be found in the attempt to integrate it into a larger context. A wider perspective may even imbue the suffering with some value. How can suffering be understood (and thereby integrated) in a greater context? Logotherapy (Frankl, 1963; 1967, pp. 15-16; 1973, pp. 105-116) is a psychological approach that offers valuable guidance on how to integrate and cope with suffering and how to discover existential meaning in suffering. The emergence of the "existential turn" enables us to be open to the possible meaning of suffering in two ways in which the person still maintains his or her freedom: in *how* we suffer; and *for whom* we suffer (cf. Längle, 1987; 1994c).

The first existential approach to suffering concerns how we suffer and the myriad of possible expressions. We might deal with suffering openly and publicly or silently, in an introverted manner, by seeking others out, through sacrifice, or by condemning what we are suffering from. The second existential approach to suffering concerns our relationships: Do we relate to others in our suffering and therefore behave in a certain way so as to spare them further strain or burden, for example? Can we relate to ourselves? Can we, for example, look into our eyes and relate to how we deal with suffering? Or do we relate to God for whom we are prepared to shoulder the suffering? Frankl called these two forms of coping with suffering a "main avenue to meaning." Both relate to a highly personal category of *attitudinal values* (Frankl, 1973, pp. 44) because the value or meaning of suffering lies in the attitude an individual adopts or expresses towards the suffering. Attitudinal values are, in the final analysis, an expression of a person's deepest relationship with life. They describe how a person sees life fundamentally and whether life is conceptualised positively or negatively (cf. Längle, 1994c, p. 504).

Beyond the existential approach in both coping and integration, there is a different category of meaning to suffering. There is a metaphysical meaning, a meaning which does not depend on an individual and his or her attitude. We call it "ontological meaning" (Längle, 1994a). It derives from the totality of all that exists and represents the meaning that underlies all beings. Such meaning surpasses human knowledge and understanding. Ontological meaning is a matter of faith and faith can provide us with hope and the prospect of salvation.

In one of his early works, Frankl (1975/1946, pp. 310-333) wrote that suffering has a specific effect on the person undergoing it. If a person succeeds in enduring it and does not despair, he or she may even grow. A person may progress or develop in the spiritual dimension and possibly gain new abilities, for example. Furthermore, it is possible to grow in maturity. A person's mental and spiritual faculties can unfold, be enlarged, and be reinforced. Finally, Frankl suggested that human beings are capable of surpassing themselves (i.e., transcending themselves). Human beings have the potential for actions and attitudes they would not have believed themselves capable of before. It is precisely the feelings of distress experienced in suffering that motivate people to greater human achievements.

Frankl was forced to bear witness to indescribable suffering during his two and a half years in concentration camps. At the end of *Man's Search for Meaning* (1963), Frankl summarized his experience of suffering with the following statement, "The crowning experience of all, for the homecoming man, is the wonderful feeling that, after all he has suffered, there is nothing he needs fear any more—except his God" (p. 148). I want to conclude with another quote of Frankl's (1959) from one of his early works: "Suffering makes man clear-sighted and the world transparent" (p. 709). Suffering may open our eyes to a depth and scope that surpasses everyday life. Suffering may put the events of the world into perspective thereby reducing their felt and perceived significance to a degree that makes the physical transparent for the metaphysical.

References

Camus, A. (1955). *The myth of Sisyphus.* New York: Vintage Books

Frankl, V. E. (1957). *Grundriß der Existenzanalyse und Logotherapie. (pp. 663-736).* In V. E. Frankl, V. v Gebsattel, & J. H. Schultz, (Eds.), *Handttbuch der Neurosenlehre und Psychotherapie.* Munich, Germany: Urban & Schwarzenberg.

Frankl, V. E. (1963). *Man's search for meaning.* New York: Simon & Schuster.

Frankl, V. E. (1967). *Psychotherapy and existentialism: Selected papers on Logotherapy.* New York: Simon & Schuster.

Frankl. V. E. (1975/1946). *Anthropologische Grundlagen der Psychotherapie.* Bern, Germany: Huber.

Frankl, V. E. (1976). *The will to meaning: Foundations and applications of Logotherapy.* New York: New American Library.

Längle, A. (1987). *Sinnvoll leben.* St. Pölten, Austria: Niederöster Pressehaus.

Längle, A. (1992/1999). Die existentielle Motivation der Person. *Existenzanalyse, 16, 3,* 18-29.

Längle, A. (1994a). Sinn-Glaube oder Sinn-Gespür? Zur Differenzierung von ontologischem und existentiellem Sinn in der Logotherapie. *Bulletin GLE 11, 2,* 15-20.

Längle, A. (1994b). Lebenskultur-Kulturerleben. Die Kunst, Bewegendem zu begegnen. *Bulletin der GLE 11, 1,* 3-8.

Längle, A. (1994c). Zur Bewältigung von Angst und Schmerz bei schwerer Krankheit. *Der Praktische Arzt, 48, 708,* 498-505

Längle, A. (1999) Existenzanalyse – Die Zustimmung zum Leben finden. *Fundamenta Psychiatrica 12,* 139-146.

Längle, A. (1992/1999b). Die existentielle Motivation der Person. *Existenzanalyse 16, 3,* 18-29.

Längle, A. (2001). *Lehrbuch der Existenzanalyse – Bd. 1: Grundlagen und Einführung.* Vienna, Austria: GLE-Verlag.

Längle, A. (2002a). *Wenn der Sinn zur Frage wird.* Vienna, Austria: Picus.

Längle, A. (2002b). Die Grundmotivationen menschlicher Existenz als Wirkstruktur existenzanalytischer Psychotherapie. *Fundamenta Psychiatrica 16, 1,* 1-8.

Längle, A. (2003). The art of involving the person: Fundamental existential motivations as the structure of the motivational process. *European Psychotherapy 4, 1,* 25-36.

Editors' Note

Translation by Godela von Kirchbach, Geneva. English assistance by Britt-Mari Sykes, University of Ottawa.

The Positive Psychology of Suffering and Tragic Optimism

PAUL T. P. WONG

Abstract

The paper proposes the need for a positive psychology of suffering with an emphasis on meaning, spirituality, and tragic optimism. Viktor Frankl's (1985) tragic optimism (TO) posits that one can remain optimistic in spite of tragic experiences. Extending Frankl's construct, Wong's (2001) existential-humanistic model of TO postulates that the only kind of hope that can stand the harsh blows of reality needs to contain five key ingredients: (a) acceptance of what cannot be changed, (b) affirmation of the value and meaning of life, (c) self-transcendence, (d) faith in God and others, and (e) courage to face adversity. The chapter also briefly describes the Life Attitudes Scale (LAS) as a valid and reliable measure of TO. Finally, it identifies the characteristics of a mature positive psychology with TO as a prototype.

In the depth of winter, I finally learned that there was within me an invincible summer.
Albert Camus

The only genuine hope is hope in what does not depend on ourselves, hope springing from humility and not from pride.

Gabriel Marcel

Deep unspeakable suffering may well be called a baptism, a regeneration, the initiation into a new state.

George Elliot

The mind is its own place and in itself, can make heaven of Hell and hell of Heav'n.
John Milton

Show me a hero and I'll write you a tragedy.

F. Scott Fitzgerald

The five quotes above express very well the essence of what I am trying to say: Enduring hope can only rise from the ashes of death and despair, and authentic joy is often born in the crucible of suffering. These ideas may sound foreign to those who live a pampered, privileged life, but resonate with those who have survived devastating tragedies.

In the past few years, whenever I told people that my primary research interest was in the positive psychology of suffering, invariably I got a puzzled, incredulous response. Some reacted strongly: "How can suffering be positive?" Many well-intentioned positive psychologists have repeatedly tried to set me straight by telling me that suffering and negative emotions are beyond the parameters of positive psychology, which is a "science of positive subjective experiences, positive traits, and positive institutions" (Seligman & Csikszentmihalyi, 2000, p. 5).

Resistance towards negative emotions and experiences come from both a narrow interpretation of the above tenets of American positive psychology and a culture obsessed with personal happiness and success. In a society of consumerism and narcissism, happiness has become an end in itself and suffering is regarded as Public Enemy No. 1. In sum, the good life is equated with a happy life.

Schumaker (2007) has provided a provocative critique of the current happiness craze and proposed a deeper interpretation of happiness. Citing James Poniewoziks' *Time* magazine article "The Art of Unhappiness," Schumaker commented we need to be directed towards "the sobering truth that loss, pain, sacrifice, and disappoint-ment are the grounds from which happiness grows" (p. 130). This paper argues for a broader perspective of positive psychology that incorporates such negative realities of life, a view that has also been advocated by Christopher Peterson (2004).

NEED TO BROADEN POSITIVE PSYCHOLOGY

The tragic event of 9/11 has posed a serious challenge to American positive psychology. Many of the survivors are struggling with grief and pain. Posttraumatic stress disorder (PTSD), depression, and anxiety have been on the increase. We have entered a new era of vulnerability and fear. Americans have begun to develop a tragic sense of life, which is all too familiar to people living in two-thirds of the world.

What do we say to those whose lives have been devastated, and to those who have struggled with their gaping wounds? What do we say to those living in Iraq where terror and death are everywhere? What do we say to the thousands who die of AIDS and poverty each day in Africa? The gospel of happiness and success sounds hollow to those who are struggling daily to survive in a living hell; they can neither control nor understand the negative forces that are destroying their lives.

Indeed, life is full of suffering, as Buddhism has proclaimed. Human beings are indeed suffering beings, as Frankl (1986) has repeatedly claimed. Human history is drenched in blood and tears. All the progress in science and technology has not reduced global suffering; the weapons have become more lethal, the problem of global warming has worsened, and the gap between the haves and the have-nots has widened. The state of the world is not good. What is happening around us makes us sad and angry, unless we choose to ignore the bleak realities.

The acid test of any model of positive psychology is how it fares in boundary situations of suffering. Positive psychology needs to work for the good times and bad times, and for both the privileged class and the underclass. The tragic optimism (TO) of Viktor Frankl provides a promising direction towards such a mature positive psychology.

A CASE FOR TRAGIC OPTIMISM

It took the horror of Nazi death camps for Viktor Frankl (1985) to discover the power of TO. He defined TO as "an optimism in the face of tragedy" (p. 162). His chapter, entitled "A case for tragic optimism"

> addresses present day concerns and how it is possible to "say yes to life" in spite of all the tragic aspects of human existence. To hark back to its title, it is hoped that "optimism" for our future may flow from the lesson learned from our "tragic" past. (p. 17)

He demonstrated this overlooked but important dimension of hope in Nazi concentration camps: All the horrors of atrocities, all the dehumanizing deprivation and degradation, and all the pains inflicted on him by his tormentors, could not strip him of his human dignity and his abiding hope in the meaning and value of life. His own defiant spirit and courage in the most hopeless, helpless situation bore witness to the power of TO.

After surviving the Holocaust, Frankl (1985) eloquently discussed the critical nature of attitude toward suffering. He was not willing to engage in what he called false illusions or artificial optimism. An optimistic attitude was literally a posture, a stance to be embraced in the face of terror. He has taught us that whatever the sufferings we may endure and however oppressive and grim the situation may be, we can always choose the stance we take towards our suffering:

> Man can preserve a vestige of spiritual freedom, of independence of mind, even in such terrible conditions of psychic and physical stress. We who lived in concentration camps can remember the men who walked through the huts comforting others, giving away their last piece of bread. They may have been few in number, but they offer

> sufficient proof that everything can be taken from a man but one thing: the last of the human freedoms—to choose one's attitude in any given set of circumstances, to choose one's own way. (Frankl, 1985, p. 86)

> He may retain his human dignity even in a concentration camp. Dostoevsky said once, "There is one thing that I dread: not to be worthy of my sufferings." These words frequently came to my mind after I became acquainted with those martyrs whose behavior in camp, whose suffering and death, bore witness to the fact that the last inner freedom cannot be lost. It can be said that they were worthy of their sufferings; the way they bore their suffering was a genuine inner achievement. It is this spiritual freedom—which cannot be taken away—that makes life meaningful and purposeful. (Frankl, 1985, p. 87)

To realize that one is trapped in an underground mine or locked up in a torture chamber naturally makes one feel pessimistic and depressed. But enters TO, and the equation changes: There is always hope in hopeless situations. People can be both realistically pessimistic and idealistically optimistic at the same time (Wong, 2001a). They can feel the pain and experience the terror, but at the same time they can still celebrate the fact of being alive and cling to the belief that as long as there is life, there is hope. Unlike other kinds of hope, TO cannot be crushed by adversities or catastrophes, because like true gold, it is purified in the crucible of suffering and rooted in an abiding inner value. Frankl (1985) aptly added: "The consciousness of one's inner value is anchored in higher, more spiritual things, and cannot be shaken by camp life" (p. 83).

Tragic optimism can even be extended to one's worldview of society and the human condition. For example, in an interview with Cromartie (1998) about race in America, Stanley Crouch, a brilliant black writer, claimed "I am much more optimistic than a lot of other people, but my optimism is what I always refer to as 'tragic optimism.' It's an optimism that accepts the horror of life, the horror of the past, the horror of the present." Fully aware of the history of oppression and the current struggles of black people in America, Crouch has chosen to take the stance of TO.

COMPONENTS OF TRAGIC OPTIMISM

Based on Frankl's writings, I have identified five essential components that comprise TO: (a) acceptance of what cannot be changed, (b) affirmation of the meaning and value of life, regardless of circumstances, (c) self-transcendence in serving a higher purpose, (d) faith or trust in God and others, and (e) courage to face adversity. These components can also be found in clinical literature on trauma as well as in larger literature of humanities.

After 9/11, the same five components were also evident in many speeches, prayers, interviews, testimonies, and more importantly in the actions of the rescue workers, survivors, and fellow citizens. What sustained the New Yorkers and all Americans in their darkest hours was their affirmation of the inherent value of liberty, justice, and the meaning of life. In spite of acceptance of the grim reality and the devastating losses, so many still maintain faith—faith in the miracles that their loved one may still be alive, faith in reunion in heaven, faith in the eventual triumph of justice and goodness over evil, faith in the American ideals, and faith in God. Thousands gave themselves sacrificially, and many had literally given their own lives, in their effort to rescue others. No word has been summoned more often than "courage"—"courage to combat pain," "from the depth of tragedy to the height of courage," and the "courage and resolve to persevere." Together, these sentiments weave a glorious tapestry of the meaning of TO.

Acceptance of What Cannot be Changed

Acceptance of reality is the defining characteristic of TO. By definition, TO depends on confronting and accepting reality as experienced, no matter how painful and gloomy. Acceptance also encompasses one's past traumas and possible future tragic events. Tragic optimism differentiates itself from other models of optimism by incorporating acceptance as an essential component of hope. Unless and until one fully accepts the dark sides of life and a pessimistic assessment of grim reality, without delusional or defensive attribution, one cannot discover TO. All other components of TO become possible because of acceptance.

One of the most widely accepted assumptions is that a sense of reality is the hallmark of mental health. "Acceptance has deep roots in the history of psychology and psychotherapy. Psychoanalysis, existential psychotherapy, cognitive-behavioral therapy, and humanistic treatment all require the client to confront, approach, or endure the pain that is part of life," (Sanderson & Linehan, 1999). Recent research findings also show that acceptance of reality is a major dimension of well-being and happiness (Ryff & Keys, 1995; Wong, 1998).

The present model of TO simply states that enduring hope must be based on a realistic assessment of reality, no matter how pessimistic the prospect. However, the benefits of acceptance are dependent on the concomitant presence of positive beliefs and attitudes, such as affirmation.

The psychological benefits of acceptance in terminal illness cases have received empirical support. For example, in one study examining the concept of empowerment in cancer patients in China, Mok (2001) discovered that acceptance is an integral part of empowering clients to find meaning and connectedness:

> In becoming empowered, the participants were also reconstructing their beliefs of the world, which affected how they viewed their relationships, themselves, and their health problem. It was completely unrealistic for the patients to presume that they could reverse the illness situation. By reframing and reinterpretation of the illness, these patients looked at cancer from a more positive perspective and tolerated the situation more easily. They found that, although they cannot change the course of the illness, they have the freedom to choose how they view it. (p. 72)

In Mok's study, it was also found that acceptance of illness was tied into the traditional Chinese cultural beliefs of harmony with the universe and Taoist teaching of *wu wei* (which literally means "do-nothing"). By looking at some aspects of Chinese culture, that one can see that Harmony with heaven, or surrender to the way of Nature, allows Chinese people to cope with many uncontrollable troubles, without sinking into despair (Chen, 2005).

It needs to be pointed out that acceptance means to honestly confront the seriousness of our situation. It does not mean giving up one's hope, but it means that one will not bang one's head against the brick wall. Acceptance is not simply acknowledging our predicament and hopeless state, but at the same time, making the heroic choice to live and endure with dignity and optimism.

The Serenity Prayer, which has been credited to the late American theologian Reinhold Niebuhr, says it well: "God, grant me the serenity to accept the things I cannot change." Frankl (1985) has shown that accepting the harsh reality of life and facing the world in all its evils is the pathway to achieving serenity and rebuilding a shattered life.

> Once the meaning of suffering had been revealed to us, we refused to minimize or alleviate the camp's tortures by ignoring them or harbouring false illusions and entertaining artificial optimism. Suffering had become a task on which we did not want to turn our backs. We had realized its hidden opportunities for achievement. (p. 99)

When false hope eventually gives way to realistic pessimism, one is faced with two choices: Either one sinks into depression, or embraces TO. Acceptance involves a double-affirmative: saying Yes to suffering and death, and saying Yes to meaning and life. Suffering intensifies hope, when acceptance is coupled with affirmation.

Affirmation of the Inherent Meaning and Value of Life

Affirmation of the inherent value of life and meaning represents the first positive step towards coping with traumas and rebuilding shattered assumptions. It is the turning point from the negative affect of realistic pessimism towards a positive affect in affirming the positive value of being alive. Dunbar, Mueller, Medina, and Wolf (1998) investigated the accounts of women living with HIV/AIDS to see how they were coping with their illness. The authors decry the disproportionate amount of literature that speaks of the devastation of AIDS on the individual and leaves out the stories of people who have been motivated to live healthier, fuller lives because of AIDS:

> The vastly disproportionate focus of the existing literature on negative aspects of HIV, with only a few more recent studies on coping, is unjustified. By failing to recognize the growth some women with HIV have created in themselves, social work professionals can inadvertently minimize the personal strengths and power of their clients. (Dunbar, et al., 1998, p. 146)

The authors found that after interviewing 34 women about their experiences living with HIV/AIDS, 28 responded that they had experienced unexpected positive outcomes related to their disease. Of the positives mentioned, affirmation of life was a common factor:

> Many women who spoke of reckoning with death described a subsequent discovery of the will to live. Affirming life in the face of a fatal illness is profound, for in the face of death, life takes on a different meaning. Ironically, it was the participants who decided to live consciously and fully who seemed to experience the greatest grief. One participant described a period of depression in which she tried to numb herself with excessive substance use. She came out of her depression slowly as a result of affirming her will to live. (Dunbar et al., 1998, p. 152)

The affirmation of life is the cornerstone of TO. Without firmly believing in the possibility of meaning in all aspects of human existence, without believing in the intrinsic value and dignity of human life, it would be difficult to experience optimism in the face of tragedy. The following quote is a shining example of such affirmation.

> I told my comrades (who lay motionless, although occasionally a sigh could be heard) that human life, under any circumstances, never ceases to have a meaning, and that this infinite meaning of life includes suffering and dying, privation and death. I asked the poor

creatures who listened to me attentively in the darkness of the hut to face up to the seriousness of our position. They must not lose hope but should keep their courage in the certainty that the hopelessness of our struggle did not detract from its dignity and its meaning. (Frankl, 1985, p. 104)

Tragic optimism is meaning oriented and value based. Thus, TO is predicated on affirming a deeply cherished set of core values, which serve as sources of meaning; these may include achievement, intimacy, self-transcendence, self-acceptance, and religion/spirituality (Wong, 1998). Tragic optimism is unshakable to the extent that these inner values and meanings are deep and secure. For example, Frankl's love for his wife and his intimate, internal dialogues with her endowed his existence with meaning and hope. He concluded: "Love goes very far beyond the physical person of the beloved. It finds its deepest meaning in his spiritual being, his inner self" (Frankl, 1985, p. 58).

Achievement, or the dream of future achievement, is another major source of meaning for Frankl in the death camp. He valued the unfinished manuscript on logotherapy. The thought of giving a public lecture on logotherapy enabled him to transcend the hopelessly oppressive death camp.

I forced my thoughts to turn to another subject. Suddenly, I saw myself standing on the platform of a well-lit, warm, and pleasant lecture room. In from of me sat an attentive audience on comfortable upholstered seats. I was giving a lecture on the psychology of the concentration camp! All that oppressed me at that moment became objective, seen and described from the remote viewpoint of science. By this method I succeeded somehow in rising above the situation, about the sufferings of the moment, and I observed them as if they were already of the past. (Frankl, 1985, pp. 94-95)

For Frankl, "meaning in life enables us to make sense of our existence despite guilt, suffering, injustice, and the inevitability of life" (Gould, 1993). Therefore, we need to discover something that is worth living and worth dying for, if we are to survive the tragedies of life. We know how to endure and survive, once we know why we exist.

As we said before, any attempt to restore a man's inner strength in the camp had first to succeed in showing him some future goal. Nietzsche's words, 'He who has a *why* to live for can bear with almost any *how*,' could be the guiding motto for all psychotherapeutic and psychohygienic efforts regarding prisoners. (Frankl, 1985, p. 97)

Self-transcendence

Self-transcendence represents an active expression of affirmation and involves the action dimension of TO. An attitude of self-transcendence invariably manifests itself in rising above self-interest and difficult circumstances in serving others. It can be directed upward in terms of serving God and doing his will; and it can also flow horizontally in terms of serving our fellow human beings. The essence of self-transcendence is self-detachment and involvement in loving God and loving our neighbors. Self-transcendence is demonstrated whenever we embrace suffering for the benefit of others (Frankl, 1985). Most religions espouse spiritual growth through transcending self-interests and serving a higher purpose (Richards & Bergin; 1997, 2000). Peterson (2000) proposed that researchers need to find out how optimism could be channeled from self-interest to concerns for others.

Transpersonal psychologists conceptualize self-transcendence as the act of identifying less with the restrictions of one's own ego personality in order to identify more with the "total self," in order to express one's existential nature in a congruent manner (Strohl, 1998). One's personality is only an outer expression of one's true "total self." According to Vaughan (1980), when one lets go of one's ego-centered perspective, and expanded sense of identity, a deeper sense of wholeness, relatedness, and connectedness is realized.

On a more practical level, stepping outside oneself to help others has been demonstrated to have an ameliorative effect. In the psychiatric rehabilitation field, for instance, it has become quite common for mental health consumers to become service providers. A recent qualitative study was conducted to examine the benefits of being a consumer-provider. In a thematic analysis of interviews with 14 such "peer providers," it was found that the peer providers benefited substantially from their work (Salzer & Shear, 2002).

Self-transcendence is related to Adler's (1964) concept of social interest. Serving others has the effect of liberating the individual from a miserable existence. For example, Frankl (1985) found it rewarding to encourage his fellow prisoners to find meaning and hope in the midst of their suffering. His ministry to the prisoners both stems from, and reinforces, his deeply held belief that meaning can be found in any situation. By attempting to restore the inner strength of others, he was strengthened. By imparting meaning to others, he found his own life enriched:

> The purpose of my words was to find a full meaning in our life, then and there, in that hut and in that practically hopeless situation. I saw that my efforts had been successful. When the electric bulb flared up again, I saw the miserable figures of my friends limping toward me to thank with tear in their eyes. (Frankl, 1985, p. 105)

All existential psychologists have come to the conclusion that transcending self-interests is one of the pathways to meaning and fulfillment (Wong, 1998). Similarly, almost all faith traditions believe that through transcending hedonistic and selfish interest, humans grow spiritually (Richards & Bergin, 1997). In self-transcendence, we lose ourselves in a higher service, and we find meaning by giving of ourselves to the world.

Self-transcendence may be conceptualized as the manifestation of TO in purposeful and goal-oriented activities. Self-transcendence represents TO in action—it is the inevitable consequence of affirmation and acceptance. If meaning is possible in the worst possible circumstances, such as the Nazi death camps, then we must act accordingly and demonstrate that there is indeed a higher purpose in our existence (Frankl, 1985).

Faith in God and in Others

Faith is crucial to TO (Wong, 2001). Tillich (1958) noted that such hope comes not from oneself but from an ultimate higher power. Trust in others becomes critical when one does not have theistic beliefs (Erikson, 1963; Capps, 1995). Capps (1995) stressed that without trust, one would not dare to hope at all. Conners, Toscova, and Tonigan (1999) wrote: "A trust in others and the sense that no matter what happens one will be fine are based on a belief in the benevolent wisdom of the universe" (p. 247).

There are numerous studies designed to measure whether certain aspects of faith have an ameliorative effect on health and well-being (Klaassen, McDonald, & James, 2005). The effect of faith and prayer on health, including seemingly deadly diseases such as cancer, has been well documented (Benson & Stark, 1996; Dossey, 1993; Matthews & Clark, 1998). Faith in God and prayer has been a source of strength and optimism to countless individuals in practically hopeless situations. It has often been said that man's adversity is God's opportunity. Faith represents a flickering light at the end of the tunnel. Often, it is the only positive expectation in an otherwise dark and hopeless world.

Frankl (1986) declared: "It is self-evident that belief in a super-meaning—whether as a metaphysical concept or in the religious sense of Providence—is of the foremost psychotherapeutic and psychohygienic importance. As a genuine faith springing from inner strength, such a belief adds immeasurably to human vitality" (p. 33).

Scheier and Carver (1985) recognized that for most people, their optimism is derived from their history of success, and confidence in their own mastery, but they also recognized that a substantial minority of people may derive their optimism from external sources. However, I would propose that most people in extreme situations beyond their control would resort to TO based on faith in God. The linkage between religion and optimism has also been pointed out by Peterson (2000), and it deserves more research attention.

Yahne and Miller (1999) referred to faith-based hope as a net that catches a person when all else fails. Such hope is vested not in oneself but in a higher power, in something more ultimate (Tillich, 1958). One example is the international 12-step tradition of Alcoholics Anonymous (1976), which emphasizes "a power outside of and greater than oneself, that is, a transcendent and in this sense spiritual power" (p. 220).

Courage to Face and Overcome Adversity

Courage encompasses the capacity to face adversity, to be true to one's convictions in spite of threats, to stand one's ground in spite of peer pressure or external force, and to survive in spite of the pain, brutality, and hopelessness of the situation. Courage may be considered the "master gland," because without it other glands will not function well. It is the pivotal point of TO—all other components hinge on courage—the heroic, defiant, human spirit. Acceptance requires courage. So does affirmation. Stepping out of our comfort zone to help others or to serve God also require the courage to be vulnerable.

We need courage to face tomorrow, courage to grow old, and courage to face sickness and death. We need courage to attempt anything, because there is always the risk of failure and oppositions. One cannot be optimistic without the courage to face an unknown and uncertain future. One cannot be optimistic about one's own competency, without the courage to take on a challenging task and risk failure.

Courage has been one of the major themes in humanistic-existential psychology (Camus, 1954, 1955; Frankl, 1985; May, 1984; Sartre 1943/1956; Tillich, 1952). But there has not been much research on courage. I have done a lot of research (Wong, 1995) on persistence. The results demonstrate that with proper training, organisms can learn endurance and resourcefulness in goal striving. Existential courage may be operationally defined as the capacity to persist in the face of adversity and failure. Based on studies of managers, Salvatore Maddi (2004) has developed a different operational definition of existential courage:

> The combined hardy attitudes of commitment, control, and challenge
> constitute the best available operationalization of existential courage.
> The hardy attitudes structure how you think about your interaction
> with the world around you and provide motivation to do difficult
> things. When they occur together, the 3 C's of hardy attitudes
> facilitate awareness that you formulate life's meaning for yourself by

the decisions you make and that choosing the future regularly, despite the anxiety of uncertainty, leads to the most vibrant life. (Maddi, 2004)

Both definitions incorporate the courage of committing one's time and energy towards an uncertain and even threatening future. The hardy attitudes of commitment, control, and challenge are manifested in behavioral persistence and resourcefulness in goal striving.

In sum, acceptance, affirmation, self-transcendence, faith, and courage are the five strands that make up the toughest rope that can endure almost any kind of stress test. When illusions, positive expectations, and self-efficacy—the bases for the kind of hopes we normally enjoy—are crushed by harsh reality, TO sets in. It is a different kind of hope. It is reality-based, solid as a rock and it works best when one has hit rock bottom. It is spirit-oriented, like the wind and the water flowing from a higher source, always reaching out and gaining strength as it goes. It is meaning centered and connected with the center of one's truest being—a set of core values and meanings that define one's identity. Finally, it is fearless and invincible, because it has overcome and transformed death.

Frankl (1985) stated that his own life in the death camps "serves as the existential validation of my theories" (p. 16). He also pointed out that survivors of the Holocaust provided further evidence—prisoners who were most likely to survive were those who had a future meaning to fulfill, and thus had a reason and purpose for living in spite of the unbearable sufferings.

TRAGIC OPTIMISM AND 9/11

In September, 2001, while I was preparing for my presentation at the Positive Psychology Summit in Washington, D.C., the unthinkable happened. From the bright morning sky, terror struck the twin towers of The World Trade Center in New York in quick succession, resulting in devastating damages and thousands of casualties. For the first time in history, on September 11, 2001, an act of war was launched against civilians on American soil, and Americans were awakened to a new reality of vulnerability. When I went to Washington on October 6th, 2001 less than a month after the fateful Black Tuesday, there was a palpable undercurrent of unease among the positive psychologists who were gathered there to present their latest findings on positive emotions and virtues. They seemed to be struggling, quietly by themselves or informally in groups of three or four, trying to find a PP answer to the challenge posed by 9/11. One of the widely accepted answers given at the Summit was "realistic courage." We were reminded by more than one speaker that realistically, the likelihood of another terrorist attack was much less than being struck by a car or a thunderbolt; therefore, there was no reason to be fearful and anxious.

My paper was entitled "Tragic optimism, realistic pessimism, and mature happiness" (Wong, 2001a), which was an elaboration of Viktor Frankl's construct of TO. I thought that Viktor Frankl's message of hope in the face of tragedies and dangers offered the best answer for the people traumatized by the losses of 9/11 who were fearful of the aftermath and the anthrax scare. But the only response I got from my audience was whether I had any hard data to support Frankl's concept of TO, as if Frankl's personal testimony and all those who bore witness to their heroic survival of the Holocaust did not count as supporting evidence.

It is amazing how psychology's obsession for crunching numbers can actually prevent us from research into the deep and profound experiences of flourishing in boundary situations. Positivism is not the only paradigm for knowledge claim. Historical, naturalistic, clinical, and narrative data are also powerful sources of psychological knowledge.

If we examine all the reports and studies on how people reacted to and coped with 9/11, we can readily identify the five components of TO. First of all, most people have come to confront and *accept* the full scope of the devastation. Many survivors said, "We know that the situation is very bleak, yet we are still looking for our loved ones, just in case." They maintained hope in spite of realistic pessimism.

There was evidence of the power of *affirmation*. Almost spontaneously, Americans across the nation, from the President to schoolchildren, affirmed their fundamental values—liberty, freedom, and the right to pursue happiness, even when the American dream had become a nightmare for many. Many had also affirmed a new sense of meaning and purpose after 9/11. They wanted to rethink their priorities and develop a more meaningful philosophy of life—family and friends mattered more than personal success.

Above all, they demonstrated the towering power of *faith* in a time of despair and sorrow. Yes, many had reacted with anger and doubts: "Where is God? How could he allow such evil to happen to my family?" Yet, in spite of their doubts and anger, they still believed in, and sought solace and strength from, God. People gathered in churches, synagogues, and mosques to pray and reflect. Faith is not the absence of doubts; it is the overcoming of doubts.

Strangers suddenly became neighbors. They all reached out to help each other. Thousands lined up for volunteer work. They wanted to do something to help. This army of eager volunteers said, "Together, we can bring hope and healing." That is *self-transcendence* in action.

All the above elements reflect courage and a defiant human spirit. It takes courage to confront the bleak reality and rebuild one's life from the wreckage. It takes courage to face an uncertain future with a newfound sense of purpose. It takes courage to going on living when the heart is aching with grief. It takes *courage* to reach out to help others in spite of their own brokenness and pain.

RESEARCH ON TRAGIC OPTIMISM

Elsewhere, I have critiqued various existing models of hope and optimism (Wong, 2007). These models of optimism are primarily based on confidence in one's own competence and expectation of positive outcomes, as long as such positive thinking squares with reality. These models contribute to effective coping, success, and well-being among healthy functioning individuals in affluent and individualistic societies, because the main thrust is on developing one's own sense of self-efficacy and pursuing personal success. Such egocentric optimism clearly reflects the American can-do attitude, but may not be appropriate for collectivistic societies. For example, Chang (2001) has found that Asians often use pessimism rather than optimism as a motivator to do well in the future.

To link expectations of positive outcomes entirely to one's own efficacy also restricts the wide range of sources of hope available, such as family, friends, God, and good luck (Wong & Reker, 1985). Lazarus (1999) has pointed out that Snyder's marriage of hope to self-efficacy (Bandura, 1997) dilutes the strength of true hope.

Another limitation of existing models is that they treat optimism and pessimism as opposite poles of the same continuum, rather than two related but independent dimensions. Lazarus (1999) argued that hope always incorporates some element of doubt and that the two constructs can coexist in healthy individuals. Peterson (2000) also contended that "optimism is not simply the absence of pessimism, and well-being is not simply the absence of helplessness" (p. 49). These comments are consistent with Frankl's construct of TO, which is predicated on the coexistence of pessimism and optimism.

Finally, a more serious limitation is that none of the existing models can be applied to extreme situations in which individuals can only expect bad events and have little or no control over the situation. For example, ethnic cleansing continues in Sudan with hundreds of thousands of refugees living in hunger and fear of being murdered. In such situations, does it give them any hope by telling them that happiness can trump suffering? Does it bring them any consolation by trying to convince them: "Don't worry, be happy?" They don't need scientific findings of studies of subjects who have never experienced starvation or faced execution; instead, they desperately need food, medicine and real "hope in hell" (Bortolotti, 2004).

Even in North America, there are individuals in extreme boundary situations. Just visit any hospice, palliative care unity, or extended care institution for the frail elderly. When getting through each day is a major achievement, there is little room for confidence in one's own self-efficacy and expectation of positive outcomes. When everything has been stripped away from them, and they are enveloped in the shadow of death, what they need is the same kind of optimism that sustained Frankl in the concentration camps.

Thus, the missing piece in the optimism literature is a model of optimism for the helpless and hopeless. Such a model would not be based on self-confidence and positive expectations, but on existential and spiritual principles (Frankl, 1985; Wong, 2001a, b).

A few graduate students and I have developed a valid and reliable instrument to measure TO (Leung, Steinfort, Vroon, & Wong, 2003). It is a 36-item self-report questionnaire called the Life Attitudes Scale (LAS). It consists of five sub-scales measuring the five components of TO.

Factorial Validity

Factorial analyses support the theoretical model postulating a five-factor solution: Acceptance, Affirmation, Courage, Faith, and Self-Transcendence. The intercorrelations among the subscales range from weak to moderate, indicating that the factors are relatively independent of each other. Also consistent with my (2001) TO model, the Acceptance subscale, which reflects realistic pessimism, is negatively correlated with other subscales, which emphasize a positive attitudes towards life in spite of a pessimistic assessment. Three separate replications of higher-order factor analyses of the means subscales further confirm the duality of the TO construct: the coexistence of heroic optimism and realistic pessimism. Therefore, the overall results on the factorial validity and factorial invariance of the LAS are satisfactory.

The Validity of the LAS

The concurrent validity studies between TO and two other optimism measures: Scheier and Carver's (1992) LOT-R, Snyder et al.'s (1996) Adult State Hope Scale, and Wong's (1998) Personal Meaning Profile (PMP) reveal positive correlations with the exception of the Acceptance subscale, which either correlates negatively or is uncorrelated with other scales. The outcomes of these studies support the dichotic construct of TO and demonstrate the convergent and discriminant validities of the LAS. The predictive validity of the LAS was demonstrated in another study which was consistent with our prediction that the LAS is a significant predictor of posttraumatic growth. This finding suggests that acceptance coupled with a meaning-and-faith-based optimism may be the underlying process of posttraumatic growth.

Tragic Optimism and the Positive Psychology of Suffering

Frankl has personally demonstrated that we can restore hope in hopeless situations through surrendering to the call of meaning. I have defined and refined the components of TO and demonstrated empirically the dialectic/paradoxical nature of TO: In our state of despair and helplessness, we discover the power of meaning and faith; in our brokenness, we hear the calling to bring healing to others; in our suffering, we encounter joy and serenity; and in our fears and vulnerability, we discover the defiant, heroic courage.

The theory and research on TO answer many of the issues raised by Peterson (2000) and suggest a new direction for optimism research as well as for positive psychology. TO is in the vanguard of developing a mature positive psychology for all humanity, including the millions who are suffering and dying each day.

Future directions in TO research should include implementing TO in developing countries (Wong, 2003), studying the defiant human spirit and courage (Wong, 1995), and applying TO in working with trauma victims and dying patients.

Tragic Optimism and Post-traumatic Growth

According to Frankl (1985), future meaning to fulfill was essential to survival and resilience: "The prisoner who had lost faith in the future—his future—was doomed. With his loss of belief in the future, he also lost his spiritual hold; he let himself decline and became subject to mental and physical decay" (p. 95).

Most of the intervention models for posttraumatic stress disorders (PTSD) emphasized the important role of meaning-based hope. For example, Herman (1992) stressed the need to integrate past trauma with future purpose. Horowitz (2001) focused on the transformative role of meaning and future plans. Janoff-Bulman (1999) emphasized the importance of restoration of shattered assumptions through restructuring one's beliefs and worldviews.

There are different consequences to trauma: (1) Many show immediate PTSD, (2) Some show delayed PTSD, (3) Some stay about the same, and (4) Some become stronger and demonstrate posttraumatic-growth, with or without therapy. The last type of reaction is most fascinating, because it testifies to both the human capacity for resilience and the important role of meaning-based TO.

Tedeschi and Calhoun (1995, 1996) suggest that there are five areas of perceived benefits or positive outcomes reported by persons who have experienced trauma (i.e., new possibilities, relating to others, personal strength, spiritual change, and appreciation of life). Interestingly, many of the concepts provided by the authors and the TO elements in this research project mutually support each other. For examples, appreciation of life is similar to affirmation of life, spiritual change is related to faith, and courage is key to personal strength.

Tedeschi and Calhoun (1995) propose that in order for one to perceive growth in the aftermath of trauma, it is crucial that one can construct or derive meaning from the traumatic experience, "when one can firmly grasp meaning and see one's life as orderly and purposeful, perceptions of control and esteem are likely to follow, and with these, a sense of well-being" (p. 40). Moreover, a person's religious beliefs and spirituality can become the pathway to meaning:

> Religion can provide higher-order schemas that can serve to preserve meaning in life even when events themselves seem senseless and tragic and... because religion deals in universal truth and enduring values, it can preserve meaning in the face of the violation of other illusions of permanence or invulnerability—that we can ward off disease; that our children will survive us; and that our homes, jobs, and fortunes are secure against crime or natural disaster. (p. 72-73)

Furthermore, aligned with the concept of self-transcendence, the authors suggest that through one's service to others, one's healing process is facilitated. However, these services must be meaningful to the person such that, "actions can serve to make events seem more manageable, but activities may be easier to engage in when it is meaningful to the actor" (p. 72). Also, a better social relationship can result from one's effort to contribute by helping others: "Part of the positive development of social relationship among survivors comes from their increased compassion, greater sensitivity to the needs and feelings of other people, and efforts directed at improving relationships" (p. 36).

As mentioned earlier, TO as measured by the LAS was positively correlated with post-traumatic growth. Also, TO served as a mediator between prior trauma and present well-being. It appears that when one's assumptive world has been shattered and denial is no longer feasible, the only type of optimism that empowers one to overcome and grow is a meaning-centered and faith-based optimism. With its unique integration of acceptance and affirmation, TO is able to provide suffering individuals with a resilient positive outlook toward life while remaining sensitive to the harsh reality. To further demonstrate the role of TO in posttraumatic growth, research has shown the following characteristics which are associated with posttraumatic-growth:

- *Acceptance*—accepting suffering as an inevitable part of life. Accept suffering as our teacher rather than our enemy—in so doing, they have acquired wisdoms about living and dying. Also accept their vulnerability and mortality. Life can be snatched away from us anytime.

- *Affirmation*—greater appreciation for life and its meaning. Appreciate life and all its possibilities. Affirm and discover the positive meaning in a difficult situation.

- *Courage*—confronting the unknown. They are prepared to pick up the pieces and re-establish themselves. They are ready to move forward with an increased sense of agency. "If I can survive this ordeal, I can survive anything." They are prepared to confront future sufferings.

- *Faith*—tapping into our spiritual resources to do the impossible. Restore faith in ultimate justice and ultimate meaning. Reaffirm their faith in a Supreme Being, who can help them when everything else fails.

- *Self-transcendence*—reaching out to others. Pain and suffering have given rise to compassion for those who suffer. They are prepared to rise above self-interests in their effort to help others.

A MATURE POSITIVE PSYCHOLOGY FOR SUFFERING

I have shown that a mature positive psychology cannot be exclusively based on positive experiences and positive affects. It must be dialectic, paradoxical, and integrative of both negative and positive experiences: Courage is not the absence of fear, but the capacity to carry on in spite of it; faith is not the absence of doubt, but the capacity to believe in spite of it, and optimism is not the absence of pessimism, but the capacity to transcend and transform it.

A mature positive psychology of suffering with TO as a prototype needs to be born of adversity and baptized by fire in order to speak to the suffering masses. The worst of times often brings out the best in us. Nothing makes hope grow stronger than setbacks and adversities, just as nothing makes the stars shine brighter than darkness. The pinnacle of human achievement, such as the conquest of Mt. Everest and the music of Beethoven, is often reached through the sacrifice of sweat and tears.

A positive psychologist capable of addressing the challenges and potentials of human existence must consider the needs of the underprivileged, suffering, and dying, the paradoxical nature of an authentic life, and the dialectic nature of positive experiences. We owe these profound psychological insights to Viktor Frankl—he has taught us how to soar above the abyss of misery to majestic heights through TO.

References

Adler, A. (1964). *Social interest: A challenge to mankind.* New York: Capricorn Books.

Alcoholics Anonymous (1976). *Alcoholics Anonymous: The story of how many thousands of men and women have recovered from alcoholism* (3rd ed.). New York: Alcoholics Anonymous World Services.

Bandura, A. (1997). *Self-efficacy: The exercise of control.* New York: W. H. Freeman

Benson, H., & Stark, M. (1996). *Timeless healing: The power and biology of belief.* New York: Scribner.

Bortolotti, D. (2004). *Hope in hell. Inside the world of Doctors Without Borders.* Buffalo, NY: Firefly Books Ltd.

Camus, A. (1954). *The rebel.* New York: Knopf.

Camus, A. (1955). *The myth of Sisyphus and other essays.* New York: Knopf.

Capps, D. (1995). *Agents of hope: A pastoral psychology.* Minneapolis, MN: Fortress.

Chang, E. C. (Ed.). (2001). *Optimism & pessimism: Implications for theory, research and Practice.* Washington, DC: American Psychological Association.

Chen, Y. H. (2005). The Way of Nature as a Healing Power. In P. T. P. Wong & L. C .J. Wong (Eds.), *Handbook of Multicultural Perspectives on Stress and Coping.* New York: Kluwer Academic/Plenum Publishers

Connors, G., Toscova, R. T., & Tonigan, J. S. (1999). In W. R. Miller (Ed.), *Integrating spirituality into treatment.* Washington, DC: American Psychological Association.

Cromartie, M. (1998, May/June). The Omni-American: Why the U.S. Constitution is like the blues, and other observations, opinions, and animadversions from Stanley Crouch. *Books & culture, a Christian review, 3.*

Dossey, L. (1993). *Healing words: The power of prayer and the practice of medicine.* San Francisco: Harper.

Dunbar, H. T., Mueller, C. W., Medina, C., & Wolf, T. (1998). Psychological and spiritual growth in women living with HIV. *Social Work, 43*(2), 144-154.

Erikson, E. H. (1963). *Childhood and society* (2nd ed.). New York: W. W. Norton.

Frankl, V. (1985). *Man's search for meaning: Revised and updated.* New York: Washington Square.

Frankl, V. (1986). *The doctor and the soul: From psychotherapy to logotherapy.* New York: Vintage Books.

Gould, W. B. (1993). *Viktor E. Frankl: Life with meaning.* Pacific Grove, CA: Brooks/ Cole Publishing.

Herman, J. L. (1992). *Trauma and recovery.* New York: Basic Books.

Horowitz, M. J. (2001). *Stress response syndromes: Personality styles and interventions* (4th ed.). Northvale, NJ: Jason Aronson.

Janoff-Bulman, R. (1999). Rebuilding shattered assumptions after traumatic events: Coping processes and outcomes. In C. R. Snyder (Ed.), *Coping: The psychology of what works.* New York: Oxford University Press.

Klaassen, D. W., McDonald, M. J., & James, S. (2006). Advances in the Study of Religious and Spiritual Coping. In P. T. P. Wong & L. C. J. Wong (Eds.), *Handbook of multicultural perspectives on stress and coping.* New York: Springer.

Chang, E. C., Tugade, M. M., & Asakawa, K. (2006). Stress and coping among Asian Americans: Lazarus and Folkman's model and beyond. In P. T. P. Wong & L. C. J. Wong (Eds.), *Handbook of Multicultural Perspectives on Stress and Coping.* New York: Springer.

Lazarus, R. S. (1999). Hope: An emotion and a vital coping resource against despair. *Social Research, 66,* 665-669.

Leung, M., Steinfort, T., Vroon, E. J., & Wong, P. T. P. (2003, August). *Life attitudes scale: Development and validation of a measurement of the construct of tragic optimism.* Paper presented at the American Pyschological Association Convention, Toronto, ON.

Maddi, S. (2004). Hardiness: An Operationalization of Existential Courage. *Journal of Humanistic Psychology, 44,* 279-298.

Matthews, D. A., & Clark, C. (1998). *The faith factor: Proof of the healing power of prayer.* New York: Viking.

May, R. (1984). *The courage to create.* New York: Bantam.

Mok, E. (2001). Empowerment of cancer patients: From a Chinese perspective. *Nursing Ethics, 8,* 69-76.

Peterson, C. (2000). The future of optimism. *American Psychologist, 55,* 44-55.

Peterson, C. (2004). *A Primer in Positive Psychology.* New York: Oxford University Press.

Richards, P. S., & Bergin, A. E. (1997). *A spiritual strategy for counseling and psychotherapy.* Washington, DC: American Psychological Association.

Richards, P. S., & Bergin, A. E. (Eds.). (2000). *Handbook of psychotherapy and religious diversity.* Washington, DC: American Psychological Association.

Ryff, C. D., & Keyes, C. L. M. (1995). The structure of psychological well-being revisited. *Journal of Personality and Social Psychology, 69,* 719-727.

Salzer, M. S., & Shear, S. L. (2002). Identifying consumer-provider benefits in evaluations of consumer-delivered services. *Psychiatric Rehabilitation Journal, 25*(3), 281-8.

Sanderson, C., & Linehan, M. M. (1999). Acceptance and forgiveness. In W. R. Miller (Ed.), *Integrating spirituality into treatment* (pp.199-216). Washington, DC: American Psychological Association.

Satre, J. P. (1956). *Being and nothingness: A phenomenological study of ontology* (H. Barnes, Trans.). New York: Philosophical Library. (Original work published 1943)

Scheier, M. F., & Carver, C. S. (1985). Optimism, coping, and health: Assessment and implications of generalized outcome expectancies. *Health Psychology, 4*, 219-247.

Scheier, M. F., & Carver, C. S. (1992). Effects of optimism on psychological and physical well-being: Theoretical overview and empirical update. *Cognitive Therapy and Research, 16*, 201-228.

Schumaker, J. F. (2007). *In search of happiness: Understanding an endangered state of mind.* Westport, CT: Praeger Publishers.

Snyder, C. R., Sympson, S. C., Ybasco, F. C., Borders, T. F., Babyak, M. A., & Higgins, R. L. (1996). Development and validation of the State Hope Scale. *Journal of Personality and Social Psychology, 2*, 321-335.

Strohl, J. E. (1998). Transpersonalism: Ego Meets Soul. *Journal of Counseling & Development, 76*, 29-35

Tedeschi, R. G., & Calhoun, L. G. (1996). The Posttraumatic Growth Inventory: measuring the positive legacy of trauma. *Journal of Traumatic Stress, 9*, 455-471.

Tedeschi, R. G., & Calhoun, L. G. (1995*). Trauma & transformation: Growing in the aftermath of suffering.* Thousand Oaks, CA: Sage.

Tillich, P. (1952). *The courage to be.* New Haven, CT: Yale University Press.

Tillich, P. (1958). *The dynamics of faith.* New York: Harper Collins.

Vaughan, F. (1980). Transpersonal psychology: Context, content, and process. In R. Walsh & E. Vaughan (Eds.), *Beyond ego: Transpersonal dimensions in psychology* (pp. 182-189). Los Angeles: Tarcher.

Wong, P. T. P. (1995). Coping with frustrative stress: A behavioral and cognitive analysis. In R. Wong (Ed.), *Biological perspective on motivated and cognitive activities.* New York: Ablex Publishing.

Wong, P. T. P. (1998). Meaning-centered counselling. In P. T. P. Wong & P. S. Fry (Eds.), *The human quest for meaning: A handbook of psychological research and clinical application* (pp. 395-435). Mahwah, NJ: Lawrence Erlbaum Associates.

Wong, P. T. P. (2001, December). A new algebra for positive psychology. *President's Column.* Retrieved May 1, 2007, from www.meaning.ca/articles/presidents_column/new_algebra.htm

Wong, P. T. P. (2001a, October). Tragic optimism, realistic pessimism, and mature happiness. Paper presented at the Positive Psychology Summit, Washington, DC.

Wong, P. T. P. (2001b, December). Living with terror: Lessons from logotherapy and positive psychology. A workshop presented at the Harvard Conference on Spirituality and Healing in Medicine. Organized by Harvard Medical School's Mind/Body Institute and The George Washington Institute for Spirituality and Health, Boston.

Wong, P. T. P. (2003, August). Tragic optimism: An existential-humanistic model. Paper presented at The American Pyschological Association Convention, Toronto, ON.

Wong, P. T. P. (2007). Viktor Frankl: Prophet of hope for the 21st century. In A. Batthyany & J. Levinson (Eds.), *Anthology of Viktor Frankl's Logotherapy*. Phoenix, AZ: Zeig, Tucker, & Theisen Inc.

Wong, P. T. P., & Reker, G. T. (1985). Optimism and well-being across the life-span. Paper presented at the Canadian Association on Gerontology, Hamilton, ON.

Yahne, C. E., & Miller, W. R. (1999). Evoking hope. In W. R. Miller (Ed.), *Integrating spirituality into treatment* (pp. 217-233). Washington, DC: American Psychological Association.

Wisdom, Religiosity, Purpose in Life, and Attitudes toward Death

MONIKA ARDELT

Abstract

A major psychological task in old age is to come to terms with the finitude of life. This study tests the relationships between wisdom, religiosity, purpose in life, and attitudes toward death, using a sample of 123 community-dwelling older adults (56+) living in north central Florida. Wisdom was defined as a combination of cognitive, reflective, and affective personality qualities. Controlling for socioeconomic status, gender, race, and the other variables in the model, multivariate regression analyses show that wisdom has a negative effect on death anxiety and escape acceptance of death, and intrinsic religiosity has a positive effect on approach and escape acceptance of death. Extrinsic religiosity is positively related to fear of death, death avoidance, and neutral acceptance of death. Purpose in life is unrelated to attitudes toward death if wisdom is included in the model, but it is negatively related to fear of death and death avoidance if wisdom is excluded. Similarly, wisdom is negatively related to death avoidance if purpose in life is eliminated from the model.

One of the major psychological tasks in life and particularly in old age is to make sense of death and dying. Erikson (1963) proposed that a person's life can be subdivided into eight different stages or developmental tasks. In old age, people have to come to terms with their life and the "inalterability of the past" (Erikson, Erikson, & Kivnick, 1986, p. 56). If they are able to look back without any major regrets and are satisfied with the way they have lived and what they have accomplished, integrity can be achieved. The successful resolution of that last crisis, integrity versus despair, supposedly results in wisdom which, according to Erikson (1964), "is detached concern with life itself in the face of death itself" (p.133). Wise elders are able to maintain the integrity of experience while at the same time acknowledging the physical deterioration of the body and the nearing of death.

Using a sample of 123 community dwelling older adults (56+) living in north central Florida, this research examines three personality qualities that are often assumed to alleviate death anxiety and negative attitudes toward death: wisdom, religiosity, and a feeling of purpose in life (Tomer & Eliason, 2000a). Attitudes toward death are assessed by the Death Attitude Profile–Revised (Wong, Reker, & Gesser, 1994), a multidimensional construct that measures fear of death, death avoidance, and death acceptance. Death acceptance, in turn, is assessed by three components: neutral acceptance of death (death is accepted as a fact of life), approach acceptance of death (death is perceived as a gateway to a blissful afterlife), and escape acceptance of death (death is considered an escape from a dreadful existence).

Wisdom is defined as a combination of cognitive, reflective, and affective personality characteristics (Ardelt, 1997, 2000; Clayton & Birren, 1980). This basic and parsimonious definition of wisdom is compatible with most intrinsic theories of wisdom (e.g., Clayton & Birren, 1980; Holliday & Chandler, 1986; Sternberg, 1990) and with extrinsic theoretical approaches that follow the wisdom traditions of the East (Takahashi, 2000). Wise people tend to look at phenomena and events from many different perspectives to overcome subjectivity and projec-tions (reflective dimension) and to discover the true and deeper meaning of phenomena and events (cognitive dimension). This process tends to result in a reduction of self-centeredness, which is likely to lead to a better understanding of life, oneself, and others and, ultimately, to an increase in sympathy and compassion for others (affective dimension). Hence, a wise person comprehends that physical deterioration is but another part of life, a fact that can neither be ignored nor denied. Wise people are expected to be unafraid of death because they understand the true nature of existence, have lived a meaningful life, and, therefore, are able to accept life as well as death (Tomer & Eliason, 2000a). However, so far, the relation between wisdom and attitudes toward death has not been empirically tested (Kastenbaum, 1999).

Similarly, the main task of religion is to make sense of life and death (Wong, 1998). Carl Jung (1969) observed that most religions could be considered "complicated systems of preparation for death" (p. 408). Moreover, religious people are presumed to be less afraid of death because they often believe that they will be rewarded for their religious behavior in the afterlife (Templer, 1972). Yet, there are important differences between *intrinsic* and *extrinsic* religiosity.

Intrinsic religiosity can be defined as a way of life and a commitment of one's life to God or a higher power. Every event is viewed through the religious lens, which provides meaning (Donahue, 1985) and establishes what Berger (1969) called "an all-embracing sacred order" (p. 51). Extrinsic religiosity, by contrast, is more superficial and ego-driven. According to Donahue (1985) it can be defined as a "religion of comfort and social convention, a self-serving, instrumental approach shaped to suit oneself" (p. 400).

Studies generally indicate a negative association between intrinsic religiosity and death anxiety, whereas the association between extrinsic religiosity and death anxiety is not necessarily significant (e.g., Fortner, Neimeyer, & Rybarczyk, 2000; Rasmussen & Johnson, 1994; Templer, 1972; Thorson & Powell, 1990; Tomer & Eliason, 2000b). In fact, Donahue (1985) reports a positive relation between extrinsic religiosity and fear of death based on a meta-analysis of the literature.

Finally, one might suspect that older people whose lives do not appear to be worth living due to physical and/or emotional strain would welcome death the most (Wong, 2000). However, past evidence suggests that, paradoxically, those elders who have found meaning and purpose in life tend to be less afraid of death and more ready to let go (Fortner, Neimeyer, & Rybarczyk, 2000; Nicholson, 1980; Quinn & Reznikoff, 1985; Tomer & Eliason, 2000b; Wong, 2000). Tomer and Eliason (2000b) speculate that "having a strong sense of one's life as meaningful may encourage an appraisal of death as an unavoidable price that one has to pay for a meaningful life and may encourage one to focus on one's life and important life goals" (p. 147).

In the present study, the following hypotheses are tested. Hypothesis 1: Wisdom is negatively related to fear of death and death avoidance, but positively related to neutral acceptance of death. No predictions are made regarding the association between wisdom and approach and escape acceptance of death. Because wise older people are assumed to understand the true and deeper meaning of life and, hence, able to accept life as it is, including physical deterioration and the existence of death, they are likely to accept death as a fact of life but unlikely to be afraid of death or to avoid any thoughts about death. However, not all wise elders might believe in a blissful existence after death, and they also might not conceive of death as a relief from a dreadful existence.

Hypothesis 2: Intrinsic religiosity has a negative effect on fear of death and death avoidance and a positive effect on neutral, approach, and escape acceptance of death. Older adults who have devoted their lives to God or a higher power and who believe in a blissful life after death should neither be afraid of death nor try to avoid thinking about death. On the contrary, those adults should look forward to a life after death that promises to be much better than their current existence, and they should not hesitate to accept death as a fact of life.

Hypothesis 3: Extrinsic religiosity is unrelated to attitudes toward death or might even be positively related to fear of death. Religion that is primarily based on self-interest rather than religious devotion to a higher cause is not expected to reduce fear of death or death avoidance or to increase neutral, approach, or escape acceptance of death.

Hypothesis 4: A sense of purpose in life has a negative effect on fear of death, death avoidance, and escape acceptance of death and a positive affect on neutral acceptance of death. No prediction is made with regard to the association between purpose in life and approach acceptance of death.

Older people who perceive life as meaningful might also perceive death as meaningful, which is likely to reduce their fear of death and death avoidance and to increase their neutral acceptance of death. Furthermore, elders who still feel a sense of meaning and purpose in life should be less likely to view death as an escape from a terrible world. However, a sense of purpose in life might or might not be related to the belief in a blissful afterlife. Socioeconomic status (SES), gender, and race are included as control variables in the analyses, although no predictions are made regarding the direction of the associations.[1] Some studies find a positive correlation between SES and fear of death (Pollak, 1979), whereas other researchers report a negative relation between SES and death anxiety (Nelson, 1979; Richardson & Sands, 1986). Similarly, the direction of the association between death attitudes and gender or death attitudes and race is not clear. Many studies indicate that women tend to report significantly higher levels of death anxiety than do men (Davis, Martin, Wilee, & Voorhees, 1980; Rasmussen & Johnson, 1994; Rigdon & Epting, 1985; Sanders, Poole, & Rivero, 1980; Young & Daniels, 1980), yet Fortner, Neimeyer, and Rybarczyk (2000) failed to discover a significant association between death anxiety and gender in a meta-analysis of 49 studies of older people. Correspondingly, some studies find that African Americans report greater fear of death than do Caucasians (Cole, 1979; Sanders, Poole, & Rivero, 1980; Young & Daniels, 1980), whereas other studies indicate a greater fear of death for Caucasians than for African Americans (Thorson & Powell, 1994) or no significant difference between African Americans and Caucasians with regard to death anxiety (Florian & Snowden, 1989; Marks, 1986; Pandey & Templer, 1972).

METHODS
Procedure

Initially, data collection took place between December 1997 and June 1998. Respondents were recruited from 18 close-knit social groups of older adults located in north central Florida. Group members who volunteered for the study were visited at home by a member of the research team who delivered and explained the self-administered questionnaire. The research team member also offered to conduct the interview if the respondent needed assistance in completing the survey. Ten respondents accepted this offer. All other 170 questionnaires were returned by mail in stamped, pre-addressed envelopes.

Ten months after the initial interview, all respondents with known addresses were contacted by mail for a follow-up survey. Participants who did not return the second questionnaire within two to three weeks were called by phone to remind them of the survey and to ask whether they needed assistance in filling out the questionnaire. Ultimately, 123 respondents or about 70% of the initial sample with known addresses returned the follow-up survey. All measures in this research are taken from the follow-up study with the exception of the control variables.

Sample

The sample consists of 123 Caucasian and African American older adults who range in age from 56 to 88 years with a mean and a median age of 73 years. Of the respondents, 72% are women, 80% are white, 62% are married, 82% are retired, 91% have a high school diploma, and 31% have a graduate degree.

Measures

Attitudes toward Death. The Death Attitude Profile–Revised (Wong, Reker, & Gesser, 1994) was used to assess five attitudes toward death: fear of death, death avoidance, neutral acceptance of death, approach acceptance of death, and escape acceptance of death. *Fear of death* is the mean of seven items (e.g., "I have an intense fear of death." "Death is no doubt a grim experience.") (a = .84); *death avoidance* is the average of five items (e.g., "I avoid death thoughts at all costs." "I always try not to think about death.") (a = .85); *neutral acceptance of death* is the average of five items (e.g., "Death is a natural aspect of life." "Death is neither good nor bad.") (a = .55); *approach acceptance of death* is the mean of 10 items (e.g., "I believe that I will be in heaven after I die." "I look forward to life after death.") (a = .97); and *escape acceptance of death* is the average of five items (e.g., "Death will bring an end to all my troubles." "Death provides an escape from this terrible world.") (a = .73). The scale of all the items ranges from 1 (strongly agree) through 5 (strongly disagree), which was reversed for all items before the average was computed.

Wisdom. The Three-Dimensional Wisdom Scale (3D-WS) was administered to measure the cognitive, reflective, and affective effect indicators of the latent variable wisdom (Ardelt, 1999). The 3D-WS consists of items from already existing scales as well as newly developed items. The *cognitive dimension* of wisdom assesses an understanding of life or the desire to know the truth. It is the mean of 14 items (e.g., "I often do not understand people's behavior." "Ignorance is bliss.") (a = .85). The *reflective dimension* measures a person's ability to look at phenomena and events from different perspectives and to avoid subjectivity and projections. It is computed as the average of 12 items (e.g., "I always try to look at all sides of a problem." "When I am upset at someone, I usually try to 'put myself in his or her shoes' for a while.") (a =.71). Finally, the *affective dimension* of wisdom captures the extent to which an individual develops sympathy and compassion for others and avoids negative emotions and behavior. It is measured as the average of 13 items (e.g., "Sometimes I feel a real compassion for everyone." "If I see people in need, I try to help them one way or another.") (a =.72). All items were assessed using one of two 5-point scales, ranging either from 1 (strongly agree) through 5 (strongly disagree) or from 1 (definitely true of myself) through 5 (not true of myself). The scale of the positively worded items was reversed before the average of the items was taken.

Religiosity was assessed by Allport and Ross' (1967) Intrinsic and Extrinsic Religion Scale. *Intrinsic religiosity* is the mean of 9 items (a =.89); *extrinsic religiosity* is the average of 11 items (a = .81). All items are measured on a scale ranging from 1 (strongly agree) through 5 (strongly disagree), which was reversed for all items.

Purpose in Life. A sense of purpose and meaning in life was measured by Crumbaugh and Maholick's (1964) Purpose in Life Test (King & Hunt, 1975). The scale is the mean of 9 items (a = .83) ranging from 1 (definitely true of myself) through 5 (not true of myself). The scale of the positively worded items was reversed before the average was computed.

Socioeconomic Status (SES) is the average of the longest held occupation and educational degree. *Longest held occupation* was coded by three raters using Hollingshead's Index of Occupations (O'Rand, 1982). At least two raters discussed and jointly decided on all ratings for occupations whose code designation was not clear. The scale ranges from 1 (farm laborers, mental service workers) through 9 (higher executive, large business owner, major professional). *Educational degree* ranges from 0 (no high school) through 3 (graduate degree). It was first transformed into a 9-point scale before it was averaged with occupation. For respondents without an occupation, SES reflects their educational degree. *Gender* and *race* were coded as dichotomous variables.

ANALYSIS

The factor score estimates of the latent variable wisdom were computed before the variable was included in the bivariate correlation and multiple regression analyses. The factor score estimates are an estimate of the latent variable wisdom. They are calculated by regressing the estimate of the latent variable on a weighted function of its indicators (Bollen, 1989; Jöreskog, Sörbom, du Toit, & du Toit, 1999). The resulting variable has a mean of zero and a standard deviation of one.

The latent variable wisdom was created through a confirmatory factor analysis procedure using the cognitive, reflective, and affective indicators of the 3D-WS and LISREL 8.30 (Ardelt, 1999; Jöreskog & Sörbom, 1996). The reflective dimension of wisdom had the highest factor loading with an unstandardized factor loading of .37 and a standardized loading of .84. This result is compatible with theoretical considerations that reflective thinking should promote both a deeper understanding of life and human nature and the development of sympathy and compassion for others. The factor loadings of the cognitive and affective dimensions were restricted to be equal because (a) there is no theoretical reason for one loading to be higher than the other, and (b) the X^2-difference between a model with and without this equality constraint was not statistically significant. The unstandardized factor loadings of the cognitive and affective dimensions of wisdom were .31 and their standardized loadings were .50 and .61, respectively.

RESULTS
Bivariate Correlation Analyses

Results of bivariate correlation analyses show that the correlation between fear of death and death avoidance is relatively high, the association between approach and escape acceptance of death is moderate, and no significant correlation exists between neutral acceptance of death and the other death attitudes (see Table 1). Wisdom and purpose in life are negatively related to fear of death and death avoidance, and intrinsic religiosity is positively related to approach and escape acceptance of death. By contrast, the association between wisdom and escape acceptance is negative. Extrinsic religiosity is positively correlated with fear of death and death avoidance, and negatively correlated with approach acceptance of death.

Table 1

Correlation matrix of attitudes toward death and predictor variables; pairwise selection of cases

Attitude	1	2	3	4	5	6	7	8	9	10	11	Mean	SD	n
1 Fear of death	—											2.37	.77	122
2 Death avoidance	.61*	—										2.32	.81	121
3 Neutral acceptance of death	-.13	.03	—									4.16	.41	123
4 Approach acceptance of death	.01	-.01	-.03	—								3.96	.95	122
5 Escape acceptance of death	.12	.12	.09	.44*	—							3.58	.75	123
6 Wisdom (factor score estimates)	-.46*	-.33*	-.06	.03	-.24*	—						0.00	1.0	123
7 Intrinsic religiosity	-.04	-.04	-.02	.77*	.28*	.09	—					3.94	.77	123
8 Extrinsic religiosity	.51*	.42*	.12	-.19t	.16	-.35*	-.26*	—				2.79	.74	123
9 Purpose in life	-.35*	-.30*	-.05	.15	-.11	.61*	.25*	-.25t	—			4.35	.53	119
10 SES	-.21t	-.33t	.04	-.25*	-.13	.23*	-.11	-.09	.24t	—		5.66	2.33	123
11 Gender (1 = female)	.05	-.05	-.19t	.24t	.08	.03	.27*	-.12	-.01	-.24*	—	.72	.45	123
12 Race (1 = Caucasian)	-.26t	-.31*	.14	-.11	-.20t	-.04	-.16	-.34*	-.08	-.06	-.04	.80	.40	122

* $p<0.01$; ᵗ $p<0.05$

Multivariate Regression Analyses

Multivariate regression analyses were performed to test the effects of the independent variables on attitudes toward death after controlling for the effects of the other independent variables in the model (see Table 2). As predicted in Hypothesis 1, wisdom is negatively related to fear of death but contrary to expectations, it is unrelated to death avoidance and neutral acceptance of death. In accordance with Hypothesis 2, intrinsic religiosity has a positive effect on approach and escape acceptance of death, but contrary to Hypothesis 2, it is unrelated to fear of death, death avoidance, and a neutral acceptance of death. By contrast, extrinsic religiosity is positively related to fear of death and death avoidance, but also to neutral acceptance of death, thereby partly confirming and partly rejecting Hypothesis 3. As expected, extrinsic religiosity is not associated with approach and escape acceptance of death. Contrary to Hypothesis 4, purpose in life is unrelated to attitudes toward death after controlling for the other independent variables in the models.

Table 2

Effects of wisdom, religiosity, and purpose in life on attitudes toward death; multiple OLS regression analyses with selected controls[a]

Dependent Variables	Fear of Death		Death Avoidance		Neutral		Approach Acceptance of Death		Escape Acceptance of Death	
Independent Variables	b	ß	b	ß	b	ß	b	ß	b	ß
Wisdom	-.20	-.26**	-.07	-.09	.02	.05	.00	.00	-.16	-.22*
Intrinsic religiosity	.04	.04	.03	.03	.08	.15	.97	.77***	.29	.30***
Extrinsic religiosity	.35	.33***	.25	.22**	.12	.22**	.00	.00	.10	.10
Purpose in Life	-.15	-.10	-.24	-.16	-.05	-.07	.00	.00	-.04	-.03
SES	-.03	-.10	-.10	-.29***	.01	.04	-.07	-.18***	-.01	-.04
Gender (1 = female)	.11	.06	-.20	-.11	-.18	-.20**	-.08	-.04	-.03	-.02
Race (1 = Caucasian)	-.31	-.16*	-.55	-.27***	.22	.21**	.00	.00	-.23	-.12
Adjusted R^2	.34	.32	.04	.61	.12					
n	117	116	118	117	118					

*** $p < 0.01$; ** $p < 0.05$; * $p < .10$

[a] The effects of other control variables (age, subjective health, marital and retirement status) were not statistically significant.

SES is negatively related to death avoidance and approach acceptance of death, and male and Caucasian elders are more likely than are female and African American elders to accept death as a fact of life. Finally, African Americans tend to fear and avoid thinking about death more than do Caucasians.

CONCLUSION

For the older adults in this study, fear of death and death avoidance are independent of their acceptance of death (Feifel, 1990; Wong, Reker, & Gesser, 1994). By contrast, the association between fear of death and death avoidance is relatively strong. Older adults tend to encounter death more frequently and on a more personal level than do younger adults, and they often have already accepted the fact that their own death is more than a theoretical possibility (Thorson & Powell, 2000). Hence, some older adults might have come to terms with the finitude of their life and might even look forward to a life after death and a reunion with their loved ones, while still being afraid of the unknown that death represents. Other older adults might not be afraid of death, but they also might not be convinced that there is indeed a life after death. Furthermore, neutral death acceptance is unrelated to any of the other death attitudes. As shown in Table 1, the mean of this scale is relatively high and the standard deviation is lower than for the other death attitude scales. This indicates that most of the older adults in this study accept death as a fact of life regardless of their fear of death or their belief in a blissful afterlife.

Controlling for socioeconomic status, gender, race, and the other variables in the model, multivariate regression analyses show that only wisdom has a negative effect on fear of death as predicted. However, the correlation between the 3D-WS and the Purpose in Life Test is relatively high ($r = .61$; see Table 1). Although a strong association between the two constructs is theoretically expected (Erikson, Erikson, & Kivnick, 1986), multicollinearity occurs if both measures are included in the same model. If wisdom is eliminated from the model, the negative effect of purpose in life on fear of death becomes statistically significant as anticipated. Similarly and as predicted, the negative effect of purpose in life on death avoidance becomes significant if wisdom is removed from the model and vice versa. Hence, both wisdom and a sense of purpose in life seem to be important factors in decreasing older people's fear and avoidance of death. However, both wisdom and purpose in life are unrelated to neutral and approach acceptance of death. Neither wisdom nor a sense of purpose and meaning in life appears to be required to accept death as a fact of life or to anticipate a blissful life after death.

Only intrinsic religiosity is highly and positively related to approach acceptance of death. Apparently, intrinsically religious older adults tend to believe in a blissful afterlife, which allows them to look forward to a life after death. Intrinsic religiosity is also significantly related to escape acceptance of death, although this association is much weaker than the previous one. Intrinsically religious older people, whose life is filled with physical and emotional suffering, might welcome the prospect of a blissful afterlife. Interestingly, wisdom (but not purpose in life as predicted) has a negative effect on escape acceptance of death. Wise elders might be less likely to feel that their existence is bleak or they might be less likely to see death as the solution to their problems.

Surprisingly, intrinsic religiosity is unrelated to fear of death, death avoidance, and neutral acceptance of death, whereas extrinsic religiosity has a positive effect on those death attitudes. This is consistent with an earlier meta-analysis of the literature by Donahue (1985) who also found a positive correlation between extrinsic religiosity and fear of death. Extrinsically religious people might be exposed to religious doctrine in church, but because they do not necessarily live a religiously devoted life they might be afraid of the unknown and an uncertain future after death. Due to their fear of death, they might also try to avoid thinking about death. However, extrinsic religiosity has a positive effect on neutral acceptance of death. In fact, for extrinsically religious older adults a neutral acceptance of death might be their way of dealing with the prospect of death. Although they might fear death and might try not to think about it, they nevertheless tend to accept the fact that death is an integral part of life that cannot be avoided.

Future studies are required to replicate these analyses with a larger and more representative data set of older adults. However, the analyses revealed that it is important to distinguish between intrinsic and extrinsic religiosity when studying attitudes toward death and that both wisdom and a sense of purpose and meaning in life might reduce older people's fear and avoidance of death.

References

Allport, G. W., & Ross, J. M. (1967). Personal religious orientation and prejudice. *Journal of Personality and Social Psychology, 5*, 432-443.

Ardelt, M. (1997). Wisdom and life satisfaction in old age. *Journal of Gerontology: Psychological Sciences, 52B*, P15-P27.

Ardelt, M. (1999). *Development and Empirical Assessment of a Three-Dimensional Wisdom Scale.* Paper presented at The Gerontological Society of America Annual Meetings, San Francisco.

Ardelt, M. (2000). Antecedents and effects of wisdom in old age: A longitudinal perspective on aging well. *Research on Aging, 22*, 360-394.

Berger, P. (1969). *The sacred canopy: Elements of a sociological theory of religion.* New York: Doubleday.

Bollen, K. A. (1989). *Structural equations with latent variables.* New York: John Wiley & Sons.

Clayton, V. P., & Birren, J. E. (1980). The development of wisdom across the life-span: A reexamination of an ancient topic. In P. B. Baltes & O. G. Brim Jr. (Eds.), *Life-Span Development and Behavior* (Vol. 3, pp. 103-135). New York: Academic Press.

Cole, M. A. (1979). Sex and marital status differences in death anxiety. *Omega - The Journal of Death and Dying, 9,* 139-147.

Crumbaugh, J. C., & Maholick, L. T. (1964). An experimental study in existentialism: The psychometric approach to Frankl's concept of noogenic neurosis. *Journal of Clinical Psychology, 20,* 200-207.

Davis, S. F., Martin, D. A., Wilee, C. T., & Voorhees, J. W. (1980). Relationship of fear of death and level of self-esteem in college students. *Psychological Reports, 42,* 419-422.

Donahue, M. J. (1985). Intrinsic and extrinsic religiousness: Review and meta-analysis. *Journal of Personality and Social Psychology, 48,* 400-419.

Erikson, E. H. (1963). *Childhood and society.* New York: Norton.

Erikson, E. H. (1964). *Insight and responsibility. Lectures on the ethical implications of psychoanalytic insight.* New York: Norton.

Erikson, E. H., Erikson, J. M., & Kivnick, H. Q. (1986). *Vital involvement in old age: The experience of old age in our time.* New York: Norton.

Feifel, H. (1990). Psychology and death: Meaningful rediscovery. *American Psychologist, 45,* 537-543.

Florian, V., & Snowden, L. R. (1989). Fear of personal death and positive life regard: A study of different ethnic and religious-affiliated American college students. *Journal of Cross-Cultural Psychology, 20,* 64-79.

Fortner, B. V., Neimeyer, R. A., & Rybarczyk, B. (2000). Correlates of death anxiety in older adults: A comprehensive review. In A. Tomer (Ed.), *Death Attitudes and the Older Adult. Theories, Concepts, and Applications* (pp. 95-108). Philadelphia: Brunner-Routledge.

Holliday, S. G., & Chandler, M. J. (1986). *Wisdom: Explorations in adult competence.* New York: Karger.

Jöreskog, K. G., & Sörbom, D. (1996). *LISREL 8: User's reference guide* (2nd ed.). Chicago: Scientific Software International.

Jöreskog, K. G., Sörbom, D., du Toit, S., & du Toit, M. (1999). *LISREL 8: New statistical features.* Chicago: Scientific Software International.

Jung, C. J. (1970). The soul and death. In G. Adler & R. F. C. Hull (Eds.), *The collected works of C. G. Jung: Vol. 8. The structure and dynamics of the Psyche* (2nd ed.). Princeton, N.J: Princeton University Press.

Kastenbaum, R. C. (1999). Afterworld. In L. E. Thomas & S. A. Eisenhandler (Eds.), *Religion, belief, and spirituality in late life* (pp. 203-214). New York: Springer.

King, M. B., & Hunt, R. A. (1975). Measuring the religious variable: National replication. *Journal for the Scientific Study of Religion, 14*, 13-22.

Marks, A. (1986-1987). Race and sex differences and fear of dying: A test of two hypotheses: High risk or social loss? *Omega - The Journal of Death and Dying, 17*, 229-236.

Nelson, L. D. (1979-1980). Structural conductiveness, personality characteristics and death anxiety. *Omega - The Journal of Death and Dying, 10*, 123-133.

Nicholson, J. (1980). *Seven ages. The truth about life crises - Does your age really matter?* Glasgow, Scotland: William Collins Sons & Co.

O'Rand, A. M. (1982). Socioeconomic status and poverty. In D. J. Mangen & W. A. Peterson (Eds.), *Research Instruments in Social Gerontology: Vol. 2. Social Roles and Social Participation* (pp. 281-341). Minneapolis, MN: University of Minnesota Press.

Pandey, R. E., & Templer, D. I. (1972). Use of the death anxiety scale in an inter-racial setting. *Omega - The Journal of Death and Dying, 3*, 127-130.

Pollak, J. M. (1979-1980). Correlates of death anxiety: A review of empirical studies. *Omega - The Journal of Death and Dying, 10*, 97-121.

Quinn, P. K., & Reznikoff, M. (1985). The relationship between death anxiety and the subjective experience of time in the elderly. *International Journal of Aging and Human Development, 21*, 197-210.

Rasmussen, C. H., & Johnson, M. E. (1994). Spirituality and religiosity: Relative relationships to death anxiety. *Omega - The Journal of Death and Dying, 29*, 313-318.

Richardson, V., & Sands, R. (1986-1987). Death attitudes among mid-life women. *Omega - The Journal of Death and Dying, 17*, 327-341.

Rigdon, M. A., & Epting, F. R. (1985). Reduction in death threat as a basis for optimal functioning. *Death Studies, 9*, 427-448.

Sanders, J. F., Poole, T. E., & Rivero, W. T. (1980). Death anxiety among the elderly. *Psychological Reports, 46*, 53-54.

Sternberg, R. J. (1990). Wisdom and its relations to intelligence and creativity. In R. J. Sternberg (Ed.), *Wisdom: Its nature, origins, and development* (pp. 142-159). Cambridge, U.K.: Cambridge University Press.

Takahashi, M. (2000). Toward a culturally inclusive understanding of wisdom: Historical roots in the East and West. *International Journal of Aging and Human Development, 51*, 217-230.

Templer, D. I. (1972). Death anxiety in religiously very involved persons. *Psychological Reports, 31*, 361-362.

Thorson, J. A., & Powell, F. C. (1990). Meanings of death and intrinsic religiosity. *Journal of Clinical Psychology, 46*, 379-391.

Thorson, J. A., & Powell, F. C. (1994). A revised death anxiety scale. In R. A. Neimeyer (Ed.), *Death anxiety handbook: Research, instrumentation, and application. Series in death education, aging, and health care* (pp. 31-43). Philadelphia: Taylor and Francis.

Thorson, J. A., & Powell, F. C. (2000). Death anxiety in younger and older adults. In A. Tomer (Ed.), *Death attitudes and the older adult. Theories, concepts, and applications* (pp. 123-136). Philadelphia: Brunner-Routledge.

Tomer, A., & Eliason, G. (2000a). Attitudes about life and death: Toward a comprehensive model of death anxiety. In A. Tomer (Ed.), *Death attitudes and the older adult. Theories, concepts, and applications* (pp. 3-22). Philadelphia: Brunner-Routledge.

Tomer, A., & Eliason, G. (2000b). Beliefs about self, life, and death: Testing aspects of a comprehensive model of death anxiety and death attitudes. In A. Tomer (Ed.), *Death attitudes and the older adult. Theories, concepts, and applications* (pp. 137-153). Philadelphia: Brunner-Routledge.

Wong, P. T. P. (1998). Spirituality, meaning, and successful aging. In P. T. P. Wong & P. S. Fry (Eds.), *The human quest for meaning: A handbook of psychological research and clinical applications* (pp. 359-394). Mahwah, NJ: Lawrence Erlbaum.

Wong, P. T. P. (2000). Meaning of life and meaning of death in successful aging. In A. Tomer (Ed.), *Death attitudes and the older adult. Theories, concepts, and applications* (pp. 23-35). Philadelphia, PA: Brunner-Routledge.

Wong, P. T. P., Reker, G. T., & Gesser, G. (1994). Death attitude profile-revised: A multidimensional measure of attitudes toward death. In R. A. Neimeyer (Ed.), *Death anxiety handbook. Research, instrumentation, and application* (pp. 121-148). Washington, DC: Taylor & Francis.

Young, M., & Daniels, S. (1980). Born again status as a factor in death anxiety. *Psychological Reports, 47*, 367-370.

Author Note

The research was supported by a Brookdale National Fellowship, a grant from NIH/NIA (R03 AG1485501), and a Research Initiation Project Award from the College of Liberal Arts and Sciences at the University of Florida. Special thanks go to Carla Edwards, Anna Campbell, Adeen Woolverton, Nicolette Fertakis, Stephen Mayer, Dacia Caglin, Dana Federici, Amy Monk, Brad Tripp, and Elizabeth Brown for their help at various stages of the research project. A previous version of this paper was presented at the International Conference on Searching for Meaning in the New Millennium, July 13 to 16, 2000, Vancouver, B.C.

Endnote

1. The effects of other control variables (age, subjective health, marital and retirement status) were also tested but results showed that they were not statistically significant. Those additional control variables were excluded from the analyses because they reduced the overall sample size by 17% in a listwise selection of cases.

A Death is Worth a Thousand Tellings: Transformation Through Storytelling

JANETTE E. MCDONALD

Abstract

Why do we share our intimate stories with others? When are personal stories most frequently told? What are the rewards and benefits of telling our personal stories? In the context of transforming loss and grief, this paper explores these questions and the meaning they reveal during death and dying. A major objective of the paper is to provide the readers with a deepened insight and appreciation for retelling the story of a death. In this paper I explore the phenomenon of storytelling as a narrative research methodology in the context of the dying and death processes. I also draw on the growing scholarly research on meaning as it relates to the end of life. The research section of this paper discusses two specific narrative stories that address different kinds of death: a suicide and a death of a young wife from breast cancer. A major focus of the narrative stories includes themes of meaning as described by each individual. These are discussed in detail as part of my general conclusions.

We each have our unique life story that is wrapped in a myriad of experiences and expressions and further composed of smaller, subconnecting life stories. Some life experiences lend themselves to humorous, captivating, and compelling stories that are retold hundreds of times. Some stories, for whatever reason, are shared with only a chosen few or remain in the silence of our own hearts. The telling of a story that surrounds the death of a loved one holds the potential for significant personal transformation because, in telling it, one reflects on and views the experience from a different emotional place each time it is re-told.

One's life is qualitatively different after a death or loss (Levine, 1982; McDonald, 1997). If one is able to perceive the loss through a different more meaningful lens, personal transformation is not only possible, it is probable. How one proceeds with this transformation depends on unique individual abilities. As noted in this study, the telling of a death reveals both beauty and pain, and one's capability to recognize and appreciate each of these qualities is the point at which personal meaning can be made. Hence, the death story is a place of entry for transformation in grieving, healing, and living. You will see from the content of these interviews that it clearly takes time, energy, and effort to arrive at this point.

The telling of a loved one's death confirms to both the teller and the listener that life is ephemeral, fragile, and precious. The description of the death and the experiences leading up to it reveals as much about the teller as it does about the deceased. It also provides the listener with keen insights into the lives that preceded it. Ultimately, it is the telling or retelling of a death that helps one embrace the meaning in life, and indeed suggests that a death is worth a thousand tellings.

In Western culture certain topics are difficult to discuss and may even be viewed as taboo. Kubler-Ross (1997), among a host of other scholars in the field of thanatology, asserts that we are a death-denying culture. Therefore, because the topic of death is a difficult one to discuss, its telling and retelling are precisely the reason that the story of a loved one's death is so powerful and offers a path of transformation in the first place.

This paper examines the phenomenon of story telling as a way of making meaning for those who have experienced the death of a loved one. It further suggests that personal transformation is a result of the meaning-making process. Drawing from Roemer's (1995) work on narrative and storytelling and Frankl's (1985) classic research on meaning, this paper assumes that telling the story of a loved one's death provides a deepened insight into appreciating life and death even when pain and struggle may accompany that death. The following two narrative stories will be discussed to support these concepts.

Although each story is different, this narrative study describes similar themes of meaning and transformation as expressed by the participants. Narrative research using storytelling is intended to recount as accurately as possible those stories described by the participants. Storytelling, as a method of research, is extremely personal, and while the interpretation by the researcher is also a personal rendering of descriptions, it is no less rigorous in its scholarly attempt to accurately and truthfully portray what the participants experienced.

First, to provide a brief context and to clarify terms for the readers, I wish to define these terms: *teller, listener, death story,* and *life story.* The teller is simply the person who shares the story. The listener is the person or audience who hears what the teller has to say. The death story addresses the way in which the loved one died, but also integrates a number of smaller life stories. Potentially, the death story uncovers a significant number of life events and is part of the person's larger life story. The life story is the person's total history, which can never be completely told because human life is constantly moving, developing, and evolving. As soon as a story has been told, life has continued, thereby adding more to the story, even after death.

This paper is organized as follows: four points from Roemer's (1995) work will be discussed to illustrate a place of intersection between one's personal transformative process and the experience of a loved one's death. The four points are: (a) stories connect us to other people, things, and events; (b) the context of stories is known prior to the telling; (c) most stories are family oriented; and (d) all stories are past and therefore precluded. Following Roemer's work I will draw connections to Frankl's research on meaning and meaning making as relevant to death. I will conclude with suggestions on how storytelling can function as a transformative process in resolving death, loss, and grief.

ROEMER'S WORK ON NARRATIVE AND STORYTELLING

While Roemer's (1995) work primarily offers a philosophical analysis of storytelling in the context of fictional literature and prose, it also has merit for specific storytelling at the end of a life. He notes that, "despite our knowledge, we lend ourselves to their adventures" (p. 3). I make a connection to Roemer (1995) because as we hear stories of death and loss, we grasp a sense of our own vulnerability and unpredictable future. In our storytelling and story listening our own mortality becomes hauntingly evident. Roemer (1995) identifies a significant point, that:

> death is the sanction of everything the storyteller can tell. In life, the most immediate evidence we have for the "real" or sacred is death, which constitutes our most persuasive encounter with necessity... we know we must die, and this knowledge could be said to govern us.... Death gives meaning and order to the life of the individual and to the community. It is a predicate of our existence that links the thinking of common folk to the investigations of philosophers, and informs our shared understanding of the human condition. It sanctions story as

it does relationship and morality…. As death limits and governs our existence, so it governs traditional story. We know how the story—like our lives—will end, but not generally, how the figures willingly get there. Death is indeed, the source of story's authority. (p. 84-85)

As noted by Roemer (1995) and as indicated by the stories of my participants, few events have the potential to create significant meaning in our lives like that of death. When something or someone we love or cherish is about to be taken away from us, we are forced to look more deeply at what we value in life. A death intensifies our need to refine our perspective on life and forces a reorganization of our priorities. A death reminds us that life is short. Recognizing life's brevity often motivates us to make the most of the life we have. A death indeed sanctions life.

In his 1984 preface to his classic work, Frankl (1985) seems to confirm my point. In referring to why he was motivated to compose *Man's Search for Meaning* he writes, "I had wanted simply to convey to the reader by way of a concrete example that life holds a potential meaning under any condition, even the most miserable ones." (p. 16). The stories you will hear, although not as horrendous as those from a concentration camp, may nonetheless evoke a propinquity of raw tenderness in our hearts.

Stories Connect and Unite Us

Roemer (1995) suggests that stories connect and unite us. His emphasis is primarily on the teller since his work centers on drama, prose, and poetry, but he does appear to recognize the vital role of the listener. An interesting transition occurs after one hears the death or life story that further connects one to others. The listener may choose to later become a teller of the story he has previously heard. Because of this connection all storytellers first have been story listeners, even if this may mean listening to one's own experiences and then later telling them to the world for the very first time.

Furthermore, the listener has an intimate connection with the death story in another way. The listener becomes an integral part of one's history because the dying person will not be alive to tell his own death story. We all must rely on others to tell our story after we have left this earthly plane and how much of it is fact or fiction, flattering or incriminating, public or private, vivacious or mundane depends on someone else. What we leave behind in the way of personal journals and other possessions may assist those who wish to tell our story. But eventually we relinquish the telling of our history to someone else.

Stories of death and life then are always set in the context of relationship with others. In a sense, we are never not in relationship with someone or something.

Roemer (1995) implies an analogous thought when he writes, "In narrative, no one is an island, however isolated or free he may believe himself to be" (p. 11). Roemer suggests whether we know it or not, we are always connected to someone or something else. His following quote more clearly emphasizes our inherent relationship with others:

> But while the knowledge of our mortality makes us fearful, it can also induce the concern and tenderness—not just for those close to us, but for all others—that are a distinguishing mark of our species. Mortality makes us alike: it makes us kin and can make us kind. (Roemer, 1995, p. 85)

The Context of the Story is Known

Roemer (1995) writes that in narrative one generally knows the context of the story before it has been told. For instance, long before many of us first read Shakespeare's *Romeo and Juliet* we were at least familiar with the story line; somewhere we had learned that this was a love story of two young people whose lives ended in tragedy because of feuding families. The rest of the details were acquired as we read or saw the play. A parallel can be made with the death story. When we are telling the story of our loved one, we clearly know its context. Our listener may not have the same understanding, but it is revealed to them through our storytelling.

Stories are about Families

Roemer (1995) also states that most stories are family centered and, as such, they have the capacity to "nurture and undermine, wound and heal, sustain and strangle" (p. 14). As a bereaved person tells the story, this notion becomes even more evident. Loss and illness potentially bring out the best and worst in families as they cope. As you will hear about one of the participants, her family and their unconditional love is what has sustained her throughout her grief process. The story that the other participant tells is almost completely interconnected with his family.

Stories are Past and Precluded

Whether we tell or listen to the death story we are generally aware of the outcome. The specific details may be unknown, but we are aware of the conclusion. When we attend a funeral we know at least one part of the deceased's story: That he died and that a segment of his story is past and precluded. More of the details will be unraveled as we listen to the loved one telling his story. Just as we are aware that we will have a past to our story, we know that it is precluded.

CREATING MEANING THROUGH STORIES

We live in a time when growing numbers of people tell personal stories of woe. Throughout the world many report that their lives are filled with meaninglessness despite the abundance of material wealth and prosperity (Wong & Fry, 1998). Perhaps the most disturbing phenomenon is that a significant number of youth, especially Americans, report a lack of meaning in their lives (Krasko, 1997).

This paper is primarily concerned with the written and spoken words of people and how their expressions reveal meaning in their lives. Their making of meaning then leads to their personal transformation. A superb example is found in Frankl's (1985) work. In fact, his entire account could be seen as a meaningful story in which he retells his experiences in the concentration camps. One story that holds significance for this paper involves his recollection of a vivid memory of his beloved wife. He writes:

> Occasionally I looked at the sky, where the stars were fading and the pink of the morning was beginning to spread behind a dark bank of clouds. But my mind clung to my wife's image, imagining it with an uncanny acuteness. I heard her answering me, saw her smile, her frank encouraging look. Real or not, her look was then more luminous than the sun which was beginning to rise. (p. 56-57)

This passage described not only the physical details of what that moment was like, it also revealed with poetic beauty the depth of the love he held for her. Frankl continued:

> A thought transfixed me: for the first time in my life I saw the truth as it is set into song by so many poets, proclaimed as the final wisdom by so many thinkers. The truth—that love is the ultimate and the highest goal to which man can aspire. Then I grasped the meaning of the greatest secret that human poetry and human thought and belief have to impart: The salvation of man is through love and in love. I understood how a man who has nothing left in this world still may know bliss, be it only for a brief moment. (p. 57)

In this passage the listener or reader acquires a sense of the depth of Frankl's character and what he values. One comes away from that passage knowing that truth and love are coauthors of meaning for Frankl and that the current moment, no matter what comprises it, holds tremendous power and poignancy. Specifically the reader notes that through Frankl's own admission he has gained new insight and therefore has been personally transformed by his current awareness of the present.

Meaning Making as Transformation

Although Frankl (1985) does not actually use the word *transformation* in his work, he clearly implies that finding or creating meaning in life is a transforming experience. Instead he uses such expressions as "rising or growing above" one's self to describe this transformation. In other words, transformation occurs when the meaning that has been created has fundamentally changed the individual; it has made him somehow a more complete, more full human being. In the retelling of this experience, we see that Frankl grasps what he understands as the "greatest secret that… poetry and thought" (p. 59) impart.

This passage also calls to mind an ancient Buddhist story about a man running from a charging tiger. The story goes like this: The man is running away from the tiger toward the edge of a steep cliff. As he nears the edge of the cliff, he looks down and sees more tigers at the cliff's bottom. To free himself from the ensuing tiger, he leaps for a tree branch overhanging the cliff. As the branch begins to break and the man is seconds away from falling to his fate, he notices a lovely ripe strawberry. He picks and eats it in utter bliss just before he falls. This story, somewhat like Frankl's, reminds us that even as death stares us in the face, we can embrace the present and experience a transcendent aliveness that is filled with unquestioned meaning.

Our story about our deceased loved one equips us with a similar wisdom. As we tell their stories, often in the midst of extraordinary pain, sorrow, and fear, we are given a glimmer of hope that their lives were not in vain and that somehow through their death, they are quickened. This juxtaposition between life and death heightens our awareness and transforms us because we have dared to endure loss with some sense of equanimity.

NARRATIVES REVEALED
Procedures

Two persons, one man and one woman, were asked to tell their story about their departed loved one. Four opened-ended questions were asked in order to guide them in an unobtrusive way through their narrative story. The questions were:

- What story or stories would you like me to hear?

- What story do you consider most meaningful?

- What does sharing these stories do for you?

- What advice about sharing similar stories would you give to someone else in a similar situation?

Each account was audio recorded and then transcribed and analyzed for themes of meaning. Interviews were intended to last approximately 45 to 60 minutes. Finished interviews actually lasted from 75 to 150 minutes. To ensure confidentiality, each person's name was changed. People were asked to participate based on their own willingness to tell their story about their loved one. No other stipulations for participation were required.

Each of these persons experienced a different kind of loss. In this study, the woman, Sally, tells her story of her husband's tragic suicide and its continuing effect on her family. Frank remembers his young wife's struggle and reoccurrence of breast cancer with exquisite detail and poignancy.

Sally and Peter

Sally was a soft-spoken, middle-aged Caucasian woman with a gentle demeanor whose wisdom appeared to exceed her years. I also sensed that she had a quiet strength that no doubt helped her through her ordeal. Her husband, Peter, had completed suicide three years earlier. Sally's relationship with Peter spanned over 25 years and by all measures seemed to be a very loving, healthy one. Together they had two grown children, a son and a daughter, and Peter had two children from a previous marriage. Sally was proud to mention that she still maintains a close and valued relationship with Peter's children.

As we began our interview, Sally showed me a picture of Peter. He was a very handsome man with a slender stature and thick graying hair. I remember his refined facial features and sculpted jaw line with a kindly look in his eyes. Peter could have been described as a wealthy man with several financially successful businesses. Sally said, "He was a person who seemed to have it all." He did not appear to have any significant problems with depression until he decided to sell one of his businesses. Shortly thereafter he began to experience some financial difficulties that accelerated his depression and eventual demise.

Suicide is a very difficult story to retell, which is perhaps why Sally spoke more of Peter's life and illness than of the way in which he died. However, in excruciating detail she did take a few minutes to describe how he shot himself in the throat, her first agonizing look at the sight of his body, the memory that it has forever embedded, and the many unanswered questions that will always swirl in her mind.

Today, Sally and her family are still wrestling with the settlement of Peter's estate and a legal dispute over a significant life insurance policy. It is unknown how long it will take for these matters to be rectified. Peter's death not only caused unimaginable emotional trauma and loss for Sally and her family, but it also created extreme financial hardships. Despite these very unfortunate circumstances, Sally and her loved ones appear to be coping in a reasonable and healthy way. Sally attributes this to the kind and generous support received from extended family, friends, and colleagues.

As a researcher who was given the privilege of hearing her story, I might suggest that at least part of her ability to cope is testimony to the resilience of her spirit and her desire to make some semblance of meaning from her tragedy. Neither she, nor her family members, seemed embittered or jaded by their experiences, although they understandably admitted moments of anger, regret, and sadness.

Sally's stories revealed some similar themes when contrasted to Frank's. Both began their stories by telling how they first met and fell in love with their spouses. When asked what story about Peter that Sally most wanted to share, she said in a tender, quiet tone:

> I like to tell the story of who he was when we got married.... One of the things that attracted me to him was his love of life. He loved the sunset, he loved the beach, the water, he loved flowers... he just loved life. He loved to travel. He loved people. He was very spontaneous. He would call me up and say, "Don't worry about dinner. I have something planned." And then he'd pack a picnic dinner and we would go somewhere. And then when he was really ill with depression he didn't want to do anything.

Unanswered Questions. Sally also noted that Peter was a devoted husband and father and that fact made his final act an even more difficult one to digest. Because Peter in many ways had a very good life, his suicide has left many unanswered questions. Like many family members who survive the suicide of a loved one, Sally asked herself:

> What could I have done? What did I say? What did I do or what didn't I do? You play over that last day, those 24 hours over and over again. And those answers aren't there. So you just let go of those questions. It's a continuing process. But still, when you quiet yourself and reflect on that time, you have those questions. They come back....

Sally said that Peter's actions illustrated

> how a person can change so dramatically due to an illness.... Family was very important to him... extremely. And that made it even more difficult to understand how he could end his life with four children and three grandchildren and one on the way.

Loss of Identity. Sally attributed part of the reason for Peter's death to losing his sense of identity. She said that because of the changes in his business and financial status,

> he lost a lot and what he lost I believe was his identity. One of the first things we ask people is, "what do you do?" Instead of, "tell me who you are. Tell me what you enjoy, what inspires you?" And so for Peter I think that when he lost that identity that was his downfall.

Sally shared that during Peter's memorial service her minister:

> ...talked about how hard it is for people who are successful to reveal that they have failures, especially within this community where there are expectations, where people will succeed. It is one of the most difficult things to share... you've lost or you've failed somehow. They see it as failure.

Because of the ongoing litigation and the way in which Peter died, Sally and her family have not been afforded the same luxury of closure around his death that many of us experience with loved ones who pass from this life in more natural ways. Near the end of the interview Sally reminisced:

> I wonder what my life would be like if I could have stayed in my own home, taken care of what I had and only grieved the death of Peter. What would that grief be like... to focus on the grief and not the problems that were going on. I don't know what a normal grief experience is because of all the issues I had to deal with. And I feel like I've never really had closure because of the issues that are still pending. Even his estate hasn't closed. And I still have his ashes and feel almost guilty because I haven't done anything with them yet.

Transformation. Sally said of her own transformation:

> ...just getting through this has been a journey, since my faith, which is more a spiritual faith than a religion, and being with people who are very supportive, encouraging, and loving have helped me get through this. I've become more aware of what's going on and appreciate the things like the sunset. One of the things that amazed me shortly after Peter died was how much I noticed the petal on the flower, or the leaf on a tree.

Significance of Sharing the Story. After Peter's death, Sally understood that sharing these stories had many benefits:

> From the very beginning I've been very open and think part of it is because while Peter was still living he had asked me not to share and I kept so much to myself. It was like floodgates were opened and I

didn't feel I had to protect him as much. I started sharing with people I worked with, with friends about everything. It just helped me through the grieving process. I no longer felt I had to keep everything inside and what I discovered the more I talked, the more people shared with me. I was amazed in what I heard from others about their own depression or a family member who completed suicide. So my sharing opened doors for others to share.... I really felt that I needed to share what it was like for me, so that others wouldn't have to go through that. I also felt immediately I had to do everything I could to prevent others from taking their own lives.

Sally articulated the difficulty as noted earlier about discussing death and tragedy. She described how important it was for her to relate with others during her time of sorrow:

…not everyone is comfortable sharing for different reasons, they're very private or may feel that others don't want to listen. But I would suggest that they talk, that they find people they can talk to and not worry about whether they're going to be upset.... If you talk to the right people they can be comfortable.... They know their role is not to keep you from crying or keep you from thinking about the past, but their role is to just listen. The key is to find somebody or people who are good listeners who have experienced a death. I've found that when I've talked to others who have lost a loved one that there are a lot of similarities. It's somewhat comforting to know that others have felt the way you've felt.

In Sally's closing quote, she demonstrates her own unique transformation by noting that she is redefining her life without Peter:

Sometimes when I share my story it's almost like I'm sharing someone else's story… trying to discover who I am without my husband… almost looking at it as an opportunity to redefine myself… and there are times when I'm trying to find too much meaning and all I need to do is just live.

The most touching part of Sally's story came at the very end of our interview. She described how she needed people around her and their help. Friends and people she hardly knew extended true generosity and charity. After Peter's death and news traveled that her family was experiencing financial problems, she began to receive cheques and money in the mail. Unconditional acceptance of these was very difficult for Sally because she knew she could never repay these people for their acts of kindness. She and Peter were members of a social class where they were usually in the role to extend such generosity. To be on the receiving end of this kind of charity was very humbling. My sense is that Sally is far too modest of a woman to admit that this part of her story was a tribute to her character and the kind of people both she and Peter had been.

Frank and Hannah

Frank was an executive for a large multinational corporation, in his early 40's with two young sons from a previous marriage. His ability to describe his short time together with Hannah would seem to be material for the great romantic writers. It is an understatement to say that Frank's love for Hannah was extraordinary. When asked about how he and Hannah met he said:

> …I look at it as a love story, a total love story where we were with the person we were meant to be with.… I met my soul mate. We attended this training and I looked across the room and saw this beautiful woman and this smile. I was knocked on my rear from the moment I saw her.

At this time Frank knew very little about Hannah's illness. During their first lunch together he asked if she would talk about her cancer:

> The first lunch we had we sat down and I wanted to know about her cancer. Because that had to be a focus of her life, it had to be. So as soon as we sat down I said, "I'd like you to tell me about your cancer if you're comfortable. I don't know what type of cancer it is. Can you just talk about it?" I think it caught her off guard because most people don't want to talk about those things. But I understood that was important to her. The cancer for me, for us, was something that could be out in the open.

Hannah also worked at the same multinational corporation and before meeting Frank had already survived one serious bout with breast cancer. Their relationship, although only three and half years in length, seemed as full and complete as marriages and commitments of 50 or more years. I saw their relationship as testimony to Dame Cecily Saunders famous quote, "Life is a matter of depth, not length."

Selflessness. Through the eyes of Frank, one is able to see Hannah as a tremendously selfless human being. Frank repeatedly noted her acts of kindness and generosity toward others. Early in our interview Frank shared a story about Hannah that occurred three weeks before she died. She had lent a consoling hand to a couple during their first round of chemotherapy treatment. Hannah evidently could sense their fear and trepidation and took it upon herself to offer a word of comfort. Recalling that moment, Frank said:

> ...she gets up out of her chair and without even saying a word to me, walks across the room and sits down next to them. She talks for maybe five minutes to them. I have no idea what she said, I can only guess, but she walks back and there was this look of calm on their faces. It took five minutes for Hannah to do that.... That's what she did.... In her struggling to stay alive, her concern was about the couple that comes in across the hall from her. We saw this couple the next week. It was like they were best friends. This woman came up to Hannah and it was like there was this bond that wouldn't leave. And that's just who she was.... I tell this story because it conveys who she was....

He described another story about the events of September 11, 2001, and how Hannah responded on that dreadful day:

> Hannah was still working at the time. She was in her office. She came out when she heard what was going on and there were a group of people watching TV, watching what was happening, and people were devastated. But before people really knew, really were able to grasp what was happening, in fact I think it was even before the second plane, she started crying and hugging people. She grasped the humanity of that moment and the sadness long before any one else did... after she died I opened her journal and read the entry for September 11, 2002.... In that entry she was very reflective of the year before and all those people who died a year earlier. She always ended her entries with, "here is what I've been blessed with." And one of the things she was thankful for was all the firefighters and policemen who do what they do. I know people say that, but in your journal which is all about what you are completely feeling, that's what she writes. That shows the type of person she was.

After just a few months of courtship, Hannah was diagnosed with a reoccurrence of cancer. In another riveting account Frank described the day she was informed of the cancer.

> Three days before Christmas she had gone to the doctor because she had had pain in her shoulder. She got a bone scan and she got the results and called me at work. I took the afternoon off and we both went to my apartment and just held onto each other all afternoon... and we cried and held each other.... We didn't say much at all. There was very little conversation. And then she said, "I can't burden you with my cancer."

Frank replied to her:

> You would burden me more without you in my life. If I could have
> you for three months, six months, a year, I would do it in a heart
> beat.... She chose to finish her life out with me whether it was 20
> years or 1... and we lived with hope.

Several months later, in a very private wedding ceremony on a beach, Frank and Hannah were married. A little more than a year later, she died in a hospital with Frank at her side. Frank admits that journaling has helped with his grief process: "When Hannah died I turned to writing to get my thoughts out. When I would have memories of her, I'd write because I'm fearful of losing my memories."

Faith and Suffering. Frank and Hannah clearly were good, decent, kind human beings. They were both intelligent and very thoughtful about their spiritual beliefs and convictions in the context of Hannah's dying. Frank described these along with the suffering that Hannah endured:

> As children we were not led down a certain path. We were both open-
> minded to different types of concepts from a spiritual point and had
> similar beliefs. I think she had faith that there had to be something
> beyond life. We both believed that. But you are never at a time when
> it's more important than a time like that. And at a time like that,
> doubts creep in but she had faith, and we grew together.... There
> was a journal entry in late January and she was really sick... she was
> in despair... and she did write, "I question my faith in God." But I
> think that was more a response... to her suffering.... She was more
> fearful of suffering than dying—always. What she didn't know, what
> she didn't realize, was how much she suffered before she died. She
> suffered. She really suffered.

Frank, like Sally, has questions about his loved one's death that he knows will never be answered. He discussed how he continues to struggle with the meaning that her apparent senseless suffering could have:

> Someday maybe I'll get used to the fact that there's a positive aspect
> to her death because she's not suffering anymore. And I know that's
> probably the selfless way to look at it, but right now it's still a difficult
> one for me. I quit asking why because there's no answer. I can't feel
> good today that death was her way out of suffering.... Her death
> was a good thing because she's not suffering anymore.... Well, her
> being healed would have been a better thing so that she wouldn't have
> to suffer.... That's what I hear from a lot of people, well it's good
> because she's not suffering anymore. She's in a perfect place, but you
> know what—she could have been here for 40 more years and been

healthy and then been in that perfect place. So, maybe the day will come when I can look at it with less resentment.

As a researcher and as a listener in this study, I now have some idea as to the remarkable person Hannah must have been. My hope is that I have recounted the stories accurately for my readers. Having listened to Frank's story, I wish I could have had the privilege of meeting Hannah. What I think Frank may not have grasped yet, is his own extraordinariness and humility. As I listened to him tell his story of Hannah, not only did I gain admiration, respect, and love for her, I also experienced a sense of the veracity and depth of Frank's character. In his closing remarks, he mentioned that when you have a very close relationship with someone, you become like a mirror for each other. He said, "You literally develop a new self-identity because that person you were with was a part of yourself. They were a mirror for you and who you were."

Like Frankl: Remembering Blissful Moments. One part of Frank's story reminded me of Frankl recalling the blissful memory of his own wife. Frank said, "Those moments of bliss, when I think of the first kiss she gave me, or the walk down the river with each other, it puts me back in that time. And I've never felt better than in that time."

Power of Sharing. Like Sally, Frank recognized the importance of sharing his stories:

> I would say, "Share away." I gain a sense of comfort by talking about it. And that the person I'm talking to, sees the amazing goodness of the person I was with.... Talking to you about her is just a way for me to continue to express how I feel about her.... So when I tell stories of Hannah and how we met and about the progression of her cancer— even talking about the things that are horrific in terms of the last day, the last week—for me, it's a way of dealing with those emotions.

Transformation. Near the end of our interview, Frank admitted that because of his life without Hannah, he is now experiencing a personal transformation. To preserve her memory he has started a foundation to benefit cancer patients. He frequently visits the cancer clinic where Hannah received treatments and gives beautiful bracelets to breast cancer patients in hopes of lifting their spirits. He admits:

> My experience with Hannah both when she was alive and now after she's died, I have the understanding of what these women are going through at least from a support person's perspective.... I can talk to them in an open way, in an understanding way of what they are going through. I got that from my experience with Hannah. But I

also have now, which I didn't have when Hannah was alive, a level of compassion that I never had before in my life... Every time I walk out of the clinic, I feel 100 percent better because it's an amazing thing to see goodness in people that I've never seen before. I see the goodness in people....

Despite Frank's obvious pain and sadness he admitted, "there is good that can come from this."

WHY STORIES ARE TOLD

So why do we tell stories? What do we learn from stories, and how do stories and their telling transform us? In the context of telling stories about a death, the participants in this study have artfully expressed some of their answers to these questions.

Sally and Frank have retaught us that we tell stories and listen to them to know that we are not alone. Stories help us to rekindle the flame of our loved one's life when we begin to feel it flicker from our memory. We tell stories to pass on values, traditions, and memories of events and people. We tell stories to share something of ourselves. We tell stories to preserve a sense of family, culture, and personal legacy. We tell stories for merriment and enjoyment. We tell stories to grieve. We tell stories to remember and to keep a sense of our history alive. We tell stories so we can heal and help others heal. Ultimately, we tell stories because we feel we have something of import and meaning to share. And perhaps we listen to stories for these same reasons.

Stories help Us Grieve

In a sense, the retelling of a death accommodates the grief process because it serves as a catharsis. As Sally and Frank illustrate, the teller relives the death and in some cases the life as she tells and retells the story over and over. Repetition can sooth and give solace to both the teller and the told. This may explain why traditional calling hours, wakes, funerals, memorials, delivering a eulogy, or sitting Shiva seem so important to grieving family and friends. It is a designated time created specifically for the purpose and benefit of grieved family and friends and their telling of the deceased loved one's story. At this appointed time telling the death story allows people to know that they are not alone, that other people have and will experience similar events. Although the death may have been tragic, as in both Sally's and Frank's cases, the teller may learn that one can endure this life event and future ones because one has dared to share a story with someone else who was willing to hear. While these rituals may provide comfort and solace for the storyteller who has experienced a death, such rituals may also imbue the listener.

For those who have never met the deceased, a retelling of the death is certain to reveal meaningful aspects of their life thereby allowing the deceased to live on in the hearts and memories of those who have heard their story.

CONCLUSION

In this paper I have attempted to illustrate that the telling of a death story creates meaning and can lead to personal transformation. Through the use of Roemer's (1995) work and the stories from my participants, it is clear that death can sanction a story. Furthermore, the stories told by Sally and Frank affirm the thinking of Frankl (1985): Even under miserable circumstances one can make considerable meaning.

The themes of meaning found in the stories of Sally and Frank, although different, appeared to expose similarities. Both discussed their reasons for falling in love with their spouses. Both discussed how their spouses suffered, Hannah in a more physical way and Peter in the form of an internal torment. Sally and Frank also described their own continuing personal growth and transformation: Sally in redefining herself without her husband and Frank through his ability to reach out to others and to recognize the "goodness" in new people who enter his life. And both admitted their need to share their story with others as they grieve.

For the last several minutes I have been a storyteller. Until a few moments ago you had no conception of Sally and Peter or Frank and Hannah. Yet, through the stories I have told, they now reside in your heart and memory. One of the most significant lessons this study confirmed is how necessary it is to tell our loved one's story. The greatest way to diminish another human being is not to inflict physical or emotional pain, or even death, but rather it is to silence their story.

I would like to conclude with a short story about a former faculty member I knew in graduate school. I have since lost contact with her, but she had a fond affection for narrative research and once shared a lovely metaphor that seems appropriate to mention in this context. She noted that physicists use an instrument called a cloud chamber to study subatomic particles. The amazing phenomenon is that this sophisticated instrument can never grasp the actual particle, but instead it catches the traces that are left behind. That is what storytelling does. The life experiences and events, like the subatomic particles can never again be grasped, but the traces they leave behind become the nourishment for our stories.

Perhaps when the time comes for our light to be extinguished from this life and our breath leaves the shell of our body, we can rest knowing we have seeded the beginnings of meaningful traces. In the end we hope that it can be said we have lived and died well and with meaning so that those we leave behind will have a reason for sharing our stories, for every death is worthy of a thousand tellings.

References

Frankl, V. (1985). *Man's search for meaning.* New York: Washington Square Press.

Kübler-Ross, E. (1997). *The wheel of life: A memoir of living and dying.* New York: Touchstone.

Levine, S. (1982). *Who dies?* New York: Anchor.

McDonald, J. E. (1997). The spirit of meaning through the surrender and catch of death: A phenomenological study of three hospice families (Doctoral dissertation, The Fielding Graduate Institute, 1998). *Dissertation Abstracts International, 276.*

Roemer, M. (1995). *Telling stories.* Lanham, MD: Rowman & Littlefield.

Wong, P., & Fry, P. (1998). *The human quest for meaning.* Mahwah, NJ: Lawrence Erlbaum Associates.

The Case of "Paula":
An Existentially Based Treatment
Approach to Chronic Depression

JOANNA LIPARI

Abstract

The case of "Paula" presents a multimodal existentially based treatment approach as it was applied to a case of chronic depression. This clinical case history documented the presenting problem, case history, case formulation, and treatment.

PRESENTING PROBLEM AND RELEVANT PERSONAL HISTORY

Paula,[1] a 51-year-old divorced Caucasian female, initially presented for therapy at a university clinic in a California city for ongoing symptoms of depression and anxiety related to failed career ambitions, employment stress, and difficulties with interpersonal relationships. Paula reported an extensive history of previous psychological treatment from 1973 through 1999. The university clinic records indicated that Paula first sought treatment in 1997, and participated in cognitive-behavioral treatment from January 1997 to June 1998 (38 individual sessions). This treatment was terminated when her first therapist completed her doctoral rotation and was no longer able to provide services. Paula was transferred, without a break in continuity, to a second clinic therapist who saw Paula from September 1998 to July 1999 for a total of 37 individual sessions. When the doctoral rotation was concluding for this second therapist, Paula expressed interest in continuing therapy.

In October 1999, Paula met with me; at that time I was the third therapist Paula was assigned at a university clinic. At this time, Paula reported that she was still experiencing ongoing symptoms of depression and anxiety. Paula expressed a belief that therapy was "necessary to keep [her] together" but was losing hope that she would "ever be a normal person and have a normal life." She acknowledged that antidepressant medication assisted in reducing her depressive symptoms but believed that taking the medication made her feel like a "weak person." For this reason, Paula reported that a primary goal for therapy was the discontinuation of her psychotropic medication, but she was willing to delay any decision until our therapeutic relationship had matured. Additional therapeutic goals identified by Paula included: (a) to manage and to reduce depressive and anxious symptoms, (b) to improve her ability to form and maintain interpersonal relationships, and (c) to "get to the point where I can do my art."

Because of Paula's ongoing depressive and anxious symptomatology, coupled with a history of major depressive episodes, Paula was monitored for suicidal ideation and intent on an ongoing basis throughout treatment. Twice during treatment with this therapist, Paula experienced major depressive episodes, with each lasting approximately two to two-and-a-half weeks. Although Paula denied suicidal ideation or intent during these periods, additional care was taken to ensure safety.

GOALS OF TREATMENT

Depressive and anxious symptomatology appears ubiquitous in the outpatient clinical population. Some mental health professionals suggest that cognitive approaches that have been validated through empirical research to reduce depression and anxiety should be the treatment of choice (Beck, 1995). While this point of view is not to be discounted, existential psychotherapy suggests that the reason for depression and anxiety differs with each individual though the symptoms may appear similar (Schneider & May, 1995). Further, some causes may be due less to an event or situation (e.g., death of a loved one), and more with profound questions of identity and meaning (e.g., who am I and what am I meant to do?) (May, 1958b). In fact, empirically based practitioners point to the added efficacy of cognitive therapy, when existentially oriented questions are addressed (Addis & Jacobson, 1996). Paula's persistent depressive and anxious symptomatology, despite years of counseling and extensive treatment in both cognitive-behavioral and psychodynamic therapeutic modalities, suggested that Paula's difficulties may have become chronic and part of her characterological structure. Further, one of the most salient features of her dysphoria was the anguish she experienced by not being an artist, either in the eyes of the world, or in her ability to continue creating works. The dissolution of such a core identity left Paula with little resources to handle the stresses of the present, and to reconcile difficulties from the past.

An existential perspective was adopted to explore issues of identity, meaning, and purpose. This perspective served as a base from which to integrate other theories and techniques, primarily from the domains of cognitive behavioral and psychodynamic therapies, in order to gain additional understanding of core identity issues and address the management and reduction of her depressive and anxious symptomatology. While eclecticism sometimes appears to translate as doing whatever comes to the therapist's mind, a truly eclectic approach is actually one that seeks to utilize different approaches, such as cognitive and existential therapies, in a coordinated manner (Ottens & Hanna, 1998). This approach appeared particularly relevant in that Paula made progress and some relief of symptomatology from her previous therapies. Integration of other therapeutic interventions enabled the therapist to build on what had previously been accomplished in therapy, as well as put these interventions (e.g., cognitive assignments), within a larger context that might be more meaningful to Paula.

After rapport was established, the initial goal of treatment was to attempt a phenomenological understanding of the inner world of the client (Merleau-Ponty, 1962; Schneider & May, 1995). Therapeutically, the therapist attended to three aspects of existential therapy: (a) existential neurosis, e.g., Paula's inability to see meaning in life; (b) existential "encounter," e.g., the inner experience of the relationship between client and therapist: and (c) *kairos*, or a critical decisive point when an intervention might be more readily accepted by Paula (Ellenberger, 1958). The overarching goal of this approach is to enable the client to make life choices that are based on hopes and desires for the future, rather than a capitulation to patterns from the past (Sahakian, 1976). Specifically, in Paula's case, this meant reinforcing her artistic identity while simultaneously being empathic to her need to look for work at something that was less fulfilling, but that could support her daily living needs, and, ultimately, fund her artistry. In essence, the therapeutic questions became: How can Paula merge artistry and the need to make a living, and if that is not possible, how could the therapist enable her to live constructively with existential dysphoria?

CLINICAL FORMULATION

In deciding the best formulation for Paula's treatment, this therapist considered a number of aspects of the case. At first glance, Paula would appear a good candidate for a psychodynamic (Kohutian) approach. Clinic notes from previous therapists suggested that Paula exhibited certain behaviors that were consistent with psychodynamic formulation; namely, that Paula had a fragile self-identity, a vulnerability to fragmentation under stress, and a history suggestive of arrested emotional development. In plain language, Paula often appeared like a 3-year-old, stuck squarely in the Oedipal period, in a fierce battle with the world as "mommy," both seeking approval (merger) and independence (individuation). Thus, Paula did not experience a true sense of self, but sought others to perform a mirroring self-object function. Additionally, Paula's current social support system was extremely limited. After her divorce and some failed relationships, Paula discontinued dating and socializing. Her friendships were limited and often strained, and her relations with her family members were difficult.

Although this psychodynamic conceptualization had decided merit, it did not fully capture the complete data set from this case, i.e., that Paula identified herself as an artist, but had been unable to create art for over seven years. There are two striking issues stemming from the data. First, Paula's core self was so fragile that it ceased operations (not painting), becoming disowned, and second, that the particular "self" with which she identified was dissuaded from revival because it was a "self" (the artist) that was not necessarily supported by the American culture of which Paula was a part. Existential theory is heuristic and aptly addresses this issue of personal meaning, as well as the responsibility of the individual to make choices and exercise personal freedom to create the life she or he deems is worth living (Yalom, 1980). In essence, the individual is torn between ontological anxiety (fear of the future and the unknown), and ontological guilt (regret at what might have been) in her or his struggle to become fully authentic (true to her or his own being) (Heidegger, 1962). From this theoretical perspective, the inauthentic person is one who runs away from personal and individuating choices, eschews personal freedom and responsibility, and capitulates to a worldview that may or may not be in accord with her or his own personal ideals (Heidegger, 1962). The aptness of this conceptualization for Paula is highlighted by her own continued report in clinical records that she felt "out of step" with the world around her, particularly her family, that never supported her artistic passions. Therefore, it was hypothesized that Paula's depressive and anxious symptomatology stemmed from Paula's accentuated sense of ontological guilt for what might have been, but was now too afraid to choose, resulting in an inability to tolerate ontological anxiety.

This formulation in no way negated the substantive psychodynamic formulation outlined above. In fact, an existential conceptualization only deepened the meaning and understanding of the psychodynamic one. That the two conceptualizations could operate simultaneously and be integrated into a singular approach is supported by the work of Otto Rank, who interpreted psychodynamic concepts such as attachment and individuation as being in part existential dilemmas, namely fear of death (limitedness through merger) and fear of life (anxiety about separating and individuating) (Becker, 1973). Thus, formulating Paula's case by using an existential approach appeared to be the most appropriate because it could capture the richness of Paula's difficulties as well as her phenomenological experience, while affording the therapist a flexible, structural theoretical framework with which to approach the therapeutic situation.

COURSE OF TREATMENT

Paula participated in 65 weekly psychotherapy sessions from 1999 through 2001 at the university counseling center. Diagnostically, Paula met the criteria for dysthymic disorder, early onset (300.4) and generalized anxiety disorder (300.2) within the *Diagnostic and Statistical Manual of Mental Disorder,* 4th ed. (DSM-IV). Paula also had a history of major depressive disorder, but did not meet *DSM-IV* criteria at the time of intake with this therapist.

In the first two sessions, Paula discussed her disappointment that "years of therapy" had not "fixed" her psychologically. She expressed discouragement regarding the therapeutic process, especially because she felt she had "tried so hard" to learn through the process. I suggested to Paula that there might be another way to look at therapy, rather than as being solely remedial, that is, trying to correct problems and "fix neuroses." Instead, this work might better be conceptualized as being exploratory, creative, and life enhancing. In essence, it was suggested that Paula consider therapy as chronicling the progress of becoming a "hero" in her own life.[2] Paula responded to this conceptualization by stating that it gave her a sense of renewed hope, and made her feel like she was not "damaged goods."

This initial positive response to an overarching existential concept suggested that this approach might benefit Paula. In the next two sessions, the therapist assisted Paula in exploring her thoughts and feelings about her artwork and the possible connection to her present state. Paula reported her problems stemmed from her mother, who never approved of her artistic ambitions and who "only prepared [Paula] to be somebody's wife." Paula believed that her relationship with her mother contributed to an ongoing *Weltschmerz,*[3] in that she believed what she desperately wanted most in life as an artist was impossible in a world that expected her to be "a good working stiff and somebody's wife." During an exploration of Paula's sense of personal meaning (i.e., Paula was an artist living in America), Paula revealed that she had not drawn, or painted, or created any piece of art for over seven years. She stated that when she thought of getting her art supplies out of the closet, she felt intensely "nauseous."

At this point, while the focus remained existential in that the existential issues of identity, personal meaning, freedom, and choice were central in the session, a multi-theoretical technique approach was employed to guide Paula on this journey. For example, cognitive restructuring (Meichenbaum, 1977) was introduced as a technique to actively challenge and reorient Paula's defeating self-talk. Further, because Paula's sense of self was tenuous at this juncture, techniques from Kohutian theory, such as mirroring and monitoring of disintegration anxiety and fragmentation (Wolf, 1988) provided the therapist concrete tools to assist in strengthening Paula's sense of self and enable her to forge ahead with our existential explorations. In other words, when the intensity of the existential issues made it difficult for Paula to "stay in the room" psychologically, these additional techniques and theoretical concepts would assist the therapist in providing concrete respite, as well as an opportunity to increase resiliency. Invariably, Paula would reorient through these techniques and then be willing, and, indeed, curious to proceed with deeper discussions. In subsequent sessions, Paula expressed feeling stronger, more resilient and eager, and "less like a loser," although she still experienced ongoing anxiety and depression related to work and interpersonal relationships.

As the sessions progressed, small art assignments, such as sketching on plain paper with a pencil, were initiated. During this phase of treatment, her anxiety and depressive symptoms would vary in intensity, in part due to situations regarding employment searches. By Session # 10, Paula had created her first piece of art, a pen-and-pencil drawing. This creation represented a turning point in therapy, a *kairos*. From this point forward (approximately mid-December 1999), Paula began to explore her feelings of depression and anxiety within the context of her renewing identity as an artist. This context provided Paula with the "root" she was seeking previously. She reported that before embarking on an understanding of personal meaning vis-à-vis her art, she had felt like "an amoeba swimming aimlessly in a sea of depression." Now, however, she understood her symptoms as part of a larger existential crisis. This understanding gave her a feeling of hope for the future, although she acknowledged feeling "very scared" about the challenges facing her.

During the middle phase of treatment, Paula continued creating art, although inconsistently. When experiencing anxiety and/or depression regarding the stress of work situations or interpersonal relationships, Paula would cease doing her artwork. At this point, the therapist introduced therapeutic techniques from other disciplines that were more aggressive inasmuch as Paula's sense of identity was growing in definition, strength and resiliency. The first added technique was the disputation of irrational beliefs, which is a cognitive technique from Ellis' REBT therapy (Dryden & Ellis, 1988). This technique encourages the therapist to actively dispute and challenge the client's "irrational" beliefs about herself or himself, the environment, and the future. This technique was especially useful when Paula's anxiety would be stimulated and she would devolve into ever increasing fear and worry. Introducing the disputation of irrational beliefs assisted Paula in understanding her tendency to catastrophize beyond what was most likely going to happen. Additionally, Paula would utilize catastrophizing to regress into repressive affect as a defense against the real issue. In other words, when the issue became meaningful within the session, Paula might become anxious and fearful. Because this anxiety was uncomfortable, Paula would defend against it by "giving up" and being reduced to uncontrollable crying. Certainly, Paula was experiencing pain in those moments, but that pain was also in service of defending against facing the meaningful issues that she sought to resolve.

The second added technique comes from short-term psychodynamic therapy (Davanloo, 1988). This technique places consistent pressure on a client's defenses (e.g., anything that gets in the way of the client saying what she or he is thinking and feeling), until the client's defenses are exhausted and relinquished to the authentic thoughts and feelings. This technique was especially useful with Paula in this phase of therapy because of her tendency to digress when the therapy moved into uncomfortable areas. This deflection served to derail the emotionally laden therapeutic process. By utilizing Davanloo's (1988) technique of pressuring the defenses, Paula would be able to access the meaningful material.

In October of 2000, Paula experienced a major depressive episode, precipitated by difficulties at one of her free-lance assignments, which resulted in her being terminated. Following that job, Paula found it difficult to continue seeking employment opportunities. Despite the severity of her depressive symptoms, Paula continued to work vigorously in therapy. This depressive episode was a second *kairos* in the therapeutic course. Since Paula had experienced a relatively long period of approximately one year of feeling like she was making "progress" and had renewed hope for the future, the intensity of depression from this episode made Paula even more determined to change. Therefore, she was more open both to the depth and breadth of the existential exploration, as well as to entertaining alterations in her medication, a previously resistant topic for Paula.

Prior to the onset of this depressive episode, the therapist had been concerned that Paula's complaints of gastrointestinal distress might be related to the type of antidepressant medication she was taking. After the severity of depressive symptoms abated, Paula agreed to a consultation and ongoing pro bono treatment with a psychiatrist arranged by the therapist. This psychiatrist performed a complete psychiatric evaluation on Paula and determined that in fact, the Zoloft might have been the cause of her stomach upset. Her medication was switched at that time to Prozac (20 mg). Within 3 weeks, Paula's stomach problems disappeared. In addition, Paula reported feeling "better," with improved mood consistently throughout the day. She has continued taking this medication at this dosage to the present.

At this time, Paula moved into an important new phase of existential development. She began regularly producing art. Paula also outlined hopes, dreams and goals for the future, and began to acknowledge her role as creator of her life by accepting the role of responsibility, freedom, and choice as determinants of one's life (May, 1958a). She initiated interpersonal relationships with members of her family with whom she had not spoken, most notably with a nephew. This new relationship with her nephew, his wife, and their small toddler-age child resulted in Paula experiencing a new role as "aunt" which gave her immense joy. Although Paula would experience anxiety about this deepening involvement with family members, she nevertheless continued to pursue the relationships, which have grown considerably over the past year.

In the summer of 2001, Paula experienced her second major depressive episode while in treatment with this therapist. Again, the precipitant was work related. Paula felt defeated by the stress of a deadline-laden free-lance job, and she devolved into depression. This depression lasted exactly two weeks and was markedly different from her previous depressive episodes. Paula related in therapy that she was aware that it was an "episode" while it was happening, that it was finite, and that she could "bounce back." These realizations were a major shift in Paula's previous views of herself.

During the 25 months of treatment, Paula has increasingly become more confident with her identification as an artist as well as feeling more able to handle her ongoing dysphoria and, at times, major depressive episodes. Ultimately, therapy has been about Paula learning to accept, like, and live with who she is and the world as it is, rather than remediating flawed aspects of herself to fit some imagined profile of "normal." Paula reports understanding that, though she has a tendency to become anxious and depressed, these feelings are only a facet of who she is, an attribute with which she can learn to adjust and actually use in a positive sense. As she has jokingly explained in a session, "You [the therapist] are short, and I'm depressed. So what."

CRITICAL EVALUATION

This was a challenging, rewarding, and instructive case. My overall evaluation of my handling of this case is that I have made more mistakes than I should have, made less interventions than I could have, and benefited the client more than I would have, had I not undertaken an aggressive, integrative approach. Although I would like to take credit for the immense progress this client has made, I cannot.

Her improvement has been solely through her own willingness and determination to construct a life of her own choosing.

References

Addis, M. E., & Jacobson, N. S. (1996). Reasons for depression and the process and outcome of cognitive-behavioral psychotherapies. *Journal of Consulting and Clinical Psychology, 64*(6), 1417-1424.

Beck, J. S. (1995). *Cognitive therapy: Basics and beyond.* New York: Guilford Press.

Becker, E. (1973). *Denial of death.* New York: Free Press.

Campbell, J. (1971). *A hero with a thousand faces.* Princeton, NJ: Princeton University Press.

Davanloo, H. (1988). The technique of unlocking the unconscious, Part I. *International Journal of Short-Term Psychotherapy, 3,* 123-159.

Dryden, W., & Ellis, A. (1988). Rational-emotive therapy. In K. S. Dobson (Ed.), *Handbook of cognitive-behavioral therapies* (pp. 214-272). New York: Guilford Press.

Ellenberger, H. (1958). A clinical introduction to psychiatric phenomenology and existential analysis. In R. May, E. Angel, & H. Ellenberger (Eds.), *Existence: A new dimension in psychiatry and psychology* (pp. 92-126). New York: Basic Books.

Heidegger, M. (1962). *Being and time* (J. Macquarrie & E. Robinson, Trans.). New York: Harper & Row.

Kohut, H. (1984). *How does analysis cure?* Chicago: University of Chicago Press.

May, R. (1958a). Contributions of existential psychotherapy. In R. May, E. Angel, & H. Ellenberger (Eds.), *Existence: A new dimension in psychiatry and psychology* (pp. 3791). New York: Basic Books.

May, R. (1958b). The origins and significance of the existential movement in psychology. In R. May, E. Angel, & H. Ellenberger (Eds.), *Existence: A new dimension in psychiatry and psychology* (pp. 3-36). New York: Basic Books.

Meichenbaum, D. (1977). *Cognitive behavior modification: An integrative approach.* New York: Pergamon.

Ottens, A. J., & Hanna, F. J. (1998) Cognitive and existential therapies: Toward an integration. *Psychotherapy: Theory, Research, Practice, Training, 35*(3), 312-324.

Sahakian, W. S. (1976). Philosophical psychotherapy: An existential approach. *Journal of Individual Psychology, 32*(1), 62-68.

Endnotes

1. For purposes of confidentiality and anonymity, the name of the client has been changed, with "Paula" serving as the pseudonym. Further, identifying facts in this case have also been changed to ensure confidentially.

2. The allusion is to the work of Joseph Campbell (1971), author of *Hero with a Thousand Faces* and other works regarding the use of myth. His work was made generally popular by the PBS Bill Moyer's series on television.

3. The term *Weltschmerz* was coined by Jean Paul Sartre in 1827, meaning "world pain."

Swallowed Alive by the Grief Beast: An Autobiographics of Healing

TARA HYLAND-RUSSELL

Abstract

Trauma and bereavement lead to a sense of fragmentation and disconnectedness from self, others, and the narrative threads that connect the past and the future. Writing about traumatic experiences is associated with improvements in physical and mental health. This paper explores the relationship between writing and the processing of grief in two autobiographical grief narratives and suggests using grief narratives as models to facilitate the healthy processing of grief. A practice of *autobiographics of healing* can validate feelings of loss, permit safe expression of grief, position the bereaved as witness and auditor, and facilitate healthy grieving.

I write because I cannot put aside the urgency of myself being mine known by me and intervening in that which hurts me day after day. So that I won't succumb to madness or delirium. Silenced words / absent words. I write; I weigh my words. I figure into the balance. I sink deep into myself in order to understand. (Brossard, 1988)

"I write... so that I won't succumb to madness or delirium.... I write... in order to understand," says Nicole Brossard (1988) in *The Aerial Letter*. We write to begin to know that which we do not yet know. We write to understand in the face of great pain and we write to find a way of living on despite the pain. We write to find meaning and solace. And in the end, we may meet ourselves through the writing act.

When we experience a traumatic event, one of the things that happens is that we lose a sense of the interconnectedness of life; we feel fragmented and lose our sense of significance in the world (Felman & Laub, 1992). We become disconnected from ourselves and the truths we hold about our lives. When someone close to us dies, for instance, the understanding we have held about ourselves, our relationship to that person, our future, and the rest of our lives, is broken. The ways in which we relate to the world and anticipate our lives unfolding no longer fit with the realities we are experiencing. We are bereft, disconnected not only from the physical presence of that person, but also from the invisible ties that connect us to our past and into the future—the narrative threads.

How do we go on in the face of overwhelming loss? How do we begin to negotiate a different understanding that makes some sense of the trauma? And how can we help others who face their own losses? We make sense of our lives through the stories we believe about ourselves and those around us. As Paul Ricoeur (1991) relates, "We equate life to the story or stories we tell about it. The act of telling or narrating appears to be the key to the type of connectedness that we evoke when we speak...of the 'interconnectedness' of life" (p. 77). I believe it is through finding and shaping language for the "silenced words / absent words" of loss and grief that we can find our ways back into significance and wholeness, a particular way of using language that I call an "autobiographics of healing." I read the languaged contours of grief through two works: "Hiding from the Grief Beast" (Hyland, 2002) and *lamentations* (Diehl-Jones, 1997) and suggest some implications of using language as a healing agent.

HIDING FROM THE GRIEF BEAST

"Hiding from the Grief Beast" (Hyland, 2002), a poem written soon after the death of the author's mother, offers a potent metaphor for the tangible presence of grief that threatens to overwhelm the bereaved. In an attempt to try to insulate herself from the trauma of a sudden and violent bereavement, the speaker imagines wrapping herself in the comfort of a steaming cup of coffee and the sweetness of a cherry tart:

> Small round table.
> Cherry tart oozing from
> under its brown sugar crumble.
> Steaming hazelnut vanilla coffee
> Fragrance I can wrap myself in. (Hyland, 2002, p. 28)

The comfort offered by the familiar ambience of the coffee shop is not enough, however, to insulate the speaker from the terror of her grief. The figure of the

"Grief Beast" dominates the poem; grief is figured as ravenous, monstrous, and on the prowl. The speaker fears the gaping maw of the beast that lurks, waiting to devour her, fears dissolving utterly into insignificance:

> If I concentrate on this feast-treat
> I won't see the
> black maw that is waiting for
> me on the other
> side of the table. (Hyland, 2002, p. 28)

The speaker is unable to confront her loss directly, unable to grapple with the ramifications of the loss that prompt the poem's creation, but expresses a clear need to avoid the "grief beast," fearing the violence that might erupt through a close encounter with the intense emotions that threaten to overwhelm her.

The loved one who has died is figured only through her absence in the poem; her severed relationship with the speaker is likewise unrepresented. Rather, the poem's focus is on maintaining a fragile kind of balance in the face of an unnamed loss, a balance that depends on the community of friends surrounding and supporting the speaker:

> you are the keepers
> of my soul,
> my sanity (Hyland, 2002, p. 28)

A sense of passive acceptance pervades the poem as the speaker waits upon and relies on the advice and support of friends to get her through the acute phase of bereavement. A circle of protection is drawn around the speaker, harboring her until she is ready to deal with her grief. She is aware of the grief beast's presence, but she has settled in to rest and wait, "as the beast prowls." The passive waiting experienced by the speaker and the sense of unreality that pervades the poem, as evidenced by the initial focus on the coffee and treat, are symptoms of the first stage of grief commonly experienced, that of shock (Bowlby, 1980). While the passage through grief is highly individual (Schuchter & Zisook, 1993), grieving is always situated within a sociocultural context. While our North American, Western, culture accommodates an overt and public acknowledgement of death through funerals and memorial services, the mourning period is seldom publicly marked past that point. Nor do we have well-developed symbolic or ritualistic practices to mark grieving and to assist people through the mourning process. Yet there are some languaged practices we can access to narrate our losses—those "silenced words/absent words"—that may help the bereaved move beyond through the full range of grief reactions and regain some equilibrium.

LAMENTATIONS: LANGUAGING INFANT LOSS

In *lamentations*, a sequence of linked lyric poems, Charlene Diehl-Jones (1997) turns to language as a way to cope with the premature delivery and then death six days later of her infant daughter. Diehl-Jones found language was the means through which she could meet an urgent need to locate herself and to find some meaning for the inexplicable loss that had suddenly capsized her world and turned it into a wilderness of grief. "To be overtaken by sorrow is," says Diehl-Jones (2002) in a separate article, "in a provocative way, to be hijacked by wilderness, an internal, unruly, uncivil country that is barely inhabitable by the grief-stricken... Attending to the character of this unruly interior might tell us something about the qualities of wilderness, & configuring sorrow in terms of wilderness might, in turn, open up the discourses of grief" (Diehl-Jones, 2002, p. 1).

I follow Diehl-Jones' (2002) advice to "attend to the character of this unruly interior" of grief by reading the terrain of her *lamentations* not only to become more aware of the landscape of grief but also to explore and illuminate the relationship between writing and the processing of grief.

Lamentations offers Diehl-Jones' (1997) account of mourning and constructs a song of grief, an elegy for her lost daughter and their prematurely severed relationship. A lament is "an (esp. passionate) expression of sorrow or anguish" (*The New Shorter Oxford English Dictionary*, Vol. 1., 1993, p. 1523) and the five sections of Diehl-Jones' text, "the body," "dream-texts," "storms," "prairie winter," and "lullaby," speak passionately of the layered and multivocal sorrows of the speaker's grief. Through the disconnected segments of the text, Diehl-Jones (1997) signals to us the unexpected nature of grief, its unmappable territory, and the awful place of fear that confronts us when we face our grief. Even the frontispiece and title page of each section signal to us through their physical structure the difficulty of mapping grief. The expanses of white space map the limitless terrain of Diehl-Jones' mother-grief while the ghostly subtext speaks of the deep, aching layers of her pain.

In *lamentations'* (Diehl-Jones, 1997) opening sequence, subtitled "the body," the mother approaches her grief for her infant daughter through a failure of language. The speaker simultaneously focuses on her maternal body's connection with her unborn child and the insufficiency of language to encompass or adequately express the loss of her child:

> like a child's toy a body
> nests inside another
> the world a swaying
> preposition to reorient
> the spine

...
oh daughter I
mark the loss of you
both of us ciphers now
hiding in a language we cannot
speak each day
I reinvent
a world without (Diehl-Jones, 1997, p. 3)

The intensely personal apostrophe "oh daughter," directs the poetic address to the absent infant and vividly conjures her presence despite the lack of sufficient language to speak grief. The ambiguity of the last phrase of the first page gestures toward the instability of the mother's relation to the exterior world, the world without, and with her grief. The object of the phrase is left unstated, "I reinvent/a world without" (Diehl-Jones, 1997, p. 3)—without her daughter, without being a mother (for how can one be a mother without a child?), and without the life together she thought they would have.

Though the speaker's identity as a mother has no firm place in language, her body understands its role and tries to protect her child, shielding her from harm, even if only through insufficient language:

motherbody curls around
the absent infant.
Invents fragile compartments to hold
the stuttering moment. (Diehl-Jones, 1997, p. 4)

"Dream-texts" follows and releases fragments of nightmarish excursions into the unruly interiors of grief. The dream-texts Diehl-Jones records are hers and the images were so painful that she did not even know if she could write them (personal communication, June 22, 2004), but it was precisely the urgent need to find a way to deal with the horrific aspects of her dreams that led her to begin shaping her grief into language. Diehl-Jones recalls: "And those are all of my nightmares. Some of them... I still find harrowing and I remember the feeling waking out of those dreams where it was this strange mix of being wrung out because it's just too awful to think of and kind of exhilarating because in a way there had been some kind of framing offered to me" (personal communication, June 22, 2004).

In one dream, a failed picnic serves raw hamburger, smeared grapes, and warm macaroni salad; in another the speaker addresses herself "madwoman/savant" as she displaces her frustrated mother-longing into the symbol of an empty carriage and her grief onto imagined onlookers:

I will spend my life pushing
an empty carriage
people will avert their eyes
mutter & weep (Diehl-Jones, 1997, p. 12)

Throughout these dream-texts, the author wrestles with the shock of under-standing her daughter's precipitous life and shortly thereafter death. Part of her emotional protest is bound up in the dilemma of being a mother who has lost a child and yet not being a mother because, after all, she doesn't have a baby. In an intensely poignant expression of lost maternity, another dream-text offers but fails to supply solace to the infant at the most fundamental and physical level:

a child weeps
inconsolable
i realize
i could nurse a child
i am awkward unpracticed
knead my breast
to coax the milk
i am expansive
maternal
& suddenly my nipple
tears off
the flesh disintegrating
into stringy pulp
in my hand (Diehl-Jones, 1997, p. 14)

This harrowing image of her disintegrating nipple speaks eloquently of the unanticipated and violent rending of the mother's bond with her infant. Psycholo-gists who study grief note that sudden, violent, unexpected, or other "unnatural" or "untimely" forms of dying like this infant death interfere with the grieving process (Rando, 1994). Higher than normal degrees of unresolved loss and "intrusive, vivid, repetitive images" obstruct the bereaved person's ability to cognitively process her loss (Middleton et al., 1993, p. 55).

When Diehl-Jones struggled with writing down the disturbing dream-images, a friend encouraged her to write the dreams as they were, to "make it as awful as it needs doing" (personal communication, July 2004). The act of writing the dreams helped Diehl-Jones to separate what was real from what was not, to capture the nightmarish feelings and to sort the feelings from the fear.

I could see that it was me and that it wasn't me.... I think that's where
it all started. I had all these terrible nightmares and... I woke up
and thought I knew everything about them and I thought I have to

make notes about them because it's too awful and these are obviously important to me.... I felt there was something sort of big to happen and I could start to see that the person who was suffering so much in the dreams was me and not me. (personal communication, June 22, 2004)

Diehl-Jones wrote to understand what was going on, and to try to manage her nightmarish visions before they overwhelmed her. What she found was that the process of writing them down helped contain her out-of-control feelings, helped her feel both "me and not me." In a very profound way, this is what autobiographics provides—a way of feeling our emotions, of accessing them and of finding a perspective that allows us to be present in the narrative but also to stand outside the narrative as a separate witness.

AUTOBIOGRAPHICS

The term *autobiographics* comes from Leigh Gilmore's (1994) work that addresses reading practices necessitated by nontraditional autobiography or life writing. Autobiographics describes:

> those elements that... mark a location in a text where self-invention, self-discovery, and self-representation emerge within the technologies of autobiography.... Autobiographics, as a description of self-representation and as a reading practice, is concerned with interruptions and eruptions, with resistance and contradiction as strategies of self-representation. (Gilmore, 1994, p. 42)

Autobiographics present fragmented, spiral, and complex iterations of ordinary lives and events and resists the representation of a singular autobiographical subject but instead figure a much more complex understanding of self in process.

Multiple and even contradictory aspects of self in process are essential notions when addressing grief, as the journey through the inhospitable terrain of grief is complex, individual, and varied. As Stephen Shuchter and Sidney Zisook (1993) note, "Grief is not a linear process with concrete boundaries but, rather, a composite of overlapping, fluid phases that vary from person to person" (p. 23). Psychologists differentiate between healthy and pathological grieving and have recently amended the "normal" time span of grief from several weeks or months to a much longer period. In fact, some investigators suggest that a "timeless" emotional involvement with the deceased (Marcia Kraft Goin, as cited in Schuchter & Zisook, 1993) reflects a healthy attachment.

If grief is indeed so complex and fluid, then it only makes sense that it requires a kind of language that is itself nonlinear, open, and multivocal. Thus the speaker in Diehl-Jones' *lamentations* is willing to allow the varied and difficult parts of her grieving self to collide within one text. She resists any impulse to impose a narrative closure on her text but admits the untameability of this wilderness of grief and the brokenness of her self and her narrative. We understand the brokenness for what it is: a loss that cannot be mended, only acknowledged and mourned. And we learn at some level that grieving is about feeling the pain, and going on despite knowing that it will not go away.

Diehl-Jones' elegy sings to us the particulars of her loss, yet her journey speaks powerfully to others and their own personal grief. She reports that each time when she delivers her text at a public reading, the audience responds with its own stories of loss:

> I am now the carrier of probably one hundred stories of lost babies. Everywhere I go when I am that writer, I have people coming up and telling me stories about miscarriages and... they are very much about beginning their own narrative project and I then become an auditor for them. (personal communication, June 22, 2004)

This very personal response to life writing is not unique to grief narratives; people are naturally called into a personal relationship with autobiographical texts, even outside the therapeutic context. For instance, every time when I teach an autographical or life writing text in my university literature class, some students inevitably write in response vividly personal accounts, often disclosing significant events for the first time. Some recent research on expressive writing suggests some of the dynamics behind this response.

Since 1986, James Pennebaker and associates have explored the effects of expressive writing on people's health and behavior. Typically experimental subjects "write about assigned topics for 3 to 5 consecutive days, 15 to 30 min. each day" (Pennebaker, 1997, p. 162), with the experimental group required to write about their "very deepest thoughts and feelings about an extremely important issue" that has affected them.

These studies have demonstrated that the simple act of writing about one's thoughts and feelings in relation to a traumatic event—death, injury, chronic illness, job loss, beginning college—is related to: improved health and well-being; a decrease in physician visits (Greenberg & Stone 1992; Greenberg, Wortman, & Stone 1996; Pennebaker & Francis 1996), positive effects on blood markers of immune function (Pennebaker et al., 1988; Esterling et al., 1990; Lutgendorf et al., 1994; Petrie et al., 1995; Christensen et al., 1996), a rise in grade point average, lower rates of work absenteeism, and a decrease in long-term distress and negative affect (Greenberg & Stone, 1992; Pennebaker & Beall, 1986; Murray & Segal, 1994).

Several theories have been offered to explain the positive effects of expressive writing, including cognitive change, habituation, and changes in working memory. "One consistent finding is that individuals who have written about emotional topics report that the experiment made them think differently about their experiences" (Campbell & Pennebaker, 2003, p. 60). Research on processing grief and traumatic experiences demonstrates the importance of cognitive appraisal. As Alfred Lange (1996) points out, "The required degree of self-confrontation is usually not achieved by merely talking about events because the most painful aspects are often avoided. Structured writing... provides an elegant and powerful method of self-confrontation" (pp. 375-6). But what is it about writing that creates this cognitive change?

It seems that when we engage in a practice of autobiographics, or engage in reading and writing practices that facilitate "self-invention, self-discovery" through "eruptions, resistance, and contradiction," we give a languaged structure to the grief and grant ourselves and others permission to explore our deepest feelings around traumatic experiences. Turning again to Diehl-Jones' *lamentations*, let's see what happens when we open ourselves to a reading practice of autobiographics.

Although it is placed near the end of *lamentations*, "prairie winter" was the first segment Diehl-Jones wrote. Its fragments are built on the expansive images of the prairie winter that had been the initial site of her grief. The images that Diehl-Jones felt, had "burrowed into [her] awareness" (private communication, July 9, 2004):

> reluctantly to settle
> into the unfamiliar bones of a melody
> distant drifts of snow
> blue in the sun
> the prairie knows by heart
> the ancient rhythms
> bitter ache sudden plenitude
> ...
> the perpetual weight of her skylover
> bellying down
> no one speaks the grace
> of winter
> shadows & grass
> barbed wire puncturing holes in the wind
> (Diehl-Jones, 1997, p. 35)

In this section the poet is only sometimes present to the fact of her loss; her grief is figured outside of her self, linked to the limitless space of the prairiescape. The images powerfully demonstrate the author's emotional estrangement from her grief as it is first carried off and then "snagged" on the sky's wake:

> a snowy owl cants off into the air
> my grief snags its wing
> stains its wake
> silver in the blue-white sky   (Diehl-Jones, 1997, p. 36)

The enormity of her loss is allowed to intrude only intermittently:

> pain requests its interval
> ventriloquy for the reluctant
> voice   one false note
> & the world folds up
> I tender my body's terrible lack
> watch fence posts march off the edge
> of the earth
> …
> drab winter birds
> skitter by accident to new patches of scrub
> pin branches in place
> the land absorbs grief
> holds it in trust
> the missing child already here (Diehl-Jones, 1997, p. 39)

Here, in Diehl-Jones' first writing of her grief, the prairie landscape sings the most potent keening, the land absorbing and holding in trust the author's grief. "I tender my body's terrible lack," she says, "tender" meaning to "offer," "present," "proffer," also to "stretch, hold forth" (*The New Oxford Shorter English Dictionary*, Vol. 2, 1993, p. 3247). The author submits her loss, tendering it to the broad prairie expanse, her focus less able to concentrate on the terrain *within* than on that *without;* her pain seemingly separates from her "numbed & wistful" self. "Tender" also means to "become tender; be affected with pity; soften; make gentle or compassionate" (*The New Oxford Shorter English Dictionary*, Vol. 2, 1993, p. 3247). And here I think Charlene Diehl-Jones gestures toward another function of the writing process: to create a means to access our emotions in a safe context and subject to our own timing; to allow ourselves to be affected with pity, softened toward our emotions; to allow ourselves gradually to feel the pain, anger, sadness, betrayal, rejection, loneliness, and loss engendered through death.

Of the bereaved, Shuchter and Zisook (1993) observe: "Faced with intense emotional anguish, a primary task is to shut off such pain. On the other hand, the disruptive changes that are the psychological and material reality of the survivor demand attention.... If the bereaved are fortunate, they will be able to regulate, or "dose," the amount of feeling they can bear and divert the rest" (pp. 30-31).

In "prairie winter," (Diehl-Jones, 1997) the land absorbs the bereft mother's grief and holds it in trust until she is ready to grapple with it, to feel its raw sting. As in the Grief Beast poem with which I began, grief is a menacing presence, but is not yet allowed its full range. Language is used in both works to dose or regulate the expression, and intense awareness, of the rawness of anguish. However, for healthy process through grief, we must at some time allow ourselves full contact with our feelings. We must allow ourselves to be "swallowed alive" by the grief beast. In *lamentations*, that occurs in the middle section, "storms."

"Storms" (Diehl-Jones, 1997) is the most fragmented portion of lamenta-tions and the most pain laden. Again, the title page signals to us the nature of the text and the emotional import behind the text, as the title is overshadowed by the welter of emotions seething beneath what is no longer a subtext, but the dominant text. The writer's potent and volatile grief pours across the page in a maelstrom of emotional turmoil:

> brain irritates comprehension folded lungs
> folding womb other stories inheld
> secrets (Diehl-Jones, 1997, p. 25)

The grieving mother "i" that has located the writer throughout the first two sections, "the body" and "dream-texts" is absent. A battery of words in bolded, staccato tercets beats out the writer's shattered being. The writer's identity is lost within the wrenching upheaval of the self abandoned, lost in grief:

> hip bone twisting a misplaced barricade
> tiny head heart of my & socket blind
> flooding poison (Diehl-Jones, 1997, p. 27)

No longer is Diehl-Jones the author keeping grief at bay. She has allowed herself to be swallowed alive by grief and she sputters out her gut-wrenching account of her descent into the maw of the beast:

> patient muscle skeleton viscera veins peel
> transparency sudden boneless afloat
> in the skin (Diehl-Jones, 1997, p. 28)

Grief is reduced to the raw and searing pain that floods in with every breath:

> mahogany cherry elm pine my father's roughened
> hands rhythmic & wood shavings sifting lungs
> rattle breath memory (Diehl-Jones, 1997, p. 29)

In "storms" Diehl-Jones grapples with the utter despair of her loss and *shows* as much as *tells* us the depths of her pain. Syntax fails. Language stutters and gasps, needing less to narrate than to graph the pain of loss, a more honest attempt to convey that which cannot be conveyed:

> blistering whiteness feathers me feather by
> feather dress & nest shapes gone body this precipice
> or vision (Diehl-Jones, 1997, p. 30)

In the graphing of the gaps that language cannot fathom, the emotion finds expression, finds weight, finds permission and a place to land. Traditional elegies have forms, shapes to contain their record of grief. Perhaps what Diehl-Jones shows us is that there is a time to abandon form to allow the expression of raw grief. There is a time to allow ourselves to be swallowed alive by the grief beast because that is the only way we can begin to heal.

Chronic and unresolved grief is related to "social or cultural 'learned' restraints on the expression of grief" (Middleton et al., 1993, p. 52). However, we can begin to shed some of our cultural constraints and can help people through their grieving by sharing texts like Charlene Diehl-Jones' (1997) *lamentations*. Such texts can help model ways of expressing grief in all its stuttering brokenness; to allow identification with the author's grief, to validate implicitly a range of feelings around death and loss; to grant permission for the expression of grief and mourning; to provide a safe, flexible and personal structure and site through which to grieve; to position the bereaved as both witness and auditor to allow the necessary distance to shape a new narrative understanding; and to access and to facilitate emotional expression to enable a healthy recovery through the stages of grief. Acknowledging the ongoing nature of grieving through a practice of autobiographics permits us and others to encounter ourselves and our losses each day, in their multiple and fragmented aspects. Others' texts will not mitigate our loss and pain, but they let us know that we are not alone in the unruly realm of grief. And they may help us to find a way to reconfigure our loss, to sing in a different register, as does Charlene Diehl-Jones (1997) when she learns to weave another song, despite her loss. And so I end with Diehl-Jones' words, a lamentation yes, but a lamentation that becomes a lullaby:

> i have wanted to speak of more
> than fear & frailty
> little one
> I have wanted to place my mother
> voice gently in your tiniest
> ear croon proof

in an upside down world
ancient songline between mother
& daughter lullabies
to weave lives
across leaps & leave takings (Diehl-Jones, 1997, p. 45)
...
i laugh for you child
you have discovered this wrecked & lovely world
against all odds
you have found
your way
i laugh
for your gifts
for your exquisite
life (Diehl-Jones, 1997, p. 49)

References

Bowlby, J. (1980). *Attachment and loss: Vol.3. Loss: Sadness and depression.* New York: Basic Books.

Brossard, N. (1988). *The Aerial Letter* (M. Wildeman, Trans.). Toronto, ON: The Women's Press.

Brown, L. (Ed.). (1993). *The new shorter Oxford English dictionary* (Vols. 1-2). Oxford, U.K.: Clarendon.

Campbell, R. S., & Pennebaker, J. W. (2003). The secret life of pronouns: Flexibility in writing style and physical health. *Psychological Science, 14*(1), 60-65.

Christensen, A. J., Edwards, D. L., Wiebe, J. S., Benotsch, E. G., McKelvey, L., Andrews, M., et al. (1996). Effect of verbal self-disclosure on natural killer cell activity moderation influence on cynical hostility. *Psychosomatic Medicine 58,* 150-155.

Diehl-Jones, C. (1997). *Lamentations.* Stratford, ON: Trout Lily.

Diehl-Jones, C. (2002, May). *Unruly Interiors: Mapping the Topography of Grief.* Paper presented at the Centre for Interdisciplinary Research in the Liberal Arts Conference, Banff, AB.

Esterling, B., Antoni, M., Kumar, M., & Schneiderman, N. (1990). Emotional repression, stress disclosure responses, and Epstein-Barr viral capsid antigen titers. *Psychosomatic Medicine 52,* 397-410.

Felman, S., & Laub, D. (1992). *Testimony: Crisis of witnessing in literature, psychoanalysis and history.* New York: Routledge.

Gilmore, L. (1994). *Autobiographics.* Ithaca, NY: Cornell University Press.

Greenberg, M. A., & Stone, A. A. (1992). Writing about disclosed versus undisclosed traumas: Immediate and long term effects on mood and health. *Journal of Personality and Social Psychology, 63,* 75-84.

Greenberg, M. A., Wortman, C. B., & Stone, A. A. (1996). Emotional expression and physical health: Revising traumatic memories or fostering self-regulation. *Journal of Personality and Social Psychology, 71,* 588-602.

Hyland, T. (2002). Hiding From the Grief Beast. *Sightlines,* Spring, 28.

Lange, A. (1996). Using Writing Assignments with Families Managing Legacies of Extreme Trauma. *Journal of Family Therapy, 18,* 375-388.

Lutgendorf, S. K., Antoni, M. H., Kumar, M. & Schneiderman, N. (1994). Changes in cognitive coping strategies predict EBV antibody titer change following a stressor disclosure induction. *Journal of Psychosomatic Research, 38,* 63-78.

Middleton, W., Raphael, B., Martinek, N., & Misso, V. (1993). In M. Stroebe, W. Stroebe, & R. Hansson (Eds.), *Handbook of bereavement: Theory, research, and* intervention (pp. 44-61). Cambridge, U.K.: Cambridge University Press.

Murray, E. J., & Segal, D. L. (1994). Emotional processing in vocal and written essays and psychotherapy. *Journal of Traumatic Stress, 7,* 391-405.

Pennebaker, J. W. (1997). Writing about emotional experiences as a therapeutic process. *Psychological Science 8*(3), 162-166.

Pennebaker, J. W. (2003). The secret life of pronouns: Flexibility in writing style and physical health. *Psychological Science,* 14(1), 60-65.

Pennebaker, J. W., & Beall, S. K. (1986). Confronting a traumatic event: Toward an understanding of inhibition and disease. *Journal of Abnormal Psychology, 95,* 274-281.

Pennebaker, J. W., & Francis, M. E. (1996). Cognitive emotional and language processes in disclosure. *Cognition and Emotion, 10,* 601-626.

Pennebaker, J. W., Kiecolt-Glaser, J. K., & Glaser, R. (1988). Disclosures of trauma and immune function: Health implications for psychotherapy. *Journal of Consulting and Clinical Psychology, 56,* 239-245.

Petrie, K. J., Booth, R. J., Pennebaker, J. W., Davison, K. P. & Thomas, M. G. (1995). Disclosure of trauma and immune response to a Hepatitis B vaccination program. *Journal of Consulting and Clinical Psychology, 63,* 787-792.

Rando, T. (1994). Complications in mourning traumatic death. In I. Corless, B. Germino, & M. Pittman (Eds.), *Dying, death, and bereavement: Theoretical perspectives and other ways of knowing* (pp. 253-271). Boston: Jones & Bartless Publishers.

Ricoeur, P. (1991). Narrative Identity. *Philosophy Today, 35*(1), 73-81.

Schucter, S., & Zisook, S. (1993). The course of normal grief. In M. Stroebe, W. Stroebe, & R. Hansson (Eds.), *Handbook of bereavement: theory, research, and intervention* (pp. 23-43). Cambridge, U.K.: Cambridge University Press.

Stroebe, M., Stroebe, W., & Hansson, R. (1993). *Handbook of bereavement: Theory, research, and intervention.* Cambridge, U.K.: Cambridge University Press.

Hardiness in Bereaved Parents Following Fetal or Infant Death

ARIELLA N. LANG
LYNNE M. MACLEAN

The death of a fetus or infant has a significant impact on many aspects of the health of bereaved parents. Critical for health professionals working with bereaved parents is the persistent question of why some family systems endure. and sometimes even thrive. when faced with normative transitions or situational stressors, while other families deteriorate and disintegrate. Researchers have tended to focus on the deleterious outcomes on the physical and psychological health and well-being of each spouse and on present and future family relationships (Mekosh-Rosenbaum & Lasker, 1995; Zeanah, Danis, Hishberg, & Dietz, 1995). In contrast, some parents report that they were able to make sense of their own existence following such a tragedy. Their loss brought them closer together and strengthened their marital relationship (Gilbert, 1996; Gottlieb, Lang, & Cohen, 1994). Although the exact situational and personal characteristics that attenuate or intensify the deleterious consequences have yet to be identified, personal resources such as hardiness have been shown to mitigate the impact of unexpected and important stressors like the death of a fetus/infant (Lang, Goulet, & Amsel, 2004; Tennen & Affleck, 1998). Hardiness may be defined as a personal resource characterized by a *sense of personal control* over the outcome of life events and hardships, such as the death of a fetus/infant, an *active orientation* toward meeting the challenges brought on by the loss, and a belief in the ability to *make sense* of one's own existence following such a tragedy (Lang et al., 2001). When situational stressors are unavoidable, the hardier person may appraise the situation differently, is more inclined to meet the challenges of life head on, is able to work through the negative effects of stress, and can actually experience personal growth in the face of adversity (Lang et al., 2001; Maddi, Koshaba, Persico, Lu, Harvey, & Bleecker, 2002).

In a recent longitudinal study of 110 bereaved couples who had experienced the death of a fetus or infant, hardiness consistently emerged as the single strongest predictor of health in bereaved mothers and fathers, both individually and as couple, over time. From a perspective of health promotion, health is a multidimensional concept, intimately connected to the family system, which is recognized as the context in which individuals learn about health (Feeley & Gottlieb, 2000). In order to enrich and complement the data gleaned from the battery of questionnaires administered in that study, audiotaped interviews were conducted with those 110 bereaved couples and formed the qualitative phase of that study. This present paper addresses the preliminary analysis from the narratives elicited in the audiotaped interviews of couples selected by their hardiness scores.

OBJECTIVES

The objectives of the qualitative phase of the study were twofold: first, to explore if and how elements of hardiness would emerge from the narratives and second, to compare the experiences and perceptions of bereaved parents (husbands and wives) with high hardiness (HH) to those with low hardiness (LH).

METHOD

Participants for the larger study (Lang et al., 2004) were recruited from seven Montreal-area university hospitals following scientific and ethical approval at each institution. Couples had experienced the loss of a baby (during pregnancy or the first year of life) within the previous 2 months, were 18 years of age or older, and were living together, within a 60 km radius of Montreal. They were visited in their homes at 2 months (T_1), 6 months (T_2), and 13 months (T_3) post-loss by an experienced nurse researcher. During each visit, couples simultaneously and independently completed a battery of questionnaires pertaining to their feelings and perceptions surrounding the loss, their relationship with their spouse, and their internal (hardiness) and external (marital and social supports) resources. Although not explicitly identified for the participants, hardiness was measured with the Lang & Goulet Hardiness Scale (LGHS) (Lang, Goulet, & Amsel, 2003), a generic 45-item instrument, which did not contain any items specific to the loss; rather it was designed to measure the three attributes of hardiness: *sense of personal control, active orientation,* and *making sense.* Following the completion of the questionnaires, couples participated jointly in a semistructured interview that was audiotaped. At T_1 couples were asked only one major question, which was about their experience with, and their perception of, their loss: "Can you tell me a little about what happened?" At subsequent visits, their reflections focused on their experiences and perceptions since the previous interview; once again, only one major question was asked: "Can you tell me about what has been happening since the last time we met?"

The audiotapes selected for this analysis were based on couples' T_1 scores on the LGHS (Lang et al., 2003), whether the interview was conducted in English, and the clarity of the voices for the purpose of transcription. Ten couples were selected; five couples, of which both husband and wife scored high on the LGHS, and five couples, of which both husband and wife scored low. The demographics in this subgroup were consistent with the larger sample (N = 110) including the type of loss that ranged from first trimester pregnancy loss to sudden infant death syndrome (SIDS). The tapes from all three time points (T_1, T_2, T_3) for each couple were transcribed verbatim. Categories were developed through an open coding process, coded into QSR/N6 and themes were analyzed using a constant comparison method. Amongst the myriad of categories identified hardiness and its components emerged from the data. As a first step, categories related to hardiness were explored with the extreme cases. Data were subjected to triangulation and disconfirmation procedures.

RESULTS AND DISCUSSION
Comparison of Couples with High and Low Hardiness

Bereaved couples in HH and LH were found to vary along the following dimensions of hardiness: *sense of personal control* and *making sense* but not along the dimension of *active orientation*. HH and LH couples discussed these issues in different ways and at different time periods in the grieving process. Even though both groups spontaneously described elements of hardiness within their narratives, HH couples generally spent considerable more time discussing themes relevant to the elements of hardiness. They expressed them more frequently and at greater length and depth than did couples with LH. Examples from HH include:

> I realize that there is nothing I could have done to change it so it wasn't in my power... it just happened and it was either we accept it and moved on or we didn't accept it and we stalled and made it more difficult for each other.

> ...the grieving process takes a long time... every month that goes by you learn something new about yourself and how much you can accept and deal with something.

HH couples were better able to attain or regain a sense of personal control. The LH couples attempted to attain it, but were often not as successful. For example:

> I asked them to wrap the baby in a blanket so I could hold her…. I didn't want to see it…. Instead they stuck her in one of the kidney dishes and put a face cloth over.

> Zero positive… ridiculous… like finding something spiritual, please! I find it ludicrously irritating that someone would want to waste their time finding something good in this situation… there is nothing good about finding your son dead in his crib… anybody who finds good in it was probably fucked up to begin with that they needed something like this to happen to find spirituality.

LH couples sometimes stayed trapped in their inability to move on, fixating on elements of the experience where they felt most out of control. They tended to stay focused on events or perceptions that caused them pain. In an examination of the coding patterns, it was evident that LH couples more often discussed themes of wanting, but not receiving, acknowledgement from others for their loss and grief, hurtful comments by others, and discussions of "the glass being half empty rather than half full."

An important finding, consistent with the larger study (Lang et al., 2004), was that the age of the baby at the time of its demise was not a distinguishing feature between the groups. Both HH and LH couples had experienced losses ranging from first trimester to SIDS. This continues to highlight the hazard of considering the baby's age in isolation of the context of the parent's perception of the event and their experience subsequently (Lang et al., 2004).

This preliminary and exploratory analysis revealed that hardiness and its components (Table 1) were evident in the narratives of each of these bereaved couples. Within the context of the total experience, couples discussed issues of *a sense of personal control, active orientation,* and *making sense* regardless of their scores on the LGHS. As their stories unfolded, elements of hardiness sprang to the forefront. The eloquence and robustness of their quotes contributed valuable insights on several fronts. First, the emergence of excerpts reflecting hardiness and its elements, without couples being questioned directly, helps to reinforce the presence and prominence of this personal resource and its conceptualization as a composite of three interdependent components (Lang et al., 2001). Moreover, it supplements the increasing evidence that personal resources may play a greater role than originally thought in the way people deal with such unexpected and important stressful situations (Campbell, Swank, & Vincent, 1991; Orr & Westman, 1990). Indeed, hardiness has been shown to be an effective personal resource, which can diminish potentially negative effects of life stress (Duquette, Kerouac, Sandhu, Ducharme, & Saulnier, 1995; Lang, et al., 2004; Maddi et al., 2002). Rather than reacting to stress only when it is unavoidable, individuals who have learned to draw this resource forth seek out change; instead of suffering the negative effects of stress, they are able to thrive in the face of adversity. The testimonials from bereaved couples in this study offer insights that help to illustrate and reinforce hardiness as an important predictor of health. Although preliminary, the results from this analysis support the notion that hardiness may help to explain differences observed in the responses of parents to the death of their baby.

Table 1
Hardiness and Its Components

SENSE OF PERSONAL CONTROL:	*ACTIVE ORIENTATION:	MAKING SENSE:
a belief in one's ability to influence the impact of a difficult situation, such as the loss of a fetus or infant through the exercise of knowledge, skill, and choice of attitude (Frankl, 1967). These elements influence the individual through the process of decision making, which may or may not be observable. The individual with a sense of personal control believes that changes brought on by life events are inevitable and provide incentives for growth.	a propensity to seek and use support as well as a willingness to consider various strategies to help cope with difficult situations, such as the death of a fetus or infant. It is a belief in the value of meeting the challenges of life head on and the inclination to do so.	an individual's propensity to find meaning in existence following an arduous event, such as the death of a fetus or infant. It is the inclination to reframe and situate the effects of a difficult situation by cognitively and/ or emotionally changing the way that they view their situation and subsequently find purpose and new meaning in existence.

*Note. There were no evident differences between HH and LH couples

STUDY LIMITATIONS AND DIRECTIONS FOR FUTURE RESEARCH

Findings from this study were part of a preliminary analysis focused on exploring the presence of hardiness in bereaved couples and to compare those with high and low LGHS scores. Further analyses over all of the data are required to achieve saturation of the concepts related to hardiness to determine if new themes emerge and to tease out how hardiness unfolds over time. Verification and triangulation are needed as well, by third party inductive coding without the concept of hardiness in mind. As well, research focusing on interventions from a variety of different treatment perspectives and health system contexts would be of interest.

In summary, elements of hardiness were present in the narratives of each bereaved couple, at each data collection point, regardless of their score on the LGHS or the age of the baby at the time of its demise. This evidence is compelling, given that the narratives were not designed to elicit aspects of hardiness and thus no specific questions pertaining to hardiness were asked during the interview. Moreover, it offers further evidence that hardiness does change over time (Lang et al., 2003; Lang et al., 2004), lending support to the argument that it is a personal resource, potentially amenable to change, and not a personality trait. This analysis was a first attempt to distinguish differences in perceived experiences between bereaving HH and LH couples. Although some differences emerged, further analyses are required.

The development of knowledge in this area is paramount for health professionals who are interested in enabling bereaved parents to draw upon and develop their hardiness in order not only to transcend the experience but ultimately to gain a sense of personal growth following the painful loss of their fetus or infant. Bereavement following the death of a child most often involves a lifelong process of grief that requires integration into the ongoing course of family health and development (Rubin & Malkinson, 2001; Shapiro, 2004). Bereavement theorists have discussed working through grief as a process of searching for and finding meaning in the loss experience (Attig, 2004; Worden, 2002). What distinguish individuals may be their life experiences as well as the manner and frequency with which they have learned to choose to draw this resource forth that influences all aspects of their life and ultimately their health. Everyone has some degree of hardiness within, which is developed over the life span and is learned to be used at different times and in different situations. Bereaved parents who learn to draw on their personal hardiness as a resource may overcome loss and perceive positive outcomes, such as personal growth and strengthening of their relationships with each other and significant others. Health professionals can enable bereaved parents to attain a sense of personal control through a variety of exercises, such as choice of attitude, an active orientation, and a willingness to consider different coping strategies. Such exercises will help them through their search for meaning following this arduous event.

References

Attig, T. (2004). Meanings of death seen through the lens of grieving. *Death Studies, 28*, 341-360.

Campbell, J., Swank, P., & Vincent, K. (1991). The role of hardiness in the resolution of grief. *OMEGA, 32*(1), 53-65.

Duquette, A., Kerouac, S., Sandhu, B. K., Ducharme, F., & Saulnier, P. (1995). Psychosocial determinants of burnout in geriatric nursing. *International Journal of Nursing Studies, 32*(5), 443-456.

Feeley, N., & Gottlieb, L. N. (2000). Nursing approaches for working with family strengths and resources. *Journal of Family Nursing, 6*(1), 9-24.

Frankl, V. E. (1967). *Psychotherapy and existentialism: Selected papers on logotherapy.* New York: Washington Square.

Gilbert, K. R. (1996). "We've had the same loss, why don't we have the same grief?" Loss and differential grief in families. *Death Studies, 20,* 269-283.

Gottlieb, L., Lang, A., & Cohen, R. (1994). *Coming to terms with infant death: Changes that couples experience.* Paper presented at the International Nursing Research Conference, Vancouver, BC.

Lang, A., Goulet, C., Aita, M., Giguere, V., Lamarre, H., & Perreault, E. (2001). Weathering the storm of perinatal bereavement via hardiness. *Death Studies, 25*(6), 497-512.

Lang, A., Goulet, C., & Amsel, R. (2003). Lang and Goulet Hardiness Scale. *Death Studies, 27,* 1-30.

Lang, A., Goulet, C., & Amsel, R. (2004). Explanatory model of health in bereaved parents post fetal/infant death. *International Journal of Nursing Studies, 48,* 869-880.

Maddi, S. R., Koshaba, D. M., Persico, M., Lu, J., Harvey, R., & Bleecker, F. (2002). The personality construct of hardiness. *Journal of Research in Personality, 36,* 72-85.

Mekosh-Rosenbaum, V., & Lasker, J. N. (1995). Effects of pregnancy outcomes on marital satisfaction: A longitudinal study of birth and loss. *Infant Mental Health Journal, 16*(2), 127-143.

Orr, E., & Westman, M. (1990). Does hardiness moderate stress, and how? A review. In M. Rosenbaum (Ed.), *Learned resourcefulness: On coping skills, self-control, and adaptive behavior* (pp. 64-93). New York: Springer Publishing.

Rubin, S. S., & Malkinson, R. (2001). Parental response to child loss across the life cycle: Clinical and research perspectives. In M. S. Stroebe, R. O. Hansson, W. Stoebe & H. Schut (Eds.), *Handbook of bereavement research: Consequences, coping, and care* (pp. 219-240). Washington, DC: American Psychological Association.

Shapiro, E. R. (1994). *Grief as a family process: A developmental approach to clinical practice.* New York: The Guilford Press.

Tennen, H., & Affleck, G. (1998). Personality and transformation in the face of adversity. In R. G. Tedeschi, C. L. Park & L. G. Calhoun (Eds.), *Posttraumatic growth: Positive changes in the aftermath of crisis* (pp. 65-98). Mahwah, NJ: Lawrence Erlbaum Associates.

Worden, J. W. (2002). *Grief counseling and grief therapy: A handbook for the mental health practitioner* (3rd ed.). New York: Springer Publishing.

Zeanah, C. H., Danis, B., Hishberg, L., & Dietz, L. (1995). Initial adaptation in mothers and fathers following perinatal loss. *Infant Mental Health Journal, 16*(2), 80-93.

Mythological Perspectives on the Journey of Death

WILLIAM E. SMYTHE

Abstract

A common metaphorical image of death is as a journey, as in the mythological motif of the night sea voyage wherein the souls of the dead are transported across the waters and beyond the horizons of the visible world. This mythological motif bears some affinities to the archetypal hero's journey, in that both involve a threshold crossing into an unknown realm beyond the world of everyday reality. The present paper describes some examples of the death-as-a-journey mythological motif drawing from Celtic mythology, Tibetan Buddhism, and contemporary sources. Although the details of the journey differ in these different traditions, all point to the embodied and heroic nature of the experience.

The journey does not end here. Death is but another path, one that we all must take.

Gandalf, *The Lord of the Rings*

The final chapter of the last book of Tolkien's (1991) *The Lord of the Rings* concludes with a very memorable scene. The venerable hobbits, Bilbo and Frodo Baggins, are at the Grey Havens about to board a white sailing vessel en route to a faraway destination in the company of the Elves. If the "Grey Havens" is a rather transparent reference to old age, then the sea voyage itself would be in reference to the passage of death, something frequently represented mythologically, as a journey.

The mythological image of the night sea voyage that transports the souls of the dead beyond the horizons of the visible world is a nearly universal mythological motif. Bilbo, at 131 years of age, is extremely old, even by hobbit standards, whereas Frodo, the main hero of the epic, is much younger. This pairing of the old man on the threshold of death with the young hero is a highly significant juxtaposition of mythological motifs. It points to the heroic dimension of death and dying and to certain affinities between the journey of death and the hero's journey. Both involve a threshold crossing into an unknown realm beyond the horizons of the everyday world. It is this confrontation with the unknown that ultimately calls for mythological understanding, for myth inevitably arises to fill those metaphorical spaces that cannot be filled by any form of direct experience or rational thought.

This paper examines some mythological renderings of the journey of death from diverse cultural traditions. Although the death-as-a-journey motif appears universally, it takes quite different forms in different mythologies.

THE CELTIC BOOK OF THE DEAD

In Celtic mythology, the journey of death in its heroic aspect is frequently depicted as a sea voyage to the *otherworld,* which is commonly represented as a faraway island or series of islands across the sea, beyond the "ninth wave" that separates ordinary from divine reality (O'Connor, 2000). The oldest and most elaborate story of this kind is the tale of the voyage of Mael Dúin, which, in synoptic form, goes as follows: On the advice of a druid with whom he consults, Mael Dúin set out one day on a boat with a party of 17 men, to seek his father's murderer. The party of men is later increased to 20 when Mael Dúin's three brothers swim out to join them upon their departure. They come first to two small islands, each containing a fortress, with one man boasting to another that he had slain Mael Dúin's father. However, before Mael Dúin is able to set foot on land and engage the boastful man in battle, a great wind blows their boat out to sea. This was a punishment for the transgression of taking more men than the druid's recommended party of 17. In their drifting, they visit a series of 33 islands containing a number of fantastic beings. These may be seen to represent archetypal forms that have become detached from their concrete manifestations in the visible world and presented in elemental form. There is, for example, the island of black and white, with a brass palisade separating black sheep from white sheep; an island with four fences separating kings, queens, warriors, and maidens; an island of women; an island of black mourners; the island of laughter; and a number of other islands with extraordinary species of animals, such as giant horses, fiery swine, shouting birds, among a host of others (Rees & Rees, 1961).

Rees and Rees (1961) have suggested that the Celtic sea voyage tales preserve "the tattered remnants of an oral Celtic 'book' of the dead, which proclaimed that the mysteries of the world beyond death had been at least partially explored and the stations of the soul's pilgrimage charted" (p. 325). One important purpose of these tales was "to teach the 'craft' of dying and to pilot the departing spirit on a sea of perils and wonders" (p. 325). However, it is important to point out that the realm of the archetypes is also occasionally visited by the living, in dreams and in other special states of consciousness associated with life's turning points. Conversely, dying does not in itself guarantee access to the archetypal otherworld. Another, much more limited otherworld possibility is the House of Donn, which, similar to the Catholic purgatory, is the inevitable destination for those nonheroic souls who have not yet seen through the veil of mortality to the immortal. Like the sea voyage of Bilbo and Frodo, the Celtic sea voyage tales contain potent reminders that a meaningful death requires the right heroic attitude.

THE TIBETAN INTERMEDIATE STATE

Religious mythologies tend to emphasize the vertical movement of the dead, in contrast with the horizontal movement in the Celtic sea voyages. In the Christian tradition, for example, notions of life after death are framed in terms of the doctrine of "the resurrection of the body," according to which the souls of the dead travel in bodily form "up" into heaven and "down" into hell. These same two mythologems of verticality and embodiment are also found in Buddhism.

Tibetan Buddhism, in particular, has a very elaborate mythology of dying, consisting of a complex series of stages. Of most interest with respect to the death-as-a-journey motif is the *intermediate state* that marks the transition between lifetimes. In this state, one has a body, not a substantial or corporeal body, but one "fashioned from wind and mind" (Dalai Lama, 2002, p. 192). The colour of this incorporeal body indicates the condition of one's rebirth: If the colour is that of a burnt log, one will be reborn as a hell being; if like smoke, as an animal; if like water, as a hungry ghost; if gold, as a human being or god of desire; if white, as a god of form. The direction of movement, too, signifies one's rebirth: downward for hell-beings, hungry ghosts and animals; straight ahead for humans and gods of desire; and upward for gods of form. These manifestations are marked by various apparitions, both fearful and benign, and by a sense of loss of orientation, somewhat reminiscent of the Celtic sea voyages. The intermediate state can be avoided entirely by the most accomplished yogis, who rise from death in another type of body altogether and thereby become free from the cycle of death and rebirth (Dalai Lama, 2002).

It seems paradoxical that realms of consciousness beyond the limits of embodiment and the spatial/temporal world should nonetheless require description in these terms. This is a reflection of some fundamental limits of the mythic imagination that, for the picture language of myth, in contrast to the philosophical language of metaphysics, is grounded in what is concretely visualizable. Although we can conceive abstractly of disembodied, non-spatial/temporal forms of existence, their concrete experience is utterly inconceivable to embodied beings like ourselves. Death remains an impenetrable mystery in this respect and the best that myth can do is to point symbolically and metaphorically to what might lie beyond. Also, we have again the suggestion that the process of dying is to be taken up with a certain heroic attitude, now understood in terms of the Buddhist ideal of disciplined and dedicated practice. Similar to the Celtic legends, the fully realized hero (or yogi) undergoes a different fate after death than the ordinary person.

THE JOURNEY INTO SPACE

A common motif in modern, secular mythologies of dying is the journey into extraterrestrial space. An example is in the following account from a terminal cancer patient, who conceived her experience of dying in terms of David Bowie's "Ground Control to Major Tom":

> I feel like Major Tom. I feel like I am on a mission that has taken me to a new dimension and I will never be the same. My oncology team is my Ground Control, always there to give me my "protein pills" and to pat me on the shoulder when I "make the grade." My alienation causes me to feel like I'm "floating above the Earth." (Moller, 2000, p. 22)

This image of the lonely, alienated individual floating above the Earth, desperately clinging to life, encapsulates the existential predicament of the modern individual who, even in the face of death, feels the need to make their own meaning, with only minimal support from the "Ground Control" of their local community. Extraterrestrial space is significant in this connection, as it has no boundaries or horizons. It has thus become a quintessentially modern symbol for the world of unlimited possibilities that lies beyond the temporal world of space, time, and physical existence. It also introduces yet another direction of travel in the journey of death. In contrast with horizontal, earth-bound movement of the Celtic seas voyages or the vertical movement in the Tibetan intermediate state, this is travel *outward*, beyond the horizons of earthbound experience.

The journey into space motif is also a commonplace of near-death experiences. An example is the experience that Carl Jung (1963) reported following a heart attack in 1944:

It seemed to me that I was high up in space. Far below I saw the
globe of the earth, bathed in a gloriously blue light. I saw the deep
blue sea and the continents. Far below my feet lay Ceylon, and in the
distance ahead of me the subcontinent of India. My field of vision
did not include the whole earth, but its global shape was plainly
distinguishable and its outlines shone with a silvery gleam through
that wonderful blue light. (p. 289)

Jung then reports, with no obvious indication of alarm: "I knew that I was on
the point of departing from the earth" (p. 190). There is no desperate clinging to
life here, in contrast with the visual metaphor of the dying cancer patient. In his
vision, Jung quite deliberately turned his back to earthbound consciousness and
approached the mysterious new level of reality that he found beyond. Here we move
from the *personal* to the *transpersonal* dimensions of mythological consciousness,
from the consciously constructed visual metaphor to the unconscious archetypal
vision. Jung subsequently awoke from his vision with a profound sense of disappointment which, during the ensuing weeks, developed into a severe depression,
with the realization of his inevitable return to the "box system" of personal
consciousness. From a transpersonal perspective, personal consciousness is likened
to being isolated as if in a box suspended by a thread, with death promising entry
into another mode of consciousness.

EPILOGUE: THE GREY HAVENS REVISITED

I will resist the temptation to draw any sweeping, general conclusions from
the foregoing. Myths can provide no definite answers to dispel the mysteries
connected with death, only a few symbolic pointers to what must remain fundamentally unknown. With this in mind, I return to where I began in this paper,
with Frodo's final departure at the Grey Havens, which Tolkien (1955/1991)
describes in these words:

Then Frodo kissed Merry and Pippin, and last of all Sam, and went
aboard; and the sails were drawn up, and the wind blew, and slowly
the ship slipped away down the long grey firth…. And the ship went
out into the High Sea and passed on into the West, until at last on a
night of rain Frodo smelled a sweet fragrance on the air and heard the
sound of singing that came over the water. And then… the grey rain-
curtain turned all to silver glass and was rolled back, and he beheld
white shores and beyond them a far green country under a swift
sunrise. (p. 1007)

References

Dalai Lama (2002). *Advice on dying* (J. Hopkins, Ed. & Trans.). New York: Atria Books.

Jung, C. G. (1963). *Memories, dreams, reflections* (A. Jaffé, Ed.; R. & C. Winston, Trans.). New York: Random House.

Moller, D. W. (2000). *Life's end.* Amityville, NY: Baywood Publishing.

O'Connor, P. (2000). *Beyond the mist.* London: Victor Gollancz.

Rees, A., & Rees, B. (1961). *Celtic heritage.* London: Thames and Hudson.

Tolkien, J. R. R. (1991). *The Lord of the Rings: The return of the king.* London: HarperCollins. (Original work published 1955)

Paradigm Shifting:
Transforming Catastrophic Events

MARLA J. COLVIN

Abstract

A framework for considering the unique perspectives of others in general, and in relation to events deemed catastrophic, is provided. Various consciousness levels at which individuals operate and a primary mental schema which gives meaning to individual existence are described. Three types of catastrophes individuals experience are identified: personal, sociocultural, and cosmic. An approach is outlined wherein perspectives of those impacted by catastrophic events, rather than the practitioner's framework, determine therapeutic objectives and activities.

Some people believe that everyone thinks alike, or at least should think alike. They also believe that those who think differently are psychologically impaired, intellectually inferior, deviant, or morally wrong. That uniformity of thought may not be beneficial (e.g., cult mentality) and conceptual deviance may not be a sign of perversity or impairment (e.g., creative thought) does not occur to them. Mental health professionals generally accept the existence of cognitive diversity. They realize that perceptions and meanings vary across individuals and cultures. Nevertheless, psychological interpretations of behavior as well as treatment approaches tend to be egocentric and/or ethnocentric in nature. That is, assessment and interventions are based upon the conceptual framework of the practitioner (e.g., Jungian or cognitive behavioral) rather than that of the client. How might mental health professionals incorporate their beliefs about cognitive diversity into practice? The purpose of this paper is to provide a framework for considering the unique perspectives of others in general, and in relation to events which may be deemed catastrophic (e.g., illness, incapacitation or loss of position, possessions or relationships). An approach is outlined in which the perspectives of those impacted by events, rather than the practitioner's framework, determine therapeutic activities.

One factor that seemingly accounts for varied reactions to life events across individuals and cultures is the consciousness level at which they operate. These consciousness levels, or states of awareness, correspond to cognitive developmental levels and appear to affect an individual's capacity to perceive the scope of existence and the consequence of events for self and others. These are: *elemental consciousness, group consciousness*, and *cosmic consciousness*.

Elemental consciousness involves perceiving all things as independent and unrelated, including persons, things, events, and ideas. Since similarities are not perceived, notions of class or group membership are not comprehended. Also, neither correlational nor cause-effect relationships are recognized.

With group consciousness, class or the similarity among various elements is recognized. However, the significance of difference is not grasped. Specifically, lack of similarity to other things is viewed as inherent and the only important attribute of that which differs. Reasons underlying variation are deemed irrelevant and differences in potentialities go unrecognized. Difference is considered an indication of inferiority and a basis for exclusion. Group consciousness is awareness constrained by dichotomous thinking.

Cosmic consciousness involves discerning class and category but not as exclusive domains. Criteria for inclusion extend beyond similarity and, difference does not mean unimportant or inferior. When consciousness is cosmic, every element and group is seen to be parts of one interdependent system. And all parts of the whole are of equal significance and value. However, a perceived equivalence in significance and value does not mean that difference is overlooked. Dissimilarities in form are seen to correspond to role and functional variation required for a system's optimal functioning and survival. With cosmic consciousness, thinking is unconstricted. Absence of a dichotomous focus on similarity/difference and superiority/inferiority permits the perception of potential.

The consciousness levels at which persons operate appear to influence the significance given to various events. Specifically, from an elemental perspective, events are seen as independent and unrelated. Furthermore, only events having direct personal impact are considered significant. Event impact and the consequences of one's actions on others go unrecognized or are considered unimportant. With group consciousness some relationships are perceived, but not others. That is, only those events affecting the group with which one identifies are noticed and deemed significant. The impact of events on other groups or the system is not apprehended or considered important. With cosmic consciousness, relationship is of major significance. As such, elemental events can be seen to have a group and system impact. Cosmic consciousness is holistic and has a systems point of view.

A second factor that appears to account for variation in peoples' reactions to events may be called a *primary paradigm*. A primary paradigm is a mental framework which determines the particular significance and meaning given to subsequent events.[1] This paradigm is comprised of notions regarding identity, the nature of the universe, and the relationship between the defined self and the universe. More specifically, primary paradigms are comprised of answers given, consciously or unconsciously, to the questions: "Who am I?" "What is the nature of the universe?" and "Why am I here?" The responses given to these questions determine meaning, significance, and varied reactions to events across individuals and cultures.

Although primary paradigms are unique, each reflects the consciousness level at which its formulator operates. For example, elemental consciousness with its *egocentric* orientation is reflected in answers to questions of identity, universal nature, and their relationship, such as: "I am the center of the universe;" "The universe is comprised of objects, the worth of which is assigned by me;" and "All things in the universe exist for my use and pleasure."

Paradigms reflecting group consciousness with its *ethnocentric* orientation answer these questions as follows: "I am superior because of my membership in a group that has been designated superior by a divine or infallible authority"; "The universe is comprised of two groups: the superior/good; and the inferior/ bad. Because everyone in and everything about my group is superior/good, we deserve the best life has to offer. Everyone and everything excluded from my group is inferior/bad and undeserving of anything good or beneficial in life"; "In view of our superiority and goodness, my group accepts responsibility for uplifting the universe; changing differences until they match our perspectives, forms, and behaviors. We also have the right to terminate existence that fails to conform to our standards."

Paradigms with a cosmic perspective will have content that is *allocentric*,[2] Cosmic perspective reflects the view that everything is a significant part of one unified whole.[3] Given that they reflect a systems perspective, cosmic answers to question of identity, universal nature and their relationship it may appear vague, strange or grandiose. For example, a cosmic identity statement would be, "I am That." And, a cosmic statement about the nature of the universe would be essentially the same given the notion of a unified whole. The difference would be a subject/object reversal such as, "That I am." Finally, answers to questions about the relationship between the defined self and the universe will reflect equivalency and oneness as opposed to a self/not-self dichotomy.[4] For example, "I am All that is;" or "All that is, I am."

The aforementioned notions of consciousness levels and paradigms add to the understanding of the catastrophic experience. That is, the impact of events are not inherent. The same event may be experienced as catastrophic by some and have only a minor impact on others. These outcome variations stem from differences in: (a) foresight, (b) understanding of cause-effect relationships, and/or (c) contingency planning. As such, a catastrophe is the occurrence of an unforeseen, unfathomable, or supposedly unlikely event which is experienced as overwhelming because of an inability and/or lack of preparedness to deal with it. What is foreseen, fathomed, and considered likely depends upon individuals' consciousness level and the content of their primary paradigm.

The particular events subject to be experienced as catastrophic depend on the specific contents of an individual's primary paradigm and are too numerous to specify. However, the general type of events individuals experience as catastrophic, as a function of consciousness level, may be characterized as follows. *Personal catastrophes* are events which threaten personal existence and disrupt individual functioning. These are perceived when consciousness is elemental and orientation is egocentric. *Sociocultural catastrophes* are occurrences which impede operations and thwart the survival of a collective with which one identifies. Perception of these events requires group consciousness and an ethnocentric focus. *Cosmic catastrophes* are events which cause system-wide malfunction and threaten total extinction. To perceive these events, one requires cosmic consciousness and an allocentric orientation. Consciousness level and orientation determine the significance and meaning given to life-impacting events.

How can individuals and groups who are experiencing particular types of events as catastrophic be assisted? The tangible things needed (e.g., food, materials goods, temporary shelter) can readily be identified and made available. However, what help can be given replacing such intangibles as loss of a sense of security, loss of peace of mind, or loss of joy in living? Is a show of compassion and assistance in developing coping skills sufficient to regain balance, harmony, and joy in life? What would be involved if therapeutic emphasis were broadened to "assisting individuals who have suffered events deemed catastrophic not only to survive but thrive?"

A potentially effective approach to helping individuals thrive after catastrophic events is the notion that catastrophic experiences depend upon consciousness level and primary paradigm content rather than events per se. Events are catastrophic because individuals' consciousness levels and primary paradigms prevent them from: (a) seeing the broad scope of the universe and their relationship to it, (b) seeing and accepting certain events as possibilities, and/or (c) engaging in contingency planning. Consequently, certain circumstances leave them shocked, unprepared to function effectively, and subsequently unable to find joy in living. But, more importantly, the occurrence of an unforeseen, unfathomable, or unlikely event results in the invalidation of the primary paradigm of those impacted by it. Catastrophic events provide irrefutable evidence that one's basic notions about identity, the nature of the universe, and the relationship between these two are erroneous. As a result, the individual is left without a blueprint for decision making, effective action and joyful living. As such, given a catastrophic experience, an individual has two therapeutic needs: (a) short-term assistance with stress reduction and coping with basic life demands, and (b) long-term assistance in constructing a paradigm which contains a broader and more reliable conceptualization of self, universe, and the relationship between the two. Therapeutic objectives established and procedures used need to address both short-term needs and the more complex longer term task of cognitive restructuring.

Short-term therapeutic interventions effective in helping individuals cope following a catastrophic experience might involve providing training in progressive relaxation and stress management and include use of Rogerian techniques, such as reiteration and reflection. However, these and other short-term strategies will not be addressed since such information is readily available elsewhere.

Long-term assistance with cognitive restructuring entails promoting client awareness and understanding of the nature and functions of paradigms in general and the primary paradigm in particular. Specific therapeutic objectives include fostering client awareness and understanding that: (a) paradigms are mental constructions of reality, not reality per se; (b) primary paradigms function as a framework for making sense of experiences and for making choices; (c) indecision and confusion indicate that one's primary paradigm is no longer functional; and (d) a new primary paradigm needs to be developed, which accommodates the catastrophic experience, embraces the unknown, allows for misunderstanding, and accepts the impossible and improbable. In this regard, the therapeutic objective is assisting clients in broadening their perspectives from an elemental/egocentric perspective to a group/albeit ethnocentric perspective to a cosmic/allocentric point of view.

The long-term therapeutic objective of cognitive restructuring may be achieved using any approach that fosters a broadening of perspective with regards to identity, universal nature, and the relationship between the two. For this purpose, any number of cognitive therapeutic procedures may be useful. To these might be added the Socratic Method[5] and bibliotherapy.[6] Whatever the method and procedures, indications of the successful treatment would be: (a) client behavior reflecting movement from a narrower to a broader mental framework, (b) the occurrence of fewer unexpected events, (c) the existence of more contingency plans for dealing effectively with possible life events, and (d) the judgment of fewer life events as catastrophic.

References

Caprice, A. (Ed.). (2000). *The expanded quotable Einstein* (2nd ed.). Princeton, NJ: Princeton University.

Freud, S. (1995). Psychopathology of everyday life. In A. A. Brill (Ed.), *The basic writings of Sigmund Freud* (pp. 3-118). New York: Random House.

Piaget, J. (2000). *The psychology of the child.* New York: Basic Books.

Seeskin, K. (1987). *Dialogue & discovery: A study in Socratic Method.* Albany, NY: State University of New York.

Endnotes

1. The primary paradigm is similar to Piaget's concept of schema. It influences subsequent perception, thought, and behavior as suggested by Freud's notion of psychic determinism.

2. *Allocentric* is a term coined to express the idea that all things are at the center of the universe of which they are a part.

3. Einstein's description of a human being as "...part of the whole, called by us the Universe," is an example of a cosmic primary paradigm.

4. This self/not-self equivalency is also reflected in statements about the impact of human behavior such as, "Whatever is done to another is done to me." or "Whatever I do to another I do to myself."

5. The Socratic method is a method of inquiry which uses questioning to reveal underlying assumptions and uncover truth by exposing errors to reason.

6. Bibliotherapy is the assignment of thought-provoking reading which is relevant to therapeutic aims.

PART FOUR

POSITIVE PSYCHOLOGY OF
GOOD WORK
AND OTHER VIRTUES

Good Work:
Where Excellence and Ethics Meet

HOWARD GARDNER

I am going to speak today about a project in which I have been involved since the mid-1990s. It is called the Good Work Project. Members of the Project believe that it is relevant to events happening in the world today—for example the meltdown of large and respected corporations in the United States as well as the subsequent dropping of the financial markets all around the world.

Let me first start with a word about my own background, and how I got into the Good Work Enterprise. I am, by training, a psychologist. I have worked in cognitive psychology, developmental psychology and neuropsychology. Like many psychologists I am interested in figuring out how the mind works. I have taken on quite ambitious issues, such as the nature of intelligence, of creativity, and of leadership. But I have always taken on those topics in a deliberately amoral way. I hope I have not been immoral, but I have been amoral in the sense that I have tried to understand what intelligence is, without smuggling in whether the intelligence is used benignly or malevolently. Both Goethe, the German poet, and Goebbels, the German propagandist, were very gifted in the use of the German language. Goethe used it to write great works of art. Goebbels used it to foment hatred. The intelligence was potent in each case. The uses could not have been more different.

Similarly, when it comes to leadership, both Nelson Mandela and Slobodan Milosevic are gifted leaders. They can get people in their countries to do things that might not have seemed possible. But I do not think many of us would defend Milosevic as being as ethical or as responsible a leader as Nelson Mandela. Anyway, in 1994 I and two friends, who later became colleagues, went to California to a research center called the Center for Advanced Study in the Behavioral Sciences. My two colleagues were William Damon, who is a social psychologist, and Mihaly Csikszentmihalyi, known to many of you as a person who writes about flow, and has written a book called the *Evolving Self,* which is certainly a book about personal meaning. Damon, Csikszentmihalyi, and I had gone to the Center to talk about various kinds of extraordinary individuals, people who are highly creative, people who are outstanding leaders, and people who have different kinds of intelligence. There was no imperative for us to create a project together; however, our hope was that a project would emerge from this collaboration.

Those of you who are familiar with recent United States history will know that in 1994 there was a congressional election. For the first time in 40 years the Republicans won the House of Representatives. They had a leader who immediately became very well known—his face was in all the news magazines—Newt Gingrich. What caught our attention was that Gingrich and his supporters declared that government was the enemy, and that all spheres of life are better controlled, better governed, by market forces. Now you will probably think I am about to launch into a political statement, but that is not the case.

As it turns out, the three of us, Csikszentmihalyi, Damon, and Gardner, are all over the map politically. We do not have the same political points of view. None of us has any intrinsic objection to the market. But we all felt that there were certain spheres of life that could not and should not be governed completely by market forces. For example, should only people who can afford it be allowed to have an education? Should only people who can afford it be allowed to have medical care? Speaking to people in Canada, there is certainly a very different philosophy about medical care than there is in the United States. Should only people who can afford it be able to have legal protection? So we felt that it was too facile to maintain that market forces are the best way to govern everything. They may well be the best way to govern the economy or to run a business.

Triggered by this Gingrich statement and this claim which we found peculiar, we decided to embark on a project—the study of professions, to see whether people could be highly qualified experts and at the same time show concern about their place in the community, concern such that they could make sure that everybody who wanted it could have an education, could have medical treatment, could have legal defense and so on. At the time, for various reasons we called this the "Humane Creativity Project." We wanted to know whether people could be creative, use their minds freely, generatively, productively, use "out of the box" thinking, and at the same time be humane, and use their talents in a way that displayed regard for the rest of humanity. Our hope was that a foundation—the MacArthur Foundation in particular—would give us several million dollars so that we could study different professions in the United States and perhaps elsewhere, and to see whether people could be creative and humane at the same time.

Well, life is rarely as simple as one's dreams. The McArthur Foundation had no interest in supporting our work. Nobody liked our phrase "humane creativity"; nobody knew what it meant. So we were discouraged but often out of defeat, out of a challenge, out of our frustration, something healthier can emerge.

After a while, we changed the name of our project from the Humane Creativity Project to the "Good Work Project." That term has a religious resonance; most people have at least some sense of what good work is. Rather than getting one large grant for the whole study, we ended up making a virtue of necessity. We have been carrying out many smaller projects, several of which are still very much ongoing. Indeed, the Good Work Project is now seven years old—1995 to 2002—but I still think it is in its early childhood and I expect we will be studying good work for many more years.

Now let me tell you about my plan for the rest of the talk. I am going to define good work, introduce some terminology and a framework for thinking about good work, and describe one project that was completely carried out and described in a book called *Good Work: When Excellence and Ethics Meet*. I am also going to tell you about many other facets of the project which are still ongoing and have not been written yet. Finally I will conclude with some discussion of how I think good work can be fostered. I hope these themes intersect with issues of responsibility and with issues of personal meaning. Finally, I will leave you with some closing thoughts from some very wise people.

In English the word *good* is a pun. Good has two meanings; it means "of high quality"; it also means "ethical, responsible." Good work is work that meets two criteria: It is highly expert, up to the highest standards, but at the same time it is also moral, ethical, responsible, and takes account of its social implications. Now it is certainly possible to be good in one of those senses and not the other. Let us take the practice of law. One could be a very skilled lawyer, win most of one's cases, but only take the cases of people who are very wealthy, and cut every corner in order to win. That person would be good in the first sense, but not in the second. We have another hypothetical lawyer who takes on only indigent cases, works very hard—your heart goes out to this lawyer for his or her efforts—but, unfortunately, this lawyer never wins any cases. That lawyer would be good in the second sense, but not the first sense. We looked for people who embodied both senses of goodness.

Now any particular example would be controversial, but let me mention some people whom my colleagues and I considered to be good workers. One is the recently deceased head of *The Washington Post*, Katharine Graham, who dared to publish the Pentagon papers. Another is Jonas Salk, a physician who found the polio vaccine. Another is Jackie Robinson, the baseball player who integrated baseball about 50 years ago. There is Rachel Carson, the writer who raised consciousness about ecology in the 1960s. Finally, I will mention someone probably not known to most of you, but a man who had a great influence on three authors, and to whom we dedicated our book. It is a man named John Gardner (no relation of mine) who has been a very important civic leader in the United States over the last 40 or 50 years. So there are examples of good workers, although you and I could debate whether Jonas Salk, Katharine Graham, etc., were or were not good workers. No person is above controversy in that respect.

So, how do we think about good work? Good work happens when an individual working in a profession is able to be highly skilled in that profession yet also is able to have a perennial concern of the implications of what he or she does. Nobody always does the right thing. Nobody always knows the implications of his or her work. But there is a big difference between people who think about the implications of their work all the time and try to do the right thing, and people who are indifferent to that whole set of concerns.

In analyzing good work we use three terms that I am going to introduce to you: *domain, field*, and *alignment*. The domain refers to the values of a profession. Medicine is the best example here. The domain of medicine embodies values that go back to the Hippocratic Oath—do no harm, come to the aid of somebody who is not well, do not enter into special deals or relationships with your patients. That is part of the domain of medicine. But there is also a field of medicine. The field of medicine is the current institution that is responsible for delivering health care. In the United States, parts of the field of medicine are health maintenance organizations, managed care organizations, and doctors who are working for those particular entities. The domain of medicine, i.e., the values of medicine, has not changed very much over the millennia or over the decades and centuries, but the field has changed enormously. Fifty years ago when I was young, a doctor was a man who almost always came to your house with a little black bag, took your temperature, felt your pulse, listened to your heart, told you to take two aspirin and you would be okay in the morning. It was very personalized, not at all high tech. Now, of course, at least in the United States, no doctor ever comes to anyone's home. The gender split is much more equal. Most of us belong to very large organizations where there are rules about how often you can see the doctor, how much we pay, what medicines can be prescribed, what treatments can be prescribed, and so on. The field has changed enormously.

Let me introduce the notion of alignment. A profession is well aligned when all the different stakeholders want the same thing from a profession. A profession is misaligned when the various stakeholders want things to be very different than one another. So if practitioners, the general public, the values of the domain, the current institutions, and to the extent that these are publicly traded entities, the stockholders, all want the same thing from an entity or a profession, it is very well aligned. Conversely, if a doctor wants to give everyone the treatment that he or she merits, but the HMO says he cannot see a certain person because he or she did not pay the premium or he cannot tell a patient about a cure because he or she will not pay for it or he can only see a patient for seven minutes because that is the capitation rate, then the field is pulling the doctor in a very different direction from the values of the domain. Moreover, if it is a publicly created company, as many HMOs are in the United States, what the shareholders want are not happy doctors, not good medical care, but the most money in the quarterly report. They want to have high return on their investment. So they have yet a third particular desire coming out of medicine; this is a very misaligned profession. We argue that good work is easiest to do when a profession is very fully aligned and everyone (i.e., the domain, the field, the shareholders, the stockholders, and the general public) wants essentially the same thing from a profession.

We look to see the extent to which a profession is aligned or not aligned. All alignments are temporary. No alignment is permanent. No misalignment is permanent, and if it were, the profession would stop existing and something new would come to pass. It is relatively easy to carry out good work when you are in an aligned profession but, interestingly, some of us are actually stimulated, excited, catalyzed when the domain is not well aligned. That is an interesting interaction of personality with profession.

By now you probably are very hungry for an example so I will provide one. But first let me tell you that it took us about six years to figure out exactly what question we are asking; those of you who are researchers might not be surprised because often figuring out the question is more difficult than figuring out the answer. Here is the question that the Good Work Project is designed to answer: How does a person who wants to do work that is at once excellent in quality but also responsible and ethical, succeed or fail in carrying out the good work at a time when: (a) things are changing very quickly; (b) market forces are very, very powerful and there are few, if any, counter forces; and (c) our whole sense of time and space is being radically altered by technology. Ten years ago it would have been science fiction to think that I could be giving a live talk on video to folks thousands of miles away, and that we could then have interchange. So what does it mean to do good work when everything is changing, time and space are completely altered, market forces have enormous power, and there are very few counterforces? That is the overarching question the Good Work Project is trying to answer.

In the mid-1990s, my colleagues and I said that we would like to study a dozen different professions to understand good work in those professions. We wanted to study a whole range of professions, such as the military, medicine, education, law, and the arts. But we had to start somewhere. So, for a variety of reasons we decided to start with those professions that have the most power over our minds and over our bodies. Now we could argue a bit about what those professions are, but we chose the professions of journalism and genetics. We chose journalism because journalists, writers, and news anchors, whether through the Internet, broadcast, or print, tell us what is going on in the world. So to use the current jargon, journalists give us the "memes," i.e., they give us the units of meaning, personal meaning and public meaning, which we carry around in our head.

Everybody knows about genes. Geneticists not only study our genes but increasingly they tell us about our life expectations; soon they will be advising us on what to do given the roll of the dice we have received from the genes of our biological parents, as well as various kinds of interventions like genetic therapy. So just as journalists have a lot to say about what is in our minds, geneticists have a lot to say about our bodies and our fates. Thus, we decided to nickname our study "Memes and Genes."

How do we go about doing our study? We are social scientists so we nominated journalists and geneticists who are leaders in the field and asked permission to interview them. We interviewed each nominee for about two hours. Ours is a very in-depth kind of interview with a lot of probing. We asked our subjects about a range of subjects: their goals, what they were trying to accomplish, what got in the way of that, what were the opportunities and the obstacles that they confronted in their own work, what were the big influences in their own training, who were their mentors, who were their anti-mentors (or tormenters, as we call them, because often those people have a big influence as well), to whom did they feel responsible, to what did they feel responsible, and what kind of ethical dilemmas arose in their work? These are very searching interviews and many people whom we have interviewed—we have interviewed between 700 and 800 people by now—say the interview was very helpful to them in getting some distance from themselves, or in your terms, gaining some personal meaning from the interchange.

Even though the interview lasts two hours, each interview actually takes about two weeks to complete. First, we research the people, doing them due diligence so we are well informed before we speak to them. Then we have it all transcribed. The transcripts run from 30 to 50 single-spaced pages. Then we code them using a very elaborate coding system; codification takes the most time. We put the transcripts online using NUD*IST, a qualitative software system. This gives us instant access to all kinds of information about our subjects. So, if just to be cute about it, you wanted to know how many second- born, left-handed journalists had anti-mentors, we could tell you because that information is available online. If nothing else, this project consists of an incredible archive of what busy professionals from the United States think about their work life at the beginning of the twenty-first century. We hope that in the future people will make good use of the information that we have gathered.

Let me move now to the results of the study of journalism and genetics. The study was completed in 1999. That is important to note because if the study were carried out today, I think already we would have somewhat different results. Basically, we found that two fields could not be more different from each other than these two professions. Genetics in 1997, 1998, and 1999, was a beautifully aligned profession. Journalism, on the other hand, was a massively misaligned profession. What does that mean practically? It means that geneticists loved what they were doing. They could not wait to get up in the morning. No geneticist we interviewed talked about leaving the area of genetics. Why is that? According to our analysis, at that time everybody wanted the same thing from genetics. Everybody wanted to live longer, be healthier, and make sure we knew as much as we could about how the body worked. Thus, the profession had very little tension.

While this alignment did not guarantee that people could do good work, it made it much easier because nobody was giving the geneticists any signals other than "go for it." In fact, when we asked geneticists what obstacles there were in their work, often they said the only obstacle lay in themselves: Sometimes they did not work as hard as they should or got diverted. It was an amazing experience to hear about for those of us who are not geneticists!

Conversely, journalists were not at all happy with the state of their trade. Very few of them felt aligned. Most of them felt that they had ideals they wanted to achieve (e.g., be fair, be objective, research stories in depth) but events had conspired to make it very, very difficult to be a good journalist. Those of you who know something about journalism will, I think, immediately understand why this is the case. In the United States, there are very few outlets that are owned by individuals with a primary interest in the news. They are almost all owned by large conglomerates who are not journalists themselves. They are entrepreneurs who string together different kinds of companies and they are interested in one thing—the bottom line. We have a line about television in America, "if it bleeds it leads." If you ever watch local news television in the United States it is often about a murder or a rape or some other kind of violent act. I am not saying that these incidents should not be reported, but they are hardly the most important stories in the light of eternity. Because people find that the sensational keeps the audience "glued to the tube" or buying newspapers, it becomes the operant principle in journalism. Harold Evans was the editor of both the *London Times* under Murdoch, then of the *Daily News* in New York under Mort Zuckerman. Evans has said the problem for American newspapers is not to stay in business—their profits are higher than ever. Their problem is to stay in journalism. This is the frustration of the journalists because they want to do good work but very much feel thwarted.

In the book *Good Work* we talk about the various things that make it difficult for journalists to carry out good work. For example, many journalists would like to carry out investigative reporting, but increasingly they are told they cannot do so. Why? First, it is expensive; second, it may not yield anything; and third, it might yield something that is critical of a chief advertiser. As the line between the business office, the marketing office, the advertising office, and the reporting in the editorial offices gets blurred, it becomes more and more difficult to carry out good journalism.

Interestingly, 50 years ago people said that the problem with American journalism was its parochial nature—newspapers were owned by families in cities—and it would be much better if they were publicly traded companies. That analysis could not have been more wrong. Now, essentially all the good newspapers in the United States are owned by families: the *New York Times* by the Sulzberger family, the *Washington Post* by the Graham family, and so on. It means these families have a large, if not majority, interest in the newspaper, and that they have influence about what is in it. If they feel the newspaper should be doing investigative reporting, they will support it even if it means they lose money. Publicly traded companies are in a different situation. By way of illustration, perhaps you had the misfortune of owning Time Warner AOL stock. Many Americans do, whether they know it or not, because many pension plans are tied in with AOL. Nobody who reads an editorial in *Time* magazine feels good about the editorial because they're a stockholder. They feel good about the company if the company makes money.

Now you might say, "Well those are marketing influences in journalism and I am glad I am not a journalist." But one of the things that we discovered is that market influences are rampant throughout the United States. There is not a single profession, be it religion, philanthropy, education, or art, which is not influenced by financial and monetary and market considerations. Think of education, for instance. We now have, in the United States, not only charter schools but voucher schools. A voucher is simply a market mechanism where people are given a certain amount of money and asked to choose the schools they want. Now you might like or dislike it, but it is clearly a market kind of system. At the university level now we have for-profit companies. The largest one in the world is the University of Phoenix, operating in 48 out of 50 states. There are other for-profit companies like DeVry that sell education to people and stockholders. I am at Harvard University which was, at least up until recently, the wealthiest university in the world. I always ask, "Is it harvard.edu, or is it harvard.com?", because so many things we do at Harvard, as I am sure is also true of schools you are involved with, are very much oriented toward markets. They try to attract the best students, try to give them the most effective facilities, bid for professors, and cut down professors' teaching loads in order to attract the prominent professors. These are all market-dictated practices.

You might think that the one profession that should be immune from market forces is philanthropy. After all, in philanthropy you have the money and all you have to do is give it away. But that's not true at all. We have been studying philanthropy. Philanthropy is completely influenced now by market models. The biggest question in philanthropy is whether all your grantees are accountable. Can you prove that what they are doing has value added? Now there is nothing wrong with that attitude but it is a completely market way of doing things with a bottom line kind of mentality. So we find that market forces are ubiquitous and you might say that there have always been market forces. It is true that capitalist societies are run by market mechanisms.

In addition to the familial counter forces that I just mentioned with reference to ownership of newspapers, there have usually been very strong religious or communal or ideological counter-forces. The twentieth century was a century of "isms." Like them or not, "isms" like capitalism, socialism, and fascism, were counterforces to a purely market approach. Strong families, strong religious values, and strong community values all serve as counterforces to market forces. But as those wane in power, as they do all over the world—especially so in a time of globalization—the market flexes its muscles more than ever.

I made a comment two years ago which was incredibly prescient. I said that when the markets control everything, there is only one profession left and that is accounting. Accounting tells you whether the information about the market is accurate or not, and if the accountants can be influenced or "bought," so to speak, if they "cook the books," to use current vernacular, then essentially there is no profession. This was a prescient comment because two years ago there was no particular reason to think that accountants were as deeply flawed as we have learned that they were, with Enron and Global Crossing and WorldCom and so on, because these companies were audited by Arthur Anderson and Price Waterhouse and Peat Marwick and so on, the biggest accounting companies. It now comes clear that these accounting companies were anything but objective. They did not do due diligence. If anything, they helped to cook the books and fix the figures. So you can see the risk in a market- drenched world when even the information about the markets is no longer accurate. The reason the stock market in the United States, Nikkei in Tokyo, and the Hang Seng in Hong Kong are so low, just a percentage of where they were two years ago, is not primarily because of 9/11 and the impact on the Twin Towers. It is not even primarily because a company named Enron went bankrupt. It's because people like you and me no longer believe we should invest in stocks and because we no longer believe there is honest information about the value of those companies. In a market world, that is a very, very serious problem.

Now as I said earlier, that if we did the study of journalism and genetics in the year 2002, we might find a somewhat different picture of alignment. I can give you a few bits of evidence about that. Since 9/11, journalism has become much more important. Tabloids have less appeal. People want to know what is going on militarily in defense, with different racial and ethnic groups, anthrax, other kinds of bio-terror. Quite suddenly the news is more serious. Newspapers are devoting more attention to such topics. Monica Lewinsky, and Gary Condit, the congressman, are no longer headlines as they were before 9/11. So journalism is somewhat better aligned. There have been no miracles but it is a somewhat more embattled, look-foward profession.

Nothing bad has happened to genetics, but there are danger signs. First, there is much less money available for scientific research. Second, there have been some fatalities due to misapplied genetic therapy. This is very worrisome. Third, and I think most troublesome, it has now become clear that most research in genetics is no longer government funded, but funded by private companies or for-profit companies that have a vested interest in certain kinds of results. Moreover, these companies often ask the researchers to keep their research secret. It is often hard to get peer review in genetics research because everybody is being paid by one biochem or biotech company or another. So I see the handwriting on the wall, with respect to alignment within the area of genetics. My own prediction is that you will see much more misalignment in genetics in coming years.

I said earlier that our study has expanded in various ways. I want to mention briefly what they are because some of you may have some questions about other areas we have looked at, i.e., education and the law. Also, we have carried out a study of business that is quite interesting because the question arises, "Is business a profession?"

A second dimension is age. We have worked with youngsters as young as 10 years of age, kids gifted and talented in different domains, who see their own attitudes toward good work, and we in fact have drafted a book called *Workers in Progress* about the development of very young workers. (Author's note: *Making Good: How Young People Cope with Moral Dilemmas at Work* was published by Harvard University Press in February 2004). One of the things that is amazing is how at a very young age, just 10 or 12 years old, children are already very concerned about two things: (a) whether there will be any balance in their lives when stressed, and (b) whether they will make enough money. In light of the events of the last two years, the latter will be even a greater concern.

We are investigating people of all ages, up to what we call trustees. Trustees are wise people, such as John Gardner, to whom we dedicated our book. They are people who worry about the fate of the whole domain or even the whole society. Another example is Edward R. Murrow who was a very distinguished American journalist. He was very devoted to protecting that craft. So another dimension of our work is looking at good work at different ages, from children all the way to trustees.

The third dimension that we are just beginning is to look at good work internationally. We are under no illusion whatsoever that the United States has all the answers to good work. We were working in the United States because of convenience; it is where we live. However, we have a colleague in Scandinavia who has been working both in Scandinavian countries and in Latvia, a former communist state, and trying to investigate notions of good work in those very different political situations. We hope someday, if we could find collaborators from other countries who are interested in these issues, that we will be able to look at good work in different parts of the globe.

We also have a few other studies that we have done in the margins, so to speak. One of the studies is a lineage study. With the lineage study we find a very senior person, like Edward R. Murrow, and then we look at his or her students, grand students, and great-grand students. Our goal is to see the extent to which beliefs and values of these heads of the lineages are transmitted from one generation to another. We hope to be able to demonstrate that good work or bad work is basically conveyed from one person to another. You are likely to be a good worker if you are surrounded by good workers. You are likely to be a bad worker or a "no-good" worker if you are surrounded by people who are bad workers or "no-good" workers. Edward R. Murrow was born at the turn of the century and was a mentor for people like Walter Cronkite, who many of you know as a leading newscaster for CBS in America for many years. The Murrow generation is dying out, as is his first generation of students. But one person in one institution still carries on the Edward R. Murrow lineage. I am referring to National Public Radio, which I hope is known to many of you. The senior news analyst, Daniel Schorr, is one of the last people in the Edward R. Murrow lineage. Many of the younger people at National Public Radio who work with Schorr, I consider to be good workers. In sum, while the Good Work Project was initially an attempt to look at simply a set of professions, now we are looking at a number of related issues having to do with age, lineages, trustees, different countries, and so on.

Let me move toward the conclusion of my talk. First of all, let me give you an example of what you do when you are an aspiring good worker but it is difficult to do good work. To make it concrete, say that you are an investigative journalist. You believe that the important thing about journalism is to find out what really happened and to make it public, to soothe the afflicted and challenge the powerful. But your boss says, "We are not going to do investigative reporting any more, it is too expensive and does not yield much," and as I mentioned before, "it might threaten our chief advertisers." What can you do? Well you can quit and go and sell insurance, but you probably do not want to quit, and if you have kids and a mortgage to pay and you want to send them to higher education, at least in the United States, you probably cannot afford to quit. So one reaction you might have is just to put up with your boss. Another one is to be a guerrilla worker. That means you say, "Yes, yes, I am going to quit," but actually you keep on doing investigative reporting and sometimes you will be fired. Sometimes your boss will be fired first, in which case you are the winner. And sometimes you will get an accolade like a Pulitzer Prize that serves as a protective device. If your investigative reporting gets very much rewarded, you build a certain kind of protective shield around you. That certainly would count as good work but it is a risky kind of good work.

In our study, we are particularly interested in people who actually try to change institutions or create new institutions that allow them to do good work. In the United States now, National Public Radio is taken for granted as is C-SPAN and CNN, but these are all inventions in the last 25 years by people who felt dissatisfied with the big networks like ABC, CBS, and NBC. So, individually or corporately, these social entrepreneurs created new entities that allowed them to do good work.

You will know that in the United States now we have many charter schools. Charter schools are controversial, though not as controversial as voucher schools. Charter schools are efforts by people who say, "We do not like the way the schools are now, we are going to create our own school in our own image." Those people are often aspiring good workers. An option when you are an aspiring good worker is to quit; this is sad but some people do quit. About a third of young journalists leave journalism. Almost no young geneticist leaves genetics. Simply "Do what you're told" is the option most of us would select because it is too hard to do anything else. Say, "Yes, yes" but do what you believe is right and hope you will ask for forgiveness rather than permission. The most praiseworthy or the most courageous act, I suppose, is to try to organize your own entity that allows you to do good work.

What are the leverages that encourage good work? Interestingly enough, strong religious values often promote good work and this is independent of whether people consider themselves to be religious. We interviewed many people who had a religious background who no longer are churchgoers or even believers in God, but for whom that strong value system is very, very important. Early values are a vital contributor to good work. Another factor is what we call vertical support. Vertical support means working with supervisors, mentors, masters, leaders, and bosses who are themselves good workers, and conversely, trying to create good work in your own professional offspring. Horizontal support is support from your peers. If you are in a place with peers who try to do good work, that is going to be a positive factor. On the other hand, if you are the only person trying to do good work in a place where most people are indifferent workers or bad workers, it is going to be a real deterrent. Still, even if you have good values and you are in an organization that has a vision of good work, like the *New York Times*, the *Wall Street Journal*, and the *Washington Post*, and even if you have horizontal support, it still may be very difficult if you do not get occasional booster shots or inoculations. Experiences that remind people what it is like to do good work and help them to do it are tremendously important.

My colleague Bill Damon who was in charge of our journalism study has joined forces with two good workers in journalism, Bill Kovach and Tom Rosenstiel, to create a traveling curriculum that goes to newsrooms all over America. This curriculum discusses issues of good work and gives specific strategies of how to do good work in a time when the pressures are enormously powerful. We have no illusion that we will solve individually the problems of good work in journalism, but these kinds of inoculation booster shot experiences can, we believe, be very important for individuals in midlife, and midcareer.

In closing I want to do two things. First, I will talk about the four M's that people can do if they want to do good work, and then the five M's of people who gave me insight into what is good work.

I turn first to the four M's. The first M is *mission*. If you want to do good work, whether you are a professor, teacher, journalist, doctor, business person, or actor, you have to ask: "What is my mission, and what am I trying to accomplish in my work?" This cannot just be something written in a mission statement. It has to be something you believe in your heart. Why did you choose this particular calling?

The next M is *model*. Who do you admire, and why? Who do you look up to and say, "I would like to be a worker like them." Who do you think about and say, "What would Edward R. Murrow, Daniel Schorr, Albert Schweitzer, Jonas Salk, or Rachel Carson do in a situation like this?" Who are your anti-mentors? Who are the people you would never look up to? For example, I do not want to be like Rupert Murdoch.

So we have missions, models, and now two mirror tests. A *personal mirror test* is when I look at myself in a mirror as a worker, and ask myself if I am proud of what I see or if I am embarrassed. And if I am embarrassed by myself as a worker, what can I do so I could look at myself clearly, transparently, and not feel badly about the kind of work I do? The fourth M is the *professional mirror test*. If I look at my occupation as a whole—all teachers, all professors, all priests, all clergymen, and all business people—am I proud or embarrassed about how my profession is behaving? Even if you are doing good work, if the rest of your profession is not, perhaps you have an obligation to work on your profession as a trustee. So those are the four M's which we see as the root of good work: mission, models, personal mirror test, and professional mirror test.

Turning to the five M's, the first I will mention is Margaret Mead, whom I mentioned earlier. Margaret Mead once said, "Never condemn the small group of people who get together to do something new. Nothing important in the world has ever happened any other way." What Mead says is: if you want to do it right in your profession, do not wait for other people to do it; get together with a small group of fellow believers and go do it.

Jean Monet, the great French economist who had the idea for the European union of common market, said, "I regard every defeat as an opportunity." People who try to do good work are going to be defeated a lot; it is an uphill battle. But rather than giving up, they are challenged and energized by this nonalignment and they work even harder to try to make this come out right. The best workers we studied are people who say, "I will not know until 50 years after I am dead whether what I am pushing for is going to work out and that is exactly why I am doing what I am doing." The third M is Jean-Baptiste Molière, the French playwright. Molière has said, "You're responsible not only for what you do but for what you don't do." That is where the professional mirror test is important, especially as you get older and more influential. You ought to try to help your profession, not just keep your own house quarter.

The last two M's are sort of cheating but they are a funny sort of cheating. One is E. M. Foster, a great British novelist, whose nickname was Morgan. In his most famous utterance, Foster said, "Only connect." What we tried to do in the Good Work Project is to connect a moral sense of goodness with the expertise sense of goodness because we think it is needed in the world nowadays. If there had been more good workers in the accounting firms, we would not be in the mess that we talked about earlier. The final M is from a person local to me, Ralph Waldo Emerson, the "Sage of Concord" as he was called. Emerson memorably said, "Character is more important than intellect." I have spent most of my life studying intelligence. I am a cognitive psychologist and I am known for my theory of multiple intelligences, but I have reached a point where I realize that it does not matter in the long run how smart you are or even how you are smart. If you do not have good character, if you do not try to do the right things, it is really all going to come to naught.

References

Fischman, W., Solomon, B., Greenspan, D., & Gardner, H. (2004). *Making good: How young people cope with moral dilemmas at work.* Cambridge, MA: Harvard University Press.

Gardner, H., Csikszentmihalyi, M. & Damon, W. (2001). *Good work: When excellence and ethics meet.* New York: Basic Books.

Spirituality, Meaning, and Good Work

PAUL T. P. WONG

I have been advocating a meaning-and-spirituality orientation towards management and work since the turn of the twenty-first century, because there are many macro and micro pressures demanding a radical reorientation in terms of how we do business. The bottom-line mentality and the reward systems based on wealth and success are no longer able to meet the following new challenges:

- Increase in global competition and international trades.
- A diverse work force in multinational corporations.
- Need for multicultural competencies in management.
- Global warming and concerns about sustainable development.
- Clash of civilizations and the threats of international terrorism.
- Widening gaps between the haves and have-nots.
- Problems of injustice and chronic poverty.
- Widespread corporate scandals.
- The unraveling of community and traditional values.
- Need for social responsibility in business.
- Depersonalization of workers to increase efficiency.
- Experience of burnout due to work stress.
- Diminished loyalty in a mobile, knowledge economy.
- Valuing a positive workplace more than good pay.
- Need for rethinking personal priorities after 9/11.
- The need for balancing work and family life.

The above issues have loomed large for both managers and workers. In these turbulent and uncertain times, it is only natural for people to consider the Big Story for answers. Many are wrestling with such basic questions as: What is the meaning of life? What is the point of striving for money, which cannot buy happiness? Is there a deeper meaning and higher purpose for work? How can one experience inner peace and fulfillment?

There is now increasing recognition that workers would be more satisfied with their work and become more productive, when their existential needs for meaning and purpose are met (Terez, 2000; Taylor, 1994; Wong, 2002). Creative talents, professional competence, technological innovation, and generous compensations can no longer guarantee good work in today's volatile and chaotic business environment. Something more is needed. In short, excellence and ethics are more likely to meet (Gardner et al., 2004), when meaning and spirituality are incorporated into both personal work life and the global business system.

THE IMPERATIVE OF MEANING AND PURPOSE

Meaning and purpose are important at both the corporate and personal levels. Elsewhere (Wong, 2005), I have emphasized the need for business corporations to move beyond the bottom line and consider the higher purpose of contributing to society and uplifting humanity in all their business policies and practices. This broader humanistic view not only elevates the ethical tone of corporate cultures, but also brings a sense of significance to routine daily activities. Much has been written on how to create a work environment where meaning flourishes (Autrey, 1994; Epps, 2003; Handy, 1994; Straus, 2005; Terez, 2000; Wong, 2002a). Here is a brief summary of what management can do:

- Have a clear statement of mission and vision shared by the entire organization.
- Have a set of core values consistently implemented in all policies and practices.
- Treat workers as human beings worthy of respect rather than as instruments of production.
- Create a supportive and trusting climate.
- Give all workers a meaningful role with clear responsibility.
- Recognize, and capitalize on, each employee's strengths.
- Validate workers' contributions.
- Encourage worker engagement and initiative.
- Facilitate the positive "flow" experience at work.

At the individual level, employees also need to adopt a positive meaning orientation. According to Viktor Frankl (1986), what makes work meaningful is not work per se, but the positive attitudes and motivations people bring to their work. When workers attach a higher meaning and purpose to their work, such as making a difference in this world or serving God, even mundane work takes on new values and significance. Management science begins to recognize meaning and purpose as a powerful source of incentive and satisfaction.

SPIRITUALITY AND GOD AT WORK

Spirituality and meaning are two sides of the same coin, because both are concerned with big questions, such as worldviews, personal identity, human destiny, ultimate concerns, and an individual's place in the large scheme of things. The meaning-spirituality connection is self-evident. For example, one can derive meaning by considering one's profession or business as God's calling (Novak, 1996; Stevens, 2006). Belief in ultimate meaning and higher purpose are naturally linked to faith in a Supreme Being or God (Frankl, 1986). Apart from the references to God or Higher Power, spirituality has also been defined as the quest for meaning and the uniquely human capacity to transcend self and immediate circumstances. The revival of spiritual interest in the workplace goes hand-in-hand with the resurgence of interest in meaning and purpose, because both reflect people's deepest hunger for inner peace, fulfillment, and security.

Many in corporate America have already embraced faith at work—they believe that religion can be good for business. A search on Google and Amazon. com yields more than 200 books on spirituality and business. Some books on soul and spirit at work have been among the best sellers, such as *Saving Corporate Soul, Liberating the Corporate Soul, Spirit at Work, Jesus CEO, Working from the Heart,* and *Leading with Soul.*

Academe has also begun to take spirituality seriously. Harvard Business School is at the frontier of this new development. The prestigious American Academy of Management has recently formed a special interest group at the URL: http://aom.pace.edu/msr. An increasing number of journal articles are devoted to this topic; for example, in the field of management the URL: http://www.business.scu.edu/spirituality_leadership has become quite influential.

In many complex and ambiguous situations, religious principles provide a framework or grounding for moral decisions. Spiritual values, such as integrity, justice, compassion, and work ethics also reinforce business ethics. Sellers (2003) points out that:

> Most of the New Business values fit well into Christ's kingdom: love; honor; service and servant leadership; trust-based ("covenantal") relationships between manager and employee, rather than fear-based ones dependent on corporate hierarchy; community; environmental stewardship; creativity; cooperation; qualitative company assets like a sense of achievement; competence; ethical behavior; corporate higher purpose and responsibility; and personal fulfillment and development. (p. 39)

Religion is a current concern from yet another angle. An awareness of how different faith traditions impact business behaviors is essential in working with people from other cultures. Respect and sensitivity for other people's religious values and practices help remove communication barriers and avoid unnecessary conflicts. Since religion is one of the major ingredients of culture, multicultural competencies in management require some working knowledge of world religions.

The relevance and importance of religion in the workplace have been discussed in details elsewhere (Miller, 2006; Novak, 1996). The full benefits of spirituality are unlikely to be realized until faith is fully integrated to work. In other words, spirituality needs to be integrated with every aspect of work life, such as relationships, planning, budgeting, negotiation, compensation, etc. When such a large-scale cultural transformation takes place, one will see the following positive changes at the workplace:

- The corporation will become purpose driven and meaning centered.

- There will be a shift from a fear-based culture to a love-based culture.

- Management practices and decisions will be clearly consistent with spiritual values.

- Management will learn to truly listen to employees about their concerns and suggestions.

- Management will create a sense of community and inspire a sense of belonging.

- The work place will become a major source for personal meaning and fulfillment.

- There will be a new willingness to reflect on moral implications and social responsibility in decision making.

- Management will value employees based on who they are and what they can become.

- Management will also resort to spiritual ways of resolving conflicts. Therefore, they will be reluctant to issue ultimatums and slow to fire employees.

- There will be an improvement in morale, job satisfaction, togetherness, loyalty, and productivity.

The present spiritual movement is probably the most significant trend in management since the human-potential movement in the 1960s. It appears to be a grassroots movement, as more and more people entertain the notion that work can and should be meaningful and fulfilling. In the wake of the Enron debacle and many other destructive corporate scandals, management is also more willing to take spiritual and moral values seriously. This trend will endure, simply because it speaks to the deepest human need for meaning and spirituality. Therefore, it promises to provide a remedy to declining job satisfaction and increasing employee disengagement. Even if research fails to establish a direct link between spirituality and profitability, an enlightened business orientation still has the benefit of creating a more compassionate, caring, and ethical workplace. This alone would be good news for people who spend most of their adult lives at work.

References

Autrey, J. (1994). *Life and work: A manager's search for meaning.* New York: William Morrow & Co.

Epps, J. (2003). The journey of meaning at work. *Group Facilitations, 5,* 17–25.

Frankl, V. E. (1986). *The Doctor and the soul: From psychotherapy to logotherapy.* New York: Random House, Inc.

Gardner, H., Csikszentmihalyi, M., Damon, W. (2004). *Good work: When excellence and ethics meet.* Portland, OR: Perseus Books Group.

Handy, C. (1994). *The empty raincoat: Making sense of the future.* London: Hutchinson.

Miller, D. W. (2006), *God at work: The history and promise of the faith at work movement.* New York: Oxford University Press.

Novak, M. (1996). *Business as a calling.* New York: The Free Press.

Sellers, J. M. (2003). Utopia or kingdom come?: Discerning wheat from chaff in the new business spirituality. *Christianity Today,* February, p. 39.

Stevens, R. P. (2006). *Doing God's business: Meaning and motivation for the marketplace.* Grand Rapids, MI: Wm. B. Eerdmans.

Straus, D. (2005). How to build a collaborative environment. In S. Schuman (Ed.), *The IAF handbook of group facilitation* (pp.191-203). San Francisco: Jossey-Bass.

Taylor, S. (1994). Build to last. *Harvard Business Review,* pp. 70-72

Terez, T. (2000). *22 keys to creating a meaningful workplace.* Avon, MA: Adams Media.

Wong, P. T. P. (2002). Logotherapy. In G. Zimmer (Ed.) *Encyclopedia of Psychotherapy* (pp. 107-113). New York: Academic Press.

Wong, P. T. P. (2002a). Creating a positive, meaningful work climate: A new challenge for management and leadership. In B. Pattanayak & V. Gupta (Eds.), *Creating performing organizations: International perspectives for Indian management* (pp.74-129). New Delhi, India: Sage Publications.

Wong, P. T. P. (2005). Creating a positive participatory climate: A meaning-centered counselling perspective. In S. Schuman (Ed.), *The IAF handbook of group facilitation* (pp.171-189). San Francisco, CA: Jossey-Bass.

A Transformative Approach to Compassionate and Spiritual Care

PAUL T. P. WONG

Whenever I ask people: "Can people teach and practice business ethics without being an ethical person?" they typically shake their heads vigorously. Most people believe that ethical practices flow from one's inner moral core or ethical convictions. Not too long ago, a con artist who taught business ethics made it to the national news when he was arrested for various ethical and legal violations.

When I ask them: "Can people teach and practice compassionate care without being a compassionate person?" the answer is "No" again. They believe that compassionate practices need to be genuine expressions of one's compassion; otherwise, such perfunctory acts would be nothing more than crocodile's tears.

However, when I ask a third question: "Can people teach and practice spiritual care without being a spiritual person?" there is often an uncomfortable hesitation. The main reason for their discomfort is that they all believe that all people are spiritual, but they also know that many do not practice spirituality.

In our Second Meaning Conference Symposium on Spirituality and Health, most participants, including Dr. Christine Puchalski and Dr. Harold Koenig, answered that all people are spiritual, instead of giving a simple "yes" or "no" answer to my above line of questioning. I pressed the point further: "How about those self-professed atheists and secular materialists, who do not want to be linked to anything spiritual? How about those psychopaths, who commit brutality against other human beings?" There was an awkward silence among the participants.

My own solution to this dilemma is quite simple: Indeed, all people are spiritual by design, but only some are spiritual in practice. Although spirituality is an innate dimension of human nature, it may remain dormant in the unconscious (Frankl, 1986). In other words, since all people are wired spiritually, they all possess the capacity to become aware of their spiritual nature and incorporate it into their lives. Until that awakening takes place, they remain unspiritual in how they live their lives.

359

My main thesis is that the source of compassionate and spiritual care stems from health providers' own sense of higher purpose and spiritual experience. Therefore, our approach to spiritual care needs to move beyond a narrow focus on the mechanical, instrumental value of prayers and head knowledge about different faith traditions. The present paper calls for a transformative approach, which emphasizes the spiritual transformation of both the healer and the patient.

This paper also describes the healing wheel model of positive holistic medicine. Illness becomes the focal point of interactions between the four main components of the healing wheel: the healer, the patient, God, and the healing community. According to this model, we can maximize spiritual care only when all the healing connections are activated and the entire healing wheel is turning.

Many in health professions still cling to the traditional biomedical disease model. But there is no cure for many diseases and chronic illnesses. There is no cure for aging and dying, for examples. Genetic and medical research may prolong life expectancy, but science can never give us immortality and fulfillment.

Palliative care has taken on an increasing important role because people are living longer and more people are suffering from incurable chronic conditions. In end-of-life care facilities, such as hospices, the best "medicine" is compassion, which facilitates healing of the soul. Healing is possible even for the dying, if we provide a compassionate and spiritual caring environment, which facilitates acceptance, reconciliation, forgiveness, and hope.

Drugs are important because they can control and reduce pain, but there are no drugs for the broken hearts and wounded souls, and there is no medication for the existential anxieties of alienation, loneliness, despair, meaninglessness, and death. That is why we need compassionate and spiritual care.

NEED FOR A PARADIGM SHIFT

In addition to the limitations above, the current trends towards bureaucratic control, government regulations, materialism and consumerism further corrode the quality of our healthcare systems (Carson & Koenig, 2004). The house calls and the once trusting relationships between family doctors and patients have largely become a thing of the past. Doctors are burdened by unnecessary paperwork, worried about litigations, and pressured to treat more patients per hour.

Managed care, budget cuts, and bureaucracy have created a crisis in healthcare. Forces of depersonalization and dehumanization have driven many healthcare professionals to burnout and despair. They begin to wonder: "Why am I doing this? Why am I so unhappy? What is my calling?" Such a climate calls for a holistic, compassionate approach, which may help reignite the passion of healthcare workers and tap into the vast healing resources in faith communities.

Holistic healthcare recognizes that humans are psycho-bio-social-spiritual beings. From a Judeo-Christian or Buddhist perspective, every life is important and every individual has inherent value and dignity. Such a spiritual vision can be a powerful source of compassionate and spiritual care. For example, what motivated Mother Teresa in her compassionate care for the poor was her spiritual vision; in caring for the poor, she was serving Christ. Within the medical field, Dr. Viktor Frankl provided a good example of compassionate holistic care. His logotherapy is a useful conceptual framework for medicine as a compassionate, spiritual ministry.

DR. VIKTOR FRANKL AND LOGOTHERAPY

Dr. Viktor Frankl, a neurologist and psychiatrist of Vienna, is internationally known for his book, *Man's Search for Meaning* (1984). While incarcerated in Nazi concentration camps, he discovered the power of logotherapy, which means "healing through meaning." It can be translated as meaning-centered therapy. He considers logotherapy as a medical ministry, an important adjunct to any kind of medical treatment, because it addresses the fundamental issues of meaning and purpose of life (Wong, 2002a).

Frankl maintains that healing needs to occur at the spiritual level and that medical practice must address existential questions of suffering and death. "Man is not destroyed by suffering; he is destroyed by suffering without meaning" Frankl (1984). One of the basic tenets of logotherapy is that meaning can be found in the most horrible situations.

Apart from the quest for meaning, the medical ministry needs to awaken the defiant human spirit and ignite a sense of tragic optimism (See Wong's chapter on tragic optimism). Compassion compelled him to minister to other inmates—to restore their hope and dignity in the face of brutal oppression. He has demonstrated the importance of a deep conviction and an abiding faith. His biography has given hope and inspiration to millions of people facing suffering and death.

Dr. Herbert Benson, Founder of the Mind/Body Medical Institute at Harvard University, emphasizes mind-body medicine. He and others have shown that thinking can have a real effect on physiological functions and physical healing. In contrast, Dr. Frankl emphasizes mind-spirit-body medicine. Thinking is important, but faith and meaning are equally important. His anthropology provides the necessary theoretical underpinning for holistic medicine.

THE MEANING OF COMPASSIONATE CARE

Whether we realize it or not, all healthcare professionals are supposed to be in the ministry of compassionate and spiritual care, because medicine is a helping profession dedicated to caring for the sick and to the relief of human suffering. Without compassion and spirituality, we become managers and providers of medical services rather than medical care. Medicine without compassionate and spiritual care is like a physician without heart and soul.

Historically, those who entered the profession of medicine and nursing were primarily motivated by compassion. In modern times, many are attracted to the medical profession because of its prestige and potential to gain riches. They want to treat as many patients as possible to maximize profits. Very few are willing to make house calls, because it is not profitable. It is shocking how some doctors deliver the bad news of terminal cancer to their patients in an indifferent and even callous manner.

Compassionate care is the basis of a healing ministry. The word *compassion* means more than caring for someone. It literally means to "co-suffer"—to suffer with others and to be in solidarity with the sufferers. Henri Nouwen once said: "Compassion asks us to go where it hurts, to enter the places of pain." Similarly, Puchalski (2001) wrote: "Compassionate care calls physicians to walk with people in the midst of their pain, to be partners with patients rather than experts dictating information to them" (p. 352). It is love that compels us to reach out to the needy, to journey with the sick and suffer in spite of our own fears and needs. According to Buddhism, compassion entails more than empathy because it involves the desire to reduce the suffering of others.

Compassion makes all the difference not only in the quality of care, but also in the quality of interaction with the patients and their loved ones. Love facilitates healing and recovery. A loving doctor or caring nurse can make the bitter medicine taste sweet. Although love is intangible, its effects are very real—it can make a real difference in the patients.

However, there are limits to compassion. Without proper self-care and spiritual support, eventually we will reach a point of physical and psychological exhaustion. Being burnt out is more likely to occur in an organizational culture of mistrust, secrecy, conflict, and bureaucratic control.

In order to show unconditional love to others, we need to cultivate love and kindness in ourselves. Without proper self-care, our love for others is diminished, because we will not have much to offer, even when we want to give all of ourselves. We need rest, solitude, and renewal. The Buddhist approach to compassion and mindful meditation can be very helpful. The Christian teaching of being a channel of God's love is also important, because we need to be connected with the Source of Love, which is God, the Infinite Spirit.

To sustain compassionate care, one must return to the foundation of love over and over again. We believe that God is love and he is the source of goodness, kindness, patience, and compassion. That is why it is difficult to practice compassionate care purely at a humanistic level—one needs to tap into the spiritual resources to minimize and prevent burnout. In other words, compassionate love cannot just operate at the humanistic level; we need to recognize its spiritual source. Puchalski (2001, March) wrote:

> An increasingly common view holds that although young doctors may be excellent technicians, they often lack the humanitarian skills required to be compassionate caregivers who can communicate effectively with their patients about many issues related to their medical care, including preferences for treatment, prognosis, and the patient's lifestyle, beliefs, fears, and hopes. A critical part of such communication skills is the ability to discuss a patient's spiritual beliefs and how these beliefs affect the patient's health. (p. 33)

While agreeing with Dr. Puchalski, I want to emphasize that spiritual care is more than the application of spiritually oriented communication skills, more than being compassionate at the humanistic level. I propose that we need to explore and experience the transcendental reality and the ultimate source of healing.

THE MEANING OF SPIRITUAL CARE

According to Koenig (2001), there is a long historical tradition of connecting religion, medicine, and health care. Here is a brief overview of these connections:

- There are strong religious roots of modern medicine in the Western world.

- Religion and medicine are the two oldest healthcare professions.

- Religious groups built the first hospitals in the fourth century.

- Religious orders staffed most hospitals with nurses until the early 1900s.

- In China, early practitioners of medicine were often related to Taoism and Buddhism

- Folk religion and ancestor worship also played an important role in China.

It can be difficult to navigate the complexity of the world of spiritual healing. In addition to a multitude of faith traditions and spiritual practices, we will also encounter various self-acclaimed faith healers, who prey on those with simple faith and offer remedies with no proven medical value other than the placebo effect. Given the complexity and potential excesses of religion, it is no wonder many scientists and medical practitioners remain skeptical about any claims of the healing power of faith or religion.

Current Trends in Spirituality and Health

Recent years have witnessed a rapprochement between medicine and religion. An increasing number of medical schools in the United States have included a course on spirituality and health in their curriculum. This is based on the recognition of the important role of spirituality in health care and the need to take into account patients' personal spiritual history.

The positive contributions of religious commitment, practices, and faith to patients' well-being have been well documented in recent years (Post et al., 2000; Koenig, McCullough, & Larson, 2001). Here is a summary of the positive functions of religion/spirituality:

- Prayer contributes to healing and recovery.

- Faith improves quality of life, hope, and happiness.

- Religious beliefs affect medical decisions.

- Religious beliefs facilitate death acceptance.

- Religion/spirituality facilitate coping with chronic pain, disabilities, and terminal illnesses.

- Religious beliefs make sense of chaos and uncertainty and provide a sense of coherence and integration.

- Religion can generate a sense of spiritual well-being.

- Religious beliefs and communities can be a source of love and compassion.

A summary of some of the empirical findings on the benefits of faith include (a) greater longevity, (b) faster recovery from illness and surgery, (c) reduced stress and depression, (d) better adjustment to disability, (e) higher quality-of-life score, (f) lower blood pressure, (g) fewer cardiovascular problems, (h) fewer cases of depression and anxiety, (i) better immune functioning, and (j) healthier lifestyle.

Different from the past abuse of faith healing, the current approach to religion and spirituality is rational and scientific; it emphasizes evidence-based healing. It employs a variety of research methodologies, ranging from controlled experimental studies and clinical trials, to large surveys in order to establish the efficacy of personal faith, intercessory prayer, religious beliefs, and activities.

However, in spite of the current scientific emphasis, the primary focus of spiritual care is still on the instrumental value of religion and spirituality. This instrumental approach is based on what we say and do with our patients, such as (a) addressing patients' spiritual needs, (b) addressing patients' existential needs, (c) taking a spiritual history of patients, (d) incorporating appropriate spiritual practices, (e) involving chaplains and spiritual leaders, and (f) involving the appropriate faith community.

Puchalski (2001, March) emphasizes the importance of taking a spiritual history. She believes that asking your patient's spiritual history, what gives them meaning in life, and how they cope with their illness, may:

> ...open the door to a more trusting, deeper, and more meaningful relationship. This is at the heart of patient-centered—rather than disease-centered medicine. Physicians, by recognizing the spiritual dimension of our professional lives, can reclaim the spiritual roots of our practice—compassion and service. This is one way to bring compassion back into the art and science of medicine." (p. 35)

Puchalski's Spiritual Assessment Tool

Puchalski and Romer (2000) have developed a Spiritual Assessment Tool, which may summarized by the acronym FICA.

- F—Faith and belief: "Do you consider yourself spiritual or religious?"

- I—Importance: "What importance does your faith or belief have in your life?"

- C—Community: "Are you part of a spiritual or religious community?"

- A—Address in care: "How would you like me, your healthcare provider, to address these issues in your healthcare?"

There are certain limitations to an instrumental approach; these include the placebo effect, potential manipulation of faith healers, guilt and self-blame of patients, superstitious beliefs in certain religious rituals and practices, and the possible absence of any spiritual and emotional connection between the healer and the patient. Furthermore, a mechanical, instrumental approach of prayer reduces God to something that can be manipulated and diminishes the healing potentials of experiencing God at a deeper personal and spiritual level. For these reasons, much of the research on the efficacy of prayer can be criticized for missing the point that spirituality is relational rather than mechanical.

I propose that we need to broaden the focus and explore the potentials of spiritual transformation. Such an experiential and growth-oriented approach emphasizes spiritual transformation for both the healer and the patient. A transformative approach to spiritual care is based on who we are and how we live. It involves the healing connection and the healing presence. It can be characterized by the following:

- The healing silence—listening to the inner voice.
- The healing touch—touching the inner spirit.
- The healing connection—establishing an I-You relationship.
- The healing presence—providing a compassionate presence.
- The healing process—nurturing spiritual growth in patients.
- The healing community—building a caring community.

This transformative approach places a lot more demand on the healthcare provider than the instrumental approach, because healers not only need to possess the necessary skills, but also need to experience a spiritual transformation themselves. In spiritual matters, a deeply felt soulful experience is more important than head knowledge. Some of the characteristics of a spiritually transformed healer include (a) understanding your own spiritual needs, (b) experiencing the reality of spiritual blessings, (c) nurturing your own spirituality, (d) treating spirituality as an integral part of professional development, (e) caring for the wounded healer, (f) maintaining an I-Thou relationship with patients, (g) viewing the patient from a spiritual lens, and (h) transforming spiritual care into Divine care.

I propose that there are seven stages of spiritual transformation, which cover the entire spectrum from the initial spiritual awakening to the ongoing journey of spiritual growth.

Stages of spiritual transformation:

- Awareness of one's spiritual needs and the awakening of a spiritual quest.
- Sensitivity to the spiritual dimension of people and the transcendental reality.
- Knowledge of major faith traditions and spiritual practices.
- Developing a personal belief-meaning system.

- Taking part in a set of religious commitments or spiritual practices.

- Experiencing and living out one's religious beliefs or spiritual values.

- Becoming transformed through an ongoing spiritual quest and continued involvement with the faith community.

Transformative spiritual care involves all seven stages. To grow spiritually, health care providers need to understand their own spiritual needs and nurture their own spiritual lives as a crucial aspect of personal and professional development.

Illness provides a natural focal point to forge links between God, the healer, the healing community, and the patient. Thus, the transformative approach to spiritual care can be represented by a healing wheel.

Figure 1. The healing wheel

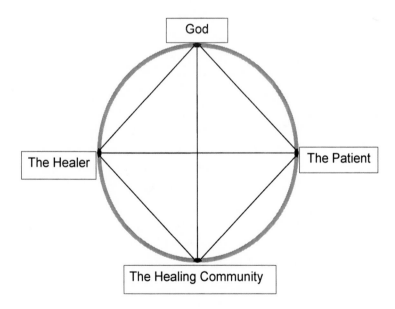

The healthcare worker needs to be spiritually transformed by God. His or her spirituality extends beyond a set of religious beliefs or spiritual practices. In fact, he or she has been renewed mentally, emotionally, and physically, and become a new creature. Her love and faith will have an impact on her patient and the healing community. There is something very calm and warm about her.

There is compassion in her tone of voice and love in her eyes. As he works with the patients, he is praying to God for wisdom and for healing. His impact on the patient works through four channels:

- His prayer moves God to touch the patient.

- His compassion contributes to a healing relationship with his patient.

- His treatment of the patient is enhanced by prayer and love.

- His healing ministry is reinforced by the healing community, who also supports the patient through prayer and other tangible expressions of love.

As a result, the patient turns to God for healing and redemption. This will complete the first circle.

God then pours out his love towards the patient. The change that takes place in the patient generates a lot of energy and excitement in the healer, who turns to God in gratitude and worship. The patient also joins the healing community, which supports the healer, who then gives thanks to God. This will complete the second circle. As the healing wheel turns over and over again, both the healer and patient are blessed, the healing community is strengthened and God is glorified.

The improbable can happen, dreams can come true, and broken lives can be made whole, when the healing wheel keeps on turning. Compassionate human encounters in the context of a supportive, validating, and trusting environment can be a powerful source of healing. The best part is that this healing process does not require money or expensive equipment, with just the human touch anointed by the spirit!

The healing wheel can be sustained to the extent that it provides meaning and purpose for both the healer and the patient. Healers find meaning and purpose in serving God and serving others. Patients rediscover the meaning of hope and love through the compassionate care received.

CONCLUSION

The healing-wheel model not only identifies the main components, but also specifies some of the processes involved in spiritual healing. It points out the need for caring for the wounded healer and for providing a healing community as the proper context for spiritual healing.

Caring for the sick and the dying can be very exhausting, especially in a nonsupportive environment. Prolonged stress can result in burnout. When this happens, healthcare workers may act cynically or callously towards the patients. Therefore, a key component of the healing wheel is broken.

Spiritual transformation is part of healthcare workers' self-care. Spiritual transformation needs to take place in the healers before it can touch the patients spiritually. That is why healthcare workers need to take time to care for their own spiritual needs. They need to spend time in solitude, in prayer, and in fellowship. They need to deepen their own relationship with God. From the perspective of Christian spirituality, Sanders (1998) emphasizes: "The only solution to all of life's complex problems is a vibrant relationship with the God of the Bible." For other faith traditions, there is a similar emphasis on spiritual discipline for transformation.

We also need a healing community to support both the healer and the patient. We cannot create such a community through the rearrangement of feng shui. We need to create a truly safe, supportive, compassionate, and nurturing environment, in which all members, both staff and patients, are encouraged to undertake a transformative journey, so that they can transform the way they look at life and death. Stanford University's Wellness Community program is a good example. Hospitals, hospices, and rehabilitation centers need to tap into the healing potentials of a vibrant healing community.

The key to success in creating a healing community hinges on leadership, because it would require a transformation of the corporate culture and organizational climate. This presentation will provide suggestions on how to create a positive and caring work place, which will serve as a healing community (Wong, 2002b).

A truly positive, holistic healthcare derives its strength from faith and conviction in times of suffering and offers compassion through self-sacrifice and surrender to God. The most important resource in healthcare is the human resource. Therefore, we need to encourage the spiritual development and transformation of healthcare workers in order to maximize their positive impact on patients in a time of budgetary cutbacks.

A truly positive, holistic healthcare is a powerful force for healing, because it flows from the heart of God and is reinforced by a healing community so that both healers and patients may have life and have it more abundantly.

References

Carson, V. B., & Koenig, H. G. (2004). *Spiritual caregiving: Healthcare as a ministry.* Radnor, PA: Templeton Foundation Press.

Frankl, V. E. (1984). *Man's search for meaning: Revised and updated.* New York: Washington Square Press.

Frankl, V. E. (1986). *The Doctor and the soul: From psychotherapy to logotherapy.* New York: Random House.

Koenig, H. G. (2001). Religion, spirituality, and medicine: How are they related and what does it mean? *Mayo Clinic Proceedings, 76,* 1189-1191.

Koenig, H. G., McCullough, M. E., & Larson, D. B. (2001). *Handbook of Religion and Health.* New York: Oxford University Press.

Post, S. G., Puchalski, C. M., & Larson, D. B. (2000). Physicians and patient spirituality: Professional boundaries, competency, and ethics. *Annals of Internal Medicine, 132,* 578-583.

Puchalski, C. M. (2001). The role of spirituality in health care. *Baylor University Medical Center Proceedings, 2001,* 352-357.

Puchalski C. M. (2001, March). Spirituality and health: The art of compassionate medicine. *Hospital Physician,* pp. 30-36.

Sanders, J. O. (1998). *A sufficient grace: Breakthrough to spiritual and emotional health.* Grand Rapids, MI: Discovery House Publishers.

Wong, P. T. P. (2002a). Logotherapy. In G. Zimmer (Ed.), *Encyclopedia of psychotherapy* (pp.107-113). New York: Academic Press.

Wong, P. T. P. (2002b). Creating a positive, meaningful work place: New challenges in management and leadership. In B. Pattanayak & V. Gupta (Eds.), *Creating performing organizations* (pp. 74-129). New Delhi, India: Sage Publications.

The Fluid Center:
An Awe-Based Challenge to Culture

KIRK J. SCHNEIDER

At the start of the cinematic marvel, *A Thousand Clowns* (1965), an unemployed comedy writer, Murray, leads his eleven-year-old nephew, Nick, to an empty Manhattan street. It is the wee hours of daylight, and as they stare into the cavernous depths, Murray suddenly turns to Nick and bellows: "In a moment you're going to see a horrible thing." "What's that?" the boy asks. "People are going to work!" Murray replies—tacitly urging Nick to broaden his horizons and transcend the complacent masses. Yet Murray's devil-may-care, multiphrenic lifestyle is not the "be-all, end-all" either, as we learn later in the movie. He, too, must hunker down in some ways, compromise, and curtail his impulses in order to live within the world, and in order to have the fuller life he seeks with Nick.

Murray's dilemma echoes the basic existential dilemma that is too often passed up today; that between our smallness (wormlikeness) and greatness (godlikeness) that is so integral to most (if not all) of our core human challenges. In this paper, I want to raise many more questions than answers about this basic human struggle between our smallness and our greatness. I want to suggest, on this millennial occasion, that the dilemma between smallness and greatness has momentous significance—not just for individual functioning, but also for our culture and, indeed, our world. Hence beyond democratism and republicanism, or capitalism and communism, beyond the petty factions of "good and bad" or "black and white" that we get ourselves into, is this epic of all battles—between our breathless possibilities and our equally daunting necessities or limitations.

How then, are we to translate this compelling insight into our everyday lives, our millennial futures? Let me suggest three ways which all lead down the same basic path: By bringing awe, carnival, and what I call the fluid center into our consciousness.

By *awe*, I mean the cultivation of the basic human capacity for the thrill and anxiety of living or, more formally, the cultivation of the capacity for humility and boldness, reverence and wonder before creation (e.g., this is the *mysterium et fascinans* that Rudolf Otto (1923/1958) speaks of in terms of the numinous); it is the capacity to be *moved*.

By *carnival*, I mean the importation of a sense of play, multi-dimensionality, and contrariety into our lives: but all within a relatively safe, supportive, and structured context. The idea here is that, ironically, the more we can play with the various "parts" of ourselves, the more deeply we can come to know ourselves: the parts of ourselves that genuinely matter.

Finally, by the *fluid center*, I mean the cultivation of all these dimensions—elasticity, pausefulness, the richest possible range of experience within the most suitable parameters of support, (or any sphere of consciousness, which has as its concern the widest possible relations to existence).

These are the same ideas that I believe Nietzsche was getting at with his "passionate people who become masters of their passion" (as cited by Kaufmann, 1968, p. 280); or Malinowski with his "freedom" as the "acceptance of the chains which suit one" (as cited in May, 1981, p. 83); or Ortega with his aspirations to a "vital design" (as cited in May, 1981, p. 93). If it does not have paradox, if it does not have contradiction, the philosopher Phillip Hallie, once intimated, "it isn't a powerful human feeling" (as cited in Schneider, 1999, p. 25).

I want to suggest that there are two pivotal settings where American, and indeed, contemporary Western, culture lacks this sense of the paradoxical, the awesome, the carnivalesque, and the fluidly centered: school and work.

In a stunningly neglected treatise, *Beyond Alienation*, Ernest Becker (1967) sets forth an equally stunningly educational proposal: the "alienation curriculum." The alienation curriculum is Becker's strategy to engage students and to animate their educational experience. In a nutshell, the curriculum teaches students how various cultures down through history have handled alienation. The curriculum inquires how various societies have estranged (e.g., humiliated, aggrandized, polarized, or fetishized) their populaces throughout history and, second, to what extent such practices relate to students' current lives. While there are many salutary dimensions to this curriculum, which would, no doubt, benefit students immensely, I would like to propose a broader and more affirming curriculum that I believe would have even greater salutary effects.

Drawing from Becker's proposal, then, I will now set forth an idea to enhance and complement the movement toward a fluid center at work, at home, and in places of worship. This proposal is for an awe-based educational curriculum.

Again, awe is defined as the capacity for the thrill and anxiety of living (the capacity to be *moved*); it is further defined as the realization of the humbling and emboldening sides of living; not as separate poles but together as integrated "wholes" of experience. In a nutshell, awe comprises an *integrated* sensibility of discovery, adventure, and boldness melded to, and in the context of, safety, structure, and support. Awe mitigates against alienation (polarization), either in the form of hyper-humility (humiliation) or hyper-boldness (arrogance).

For the awe curriculum, we might cover the Neolithic, Egyptian, Jewish, Greek-Roman, Early Christian, Medieval, Renaissance, Enlightenment-Romanticist, and industrial-technological eras; also, I would endorse studies of nonWestern (e.g., Eastern and African) contexts. Awe studies do not preclude more technical kinds of training (e.g., reading, writing, and arithmetic), but in the early years these are employed in the service of awe-based inquiry. It is only later, as students are ready to specialize, that such skills as math and science are focused upon as separate domains.

Beginning with the agrarian cultures of the Near- and Middle-East (e.g., Babylon, Greece, Egypt), then, let us look at some sample traditions and how and whether they foster awe, humility and boldness, reverence and wonder, before creation. Consider, for example, these cultures' relationships to land and nature—their religious systems (e.g., pantheism, goddess worship, and mystery cults), architecture (e.g., palaces, marketplaces, and sacred sites), art, literature, philosophy, forms of government, and transitions from agrarianism to urbanism and pantheism to monotheism. But let us not neglect the disease and pestilence in these societies—fatigue and overwork (where the average lifespan is in the 20s; the 60s if one is elite); slavery (if any), elitism, and barbarity. Let us reflect on their structure of authority (collective versus individualist, elite versus communal, and their concept of personal autonomy).

Next, we would ask students: How would these awe-inspiring (humbling and emboldening) and awe-deflating (humiliating and aggrandizing) episodes relate to their present lives, their present worlds? In what ways might they adopt or draw upon these discoveries to enhance or reform their worlds? Some possible discussion items include: What is the potential role of nature and natural environments on students' present sensibilities? What is the current significance of feminist spiritual principles (nurturance, egalitarianism)? What is the place of the sense of the sacred versus formal religion today? What is the present role of aesthetics in architecture? What are the various forms of slavery (compulsion, addiction) in today's lifestyles; what could be contemporary forms of elitism and barbarity? What is the relevance of individual versus collective authority and autonomy versus community today?

Other discussion areas could include the decadence of Rome, political rebellion and the institutional church in early Christianity, chivalry and sexuality during the Middle Ages, rationality versus religion during the Renaissance, and so on.

AWE-BASED WORK PROGRAMS

The class and income disparities in the world, particularly America, are grievous, as many readers are aware. This is a condition where in 1999, 19% of American children live in poverty (the worst rate in the developed world); where in 1992, the average American executive made 419 times what the average factory worker made; and where the top 2.7% of wage earners made as much as the bottom 100 million (Intelligence Report, Fall, 1999). It's a world where a camp counselor can, and often, does earn more than a frontline mental health worker at a home for disturbed children (personal communication, Sebastian Earl, 1999), or an information technologist makes several times the salary of a social worker, or a professional basketball player makes 10 times the wages of a teacher.

We profess to desire an engaged and invigorated populace. We say we want an informed and unified citizenry. We advertise our yen for physically and emotionally healthy children, youth who are committed to the values of work and brotherly love. Despite the rhetoric, however, we have a very puzzling way of demonstrating our concerns. How is it, for example, that our economic system is virtually tailor made to subvert our alleged values; and how is it that our morals, relationships, and lifestyles are, for all intents and purposes, contrary to our pronouncements?

The questions are: Can conventional notions of success be converted into visionary notions? Can "wealth" mean capacity for humility, reverence, and wonder (i.e., awe) before creation? While the first step toward such a transformation has already been suggested with an awe-based educational curriculum, presently, I will outline an awe-based work proposal. What if we could pass the following legislation? Suppose all nonemployer income earners in the top two percent of the American adult population and all American employers whose combined yearly individual income also exceeds the top two percent of wage earners would be offered a choice: either invest in (tax reduced) awe-based, socially responsible benefit programs or pay steep and sustained government taxes (which will in turn fulfill the same purpose). The socially responsible investment plan would roughly comprise two components: a comprehensive, universal health plan and for the employed, twice-weekly (one hour respectively) mental and physical well-being programs. The health plan would be partially subsidized by the government (from the general tax fund and the top two percent of employer and nonemployer income earners) and the well-being programs would be funded solely by the top two percent of employer income earners (or if agreed upon in advance, by an entire company). The health plan would provide generous mental and physical health benefits determined by both federal and regional authorities.

How would we get such a program implemented? First, I believe that many people, employees in particular, would welcome such an idea (especially if clearly articulated). Second, although many employers would balk at the expenditure of such a program, they would soon realize that they are all on the same playing field and that, if they want to remain in the game, they have to find a way to play, and play it well. While cost shifting (e.g., passing on expenditure costs to consumers) could be a problem, I believe that it would remain manageable because all employers in this bracket would be in the same situation, and therefore would have to keep their prices competitive. Finally, although there would likely be some suppression of incentive to become a top wage earner, employer, and entrepreneur, in the light of our proposal (especially among more materialistic types), there are three issues that I believe would mitigate this problem: (a) Everyone would be in the same boat, as previously mentioned, so jealousy, extravagant expectations, etc. would, by implication, be delimited; (b) People would soon find that there would still be room for healthy profit and wage earnings in spite of, and perhaps even in light of, the increased social consciousness at a given work setting (e.g., because of the greater social relevance of that setting's structure and product line); and (c) most, if not all, prospective workers will have undergone the awe-based educational training I alluded to earlier, and therefore would be inclined to value rather than to discount a vocational analogue of the latter.

The well-being programs would be administered by a committee comprising the employer, mental and physical health providers (e.g., psychologists, psychiatrists, general practice physicians, holistic health practitioners), and employees. The programs would be voluntary and scheduled at consistent times during eight-hour workdays. The mental well-being program could entail a wide variety of offerings, from topics of psychological and philosophical interest to those concerning spirituality and multiculturalism. The purpose of the mental well-being programs would be to promote reflection on, and where appropriate, corrective action concerning, the impact of work on employees' and employers' lives. Although such reflection and corrective action would be confined to work issues, they could address a wide variety of concerns. For example, the program might take the form of a discussion hour in which employers and employees consider the environmental relevance of their products. It could also take the form of a reflection about the need to restore pride, craftsmanship, and innovation at the worksite; or it could entail conflict mediation seminars, or forums about social values.

The mental well-being programs would need to fulfill four basic criteria. They would need to be (a) independently facilitated, (b) voluntary and non-discriminatory (i.e., protected from employer retaliation), (c) relevant to the work setting, and (d) acceptable to an employer/employee well-being committee. (For issues that fall outside these categories, other healthcare/ organizational services may be necessitated.) Finally, the well-being committee would, through one of its elected representatives, have a permanent seat on the respective company's board.

The physical well-being programs would also consist of a variety of offerings and would be administered by a physical well-being committee. The committee would consist of the employer, an elected body of employees, and a physical health expert of their choice. Activities could range from workout regimens to massage and sauna to yoga and stress-reduction exercises. There could also be provisions for a variety of programs on holistic health, exercise, nutrition, and alternative medicines. The on-staff health provider would help to monitor and, if necessary, medically advise all participants.

In addition to the above programs, there could be provisions for a range of alternative activities during the mental and physical well-being hours, from nature walks to outdoor retreats to communal projects (such as consumer satisfaction surveys). Those who choose not to partake in such activities would also have a variety of options from which to choose, from relaxing and recreating to continuing work.

Second, in order to maximize the integration of work and personal activity, four-day workweeks would be implemented. Such a period is essential for reflection, loved ones, and recreation. It also structures time for those who wish to partake in civic activities.

While it is true that about 12 hours would be subtracted from the conventional workweek, the 12 hours that would replace them should be more than enough to make up for such a loss; in fact, they should form the bedrock for a revolutionary new form of living. For in these 12 hours people would be encouraged to reflect deeply on their jobs, their lives, and the lives of those about them. The fruits of such engagement should be manifold, from enhancement of the work environment to humanization of the social terrain, and from improved vocational motivation to elevated social and moral sensitivity. The services resulting from such a transformation should also be markedly improved. There should be more services, for example, that address people's core values: such as environmentally supportive transportation programs, life-enhancing architectural arrangements, and health-affirming agricultural yields. There should be marked improvements in mental and physical health, education, and rehabilitation programs. There should be more and better medical services, with a wider range of treatment alternatives (for example, low cost, yearlong psychotherapy).

There should be pervasive improvements in recreational facilities, entertainment, and sporting events. There should be dramatically fewer overpaid executives, entertainers, and athletes, and markedly increased affordability of products and services. For example, to the extent that products become more meaningful to people, they will buy them more, which eventually should lower prices; and to the degree that entrepreneurial wealth is returned to the system that supports it, the quality and affordability of that system should also commensurately rise.

Finally, the well-being programs open up unprecedented opportunities for specialists in human service: from psychologists to physicians, philosophers to artisans, and counsellors to healers. While some may decry the ferocity of that transformation, I, and many others, would argue that it is just the counterweight necessitated today, as technicist models for living encroach upon the cultural landscape.

Awe-based prioritization should not eliminate the former technicist model; it should not erase the significant and hard-won gains of industrialization, controlling diseases, mass-producing food, and expediting information. Such a call would be sheer folly, and I do not believe many of the people urging humanistic change would seriously entertain it. However, that which an awe-based reform should bring is a deepening, a sensitizing, and a widening of our day-to-day view. It should instill the fluidity in the inert centeredness, and the flesh, bone, and heart in the pale plurality of our culture.

From this point of view, it is essential that we maintain (as Becker (1967), echoing Robert Maynard Hutchins, put it) *The Great Conversation*; and not just in the ivory tower but in the streets and suites as well. The well-being proposal releases unprecedented creative energies for individual and social expression, but, (and this is key) within the existing structures of a disciplined and committed workforce. The range of possibilities arising from the well-being forums will be rich; for not only will various companies opt for diverse presentations, but various Great Conversations within those presentations, will impact company policy-making. Put another way, The Great Conversation should lead to a continually evolving network of ideas, expressions, and sensibilities, which should result, in turn, in an ever-growing sphere of personal and vocational enhancement. Just imagine a fellow returning home from work after an exhilarating discussion about the moral import of his product line that could impact thousands of unknowing customers, not to mention the integrity of the salesman himself. Think how this state would affect his relationship with his wife, his children, and his sense of life.

The convergence of an awe-based, meaning-based, and reflection-based pause in the middle of peoples' workdays, complemented by parallel developmental and educational experiences, should have pervasive and synergistic effects on the entire ways we perceive, engage, and live out our respective days.

References

Becker, E. (1967). *Beyond alienation.* New York: George Braziller.

Intelligence Report. (1999, Fall). *Newsletter of the Southern Poverty Law Center*, p. 66.

Kaufmann, W. (1968). *Nietzsche: Philosopher, psychologist, antichrist.* New York: Vintage.

May, R. (1981). *Freedom and destiny.* New York: Norton.

Otto, R. (1923/1958). *The idea of the holy.* New York: Oxford University Press.

Schneider, K. J. (1999). *The paradoxical self: Toward an understanding of our contradictory nature.* Amherst, NY: Humanity Books.

Developmental Functions of Deferred Empathy

CHRISTINE V. BRUUN
BELINDA M. WHOLEBEN

Abstract

This study, conducted among young, middle-aged, and older adults, concerns deferred empathy (DE), which is empathy "after the fact." The developmental theory literature indicates a shift from instrumentality (e.g., achieving goals) in young adults to integrative values (e.g., inner harmony) in older adults (Ryff, 1982). Thus, it was predicted that young adults would give more instrumental examples of DE, whereas responses of older adults would be more integrative in nature. The sample included 133 adults. The Deferred Empathy Questionnaire asked each participant for a personal example, a triggering cause, and the outcome of this experience. Results indicated that young adults gave proportionately fewer integrative responses than did middle and older adults. Results of the study support the literature indicating age-related differences in instrumental and integrative thinking in adulthood. Implications are that deferred empathy may serve a significant role in helping adults accomplish important life tasks with successful aging.

Empathy is thought to be central to personal development, maturity, and well-being. Empathic concern and understanding have been linked to effective social interactions (Mead, 1934), to enhancement of the self (Kohut, 1977), to positive communication with others (Rogers, 1957), to sympathetic attributions (Regan & Totten, 1975), to mature coping (Allport, 1961; Vaillant, 1977), and to altruism (Batson, Early, & Salvarani, 1997; Eisenberg & Okun, 1996). For such an important phenomenon, it is striking that there is a dearth of research on how empathy changes through adulthood (May & Alligood, 2000). Knowing how empathy evolves through periods of adulthood would provide understanding about its functions in a developmental context.

This study, conducted among young, middle-aged, and older adults, concerns a distinct type of empathy: deferred empathy (DE), which is empathy "after the fact" (Bruun & Wholeben, 2001). Deferred empathy occurs when life experiences elicit a memory of an episode from the past in which one did not feel empathy for a target individual or group. However, as a result of the triggering experience, now there is empathy. There is active and deep emotional processing, in contrast to the previous time in which the event was thought about only from a personal perspective, or even not at all. Finally, deferred empathy is an experience that changes thinking, feeling, and/or behavior. As a retrospective re-evaluation of a former situation, deferred empathy differs from general empathy, which is usually concurrent with a present experience. We are interested in this construct from an adult developmental point of view.

Davis (1994) developed a useful multidimensional model of empathy showing its cognitive, affective, and physiological components. He explained the antecedents, mechanisms, and intrapersonal and interpersonal outcomes of empathy. Our model adapts and modifies these categories to explain the processes and content of deferred empathy. As in the Davis schema, this model includes (a) antecedent conditions, (b) mechanisms that move the re-evaluating process forward, and (c) outcomes to these processes.

First, we propose that deferred empathy begins with a stimulus event: a shared experience or an insight, either of which changes the perception of an earlier relationship with a target person or of a group. Our contention is that the stimulus event retrieves the earlier memory because it is salient and relevant to the developmental life tasks and stressors that are dominant for the person at that particular age and time. This triggering event could be the result of a critical event or from the reflection connected with life review.

Second, this event may be processed through three mechanisms: an attributional shift, cognitive dissonance, and controlled empathy. With an *attributional shift* in perspective, the individual is able to put herself in the target person's place and to regard the circumstances from this new vantage point. Life experiences and reflection may cause a role reversal, wherein the individual as observer shifts to the individual as actor. The empathizing person may then experience a self-discrepancy between her behaviors and attitudes from the past and the ways that she would currently prefer to see herself. *Cognitive dissonance* could result from a conflict between the actual and ideal self. This uncomfortable situation could provide motivation to resolve the discrepancy. It is at this point of disequilibrium, the discrepancy, that a very conscious and deliberate attempt to view circumstances from another's perspective may occur as a means of resolution. Through this form of *controlled empathy* there may be a definite effort to retrieve cues from memory and to think through the meaning and the emotion of the target person's experience.

Finally, the deferred empathy experience may ultimately result in outcome changes in behavior, thinking, and feeling in order to integrate the new perspective. The cycle might recur later in similar situations as deferred empathy is seen as an adaptive and relief-bringing strategy. Furthermore, each of these components could be bi-directional, each interacting with the other.

Because deferred empathy is, by definition, a reassessment of the past, it is often visible in life review and narratives about personal relationships. In fact, this type of empathy may, in itself, be an outgrowth of life review. In addition, deferred empathy may reflect the normative changes that occur through adulthood. The explanation of these changes in developmental theory, as well as how adults make meaning of them in life narratives, provide a helpful framework for thinking about this construct.

LITERATURE REVIEW

Erikson (1963) characterized young adulthood as a time of drawing on one's sense of self in order to consolidate intimate relationships and to work more harmoniously with others. In contrast, middle age is a time of generativity, returning the benefits one has received to younger generations, and old age is a time of wisdom, bringing meaning and coherence into the life that one has lived. Wisdom lies in accepting one's own and one's parents' imperfections, believing that each has done the best that could be done at the time. Levinson and his colleagues (1978) viewed young adulthood as a time to establish a preliminary life structure, to deepen commitments, and to seek independence. This perspective changes in midlife to re-evaluating values and goals and modifying the earlier life structure in order to develop a realistic view of self. Then, Vaillant (1977), in his 30-year longitudinal study of Harvard men, described adult development as a gradual maturing process. Whereas young adulthood is a time of building autonomy and focusing on instrumental goals of marriage and work, middle adulthood encompasses a reassessment of earlier hurts with an increase in nurturance and expressiveness. Mature coping, for Vaillant, comes with late life. Optimally for the older adult, there is less blame and bitterness and more acceptance and perspective.

Butler (1963) postulated that life review was inevitable in old age and often resulted in the wisdom and acceptance that Erikson attributed to late life. Jung (1933) viewed young adulthood as a time to live out gender-related roles. However, middle and old age were periods in which to integrate opposites, such as masculine and feminine values. Acceptance and tolerance should, ideally, increase with age. Jung thought of life review as a mechanism to gain internal psychic balance in middle-aged and older adults, a psychic balance less likely to take place in younger adults, who more typically concern themselves with external demands. For McAdams (1996), life review occurs throughout adulthood as a means of unifying experiences. Although there are theoretical differences about when life review occurs, it seems to be generally considered a means of acknowledging change in adulthood.

Research on personality changes that occur in adulthood appears to confirm the trends set forth in these theories of development. Self-perceived personality changes were noted by young, middle-aged, and older adults, based on concurrent, prospective, and retrospective ratings. The respective groups attributed high generativity to middle age and more integration and interiority to old age. Young adults predicted that they would be more accomplished in middle age (Ryff & Heincke, 1983). In a subsequent study (Ryff, 1989), subjective well-being was assessed in middle-aged and older adults. Both groups stressed the importance of being "others-oriented" and tolerant. However, for optimal functioning the middle-aged group emphasized the need for self-improvement and accomplishments, whereas the older adults stressed the importance of accepting change. Generally, there appears to be a shift from instrumentality (e.g., achieving goals) in young adults and middle age to integrative "culminant" values (inner harmony, freedom, happiness) in old age (Ryff, 1982; Ryff & Baltes, 1976). The external focus of instrumental goals and the internal focus of integrative meaning may be a fruitful dichotomy by which to evaluate the changing nature of deferred empathy in younger and older age. Both dimensions seem to be important to well-being in adulthood, respectively, in their own seasons. Wong and Watt (1991) found that only instrumental and integrative narratives in life review were representative of successful aging.

Changes in emotional development would also be relevant to the study of empathy. As adults age, they seem to grow in the ability to process emotions. Lawton, Kleban, Rajagopal, and Dean (1992) found that older adults possessed more emotional control, more stable moods, and more emotional maturity than younger adults. In addition, older adults may be better able than young adults to tolerate the tension of ambiguity and to acknowledge and express complex feelings. Instead of acting impulsively and in a retaliatory fashion, older adults may possess fuller emotional understanding and may reinterpret situations more positively (Labouvie-Vief, 1999; Labouvie-Vief, De Voe, & Bulka, 1989). Finally emotions seem to be more important and salient, and poignancy seems to increase in older adults (Carstensen & Turk-Charles, 1994). Poignancy, being a heightened awareness of inter-connections, would probably lead to an integrative type of deferred empathy.

Changes in life circumstances may also bring about a revised understanding of past relationships. Jenkins and Oatley (1996) argued that some episodes in adulthood have such emotional significance that they warrant deep self-reflection and personal change. In a similar vein, Kiecolt (1994) delineated stressors that become "critical events" and that motivate individuals to change their self-perceptions. Both emotional episodes and critical events could change identity.

Identity may be modified for adaptation in adult development. Whitbourne (1996) proposed that optimal aging requires a tension between the assimilation of experiences into an ongoing self-schema and the accommodation of self-discrepant experiences with identity changes. Randall (1996) discussed this re-evaluation process in the context of life review. He argued that "restorying" of life narratives occurs when there are discrepancies between the past and current realities. As mentioned above, life review for McAdams (1996) serves a unifying purpose across the life span, reconciling the developmental and personal changes that occur. The developmental changes experienced through adulthood seem to be registered in a personal record through life review.

Deferred empathy is a process of revising experiences and of paying attention to changes as they occur. Life review, including deferred empathy, may become a vehicle for organizing change and the different ways of viewing self and others. In this study, young, middle-aged, and older adults were asked to reflect on instances of deferred empathy. Based on the research literature concerning adult development and life review, we expected that deferred empathy would occur in all three ages but that the content and the function of the responses would vary across age groups. Based on prior findings (Ryff, 1982; Ryff & Baltes, 1976) it was predicted that young and middle-aged adults would give more instrumental examples, whereas those of older adults would be more integrative in nature.

METHOD
Participants

One hundred thirty-three participants took part in this study. There were 47 young adults (18-40 years, $M = 23.14$ years); 43 middle-aged adults (41-64 years, $M = 50.95$ years); and 43 older adults (65 years and older, $M = 73.20$ years). The sample included 104 women and 29 men. Each group included predominantly more women than men with the young adult group being comprised of 32 women and 15 men, the middle-aged group comprised of 34 women and 9 men, and the older adult group comprised of 38 women and 5 men. The young adults were undergraduate students in a small, Midwestern liberal arts college. The middle-aged and older adults were volunteers from community groups: church, civic groups, and social gatherings convened for the expressed purpose of reflecting on the concept of deferred empathy, and faculty and staff of the same Midwestern college mentioned above. The young adult group was ethnically diverse (Hispanic, African American, and Caucasian); however, the older groups were chiefly Caucasian. Also, the older groups were mainly well-educated, middle-class adults.

Measure

The Deferred Empathy Questionnaire was developed specifically for this study. The questionnaire asks for age and gender, provides a definition and example of deferred empathy, and requests from the participant a personal example, a triggering cause, and the outcome of this empathy experience. The definition is followed by two examples. One of the examples on the questionnaire is the following: "Joan recalls that she was critical and annoyed as a young girl when she had to help her slow-moving grandmother up and down stairs. Now that Joan herself is beginning to feel the effects of arthritis, she can look back on her grandmother with compassion. Because of this new understanding, she helps her aging mother with errands once a week." The final section of the measure solicits the personal experience of the participant:

- Give an example of a time when you have experienced deferred empathy.

- What prompted or triggered this feeling of deferred empathy?

- Did this experience change your thinking and/or behavior? If so, please describe these changes.

In responding to the questionnaire, the participant was allowed as much time and descriptive length as was individually preferred.

Procedure

Each small group of volunteers (e.g., church or civic group) was gathered with the intention of making clear the concept of deferred empathy. A brief description was followed by an open discussion of how this experience might occur in everyday life. The purpose of this conversation was to give the participants a feel for the meaning of the construct and to gain a sense of familiarity with it. When it appeared that the group had a working idea of how deferred empathy is a special instance of empathy in general, the questionnaires were distributed. The volunteers were given as much time as they wanted to read the definition and examples and to write about their personal examples and interpretations. When all the questionnaires had been completed and returned, the participants were given the opportunity to discuss their ideas. The exception to this procedure occurred in an undergraduate class situation. In this event, the concept was described, and students who wanted to participate completed the questionnaire and then returned them. Also, in some instances, the concept of deferred empathy was explained to an individual, who mailed the questionnaire to the experimenters upon completion (e.g., faculty members).

Scoring

The verbatim responses on the questionnaires were content analyzed. The coding system of Wong and Watt (1991) was used to differentiate instrumental from integrative responses. If an example of deferred empathy suggested that it had helped the individual solve a problem, attain a goal, or gain insight about performing a role, the response was coded as instrumental. If the example connoted the resolution of a past conflict or more interpersonal understanding, the response was coded as integrative. If a response was clearly not an example of deferred empathy, it was coded as "other" and not used. Inter-rater reliability was computed by coding a previous sample of questionnaires from young, middle-aged, and older adults similar to the ones in the present study. Raters agreed on the categories of integrative or instrumental in 70% of the cases.

RESULTS

A Chi-square test was conducted to assess whether examples of deferred empathy (instrumental or integrative) varied by age (young, middle-aged, or older adult). Results, $\chi^2(2, N = 133) = 6.855$, $p = .032$, indicated that young adults gave proportionately fewer integrative responses ($SR = -1.6$) than did middle-aged and older adults.

In additional analyses, when type of deferred empathy (instrumental or integrative) was examined by gender across all age groups, the Chi-square test indicated that men gave proportionately fewer integrative responses than did women $\chi^2(1,$ $N = 133) = 5.306, p = .021, SR = -1.5$. Also, men in the young-adult age group appeared to give fewer integrative responses than did women in the young-adult group, as well as did men and women in all other age groups. The statistical results of this analysis are not reported due to potential instability emanating from a marginal violation of expected cell frequencies for the Chi-square statistic.

DISCUSSION

This study appeared to be useful in testing the first stage of our theoretical model. We had speculated that one of the initial stimulus events that could trigger deferred empathy would be the pressing demands of a developmental task appropriate to an individual's age. As theorized, the participants in the study did, indeed, seem to give instances of deferred empathy that were congruent with the normative demands and needs of their respective points in adulthood.

The central finding in this study, that young adults gave more instrumental instances of deferred empathy compared to more integrative responses from older adults, confirmed our expectations. However, an interesting finding, contrary to expectations, was that middle-aged adults were more integrative in their responses than young adults.

Instrumentality was characterized by problem-solving, role performance, and goal attainment (Wong & Watt, 1991). The sample of young adults in this study seemed to use deferred empathy instrumentally to solve practical problems (e.g., in work, school, and families) in order to perform the roles that were required of them. An example of instrumental deferred empathy from a 19-year-old male is:

> Now I understand why my mother was always angry with me when I used her car and did not take care properly of the car. I have a car now and when my brother takes it, I act exactly like my mother did with me because the car is mine. I pay for it and, therefore you [sic] are more responsible.... Now I appreciate people's properties and I understand that one should not be angry with others when they try to protect that for which they worked hard.

This example would be consistent with Erikson's description of young adulthood as a time of forming intimate and harmonious relationships, with Levinson's theory of striving for independence with a new life structure, incorporating career and relationships, and with Vaillant's observations of building autonomy within the context of work, family, and friends.

In contrast, integrative responses were characterized by emphasis on meaning, resolution of conflicts, and interpersonal understanding (Wong & Watt, 1991).

Integration clearly was the dominant theme in deferred empathy among older adults. An example from a 75-year-old female follows:

> ...visiting my mother in a nursing home and hearing from her about our childhood and about my feelings of dislike for her... coming to realize I didn't really know what she went through as a young, divorced woman....We talked many times during her last years about her youth, my youth and [I] saw her as she had become, a lonely mom needing my love and attention. We both benefited from our empathy and understanding.

Once again, in accord with Erikson, this emphasis agreed with the developmental task in late life of finding meaning, wisdom, coherence, and self-acceptance and with Vaillant's description of more acceptance, maturity, and emotional health.

We had expected that middle-age, in the midst of careers and productivity, would be a period that would elicit instrumental types of deferred empathy. However, similar to older adults, responses coded as integrative were more the norm for the middle-aged adults. The following is an example of deferred empathy from a 47-year-old female:

> I remember being mean to my grandfather because my grandmother was mean to him. In particular, I unplugged his electric lawn mower (while he was mowing) and ran away on several occasions. As an adult, I realized that my grandmother was a very depressed woman and that she essentially mentally "abused" my grandfather by her hostile behavior to him and that what I did (thinking it was funny at the time) was part of that "abuse." I live as much by the 'Golden Rule' as possible and try to treat people fairly and at least politely. I think realizing that one person's joke is another person's nightmare made me recognize how much small actions can sometimes have larger, unintended consequences. Once my grandmother died, I tried to be as supportive and thoughtful as I could to my grandfather from a distance (since we lived far apart) and I wrote and called him regularly.

Both Levinson's characteristics of midlife as a time of reappraisal of values and of life structure and Vaillant's increase of nurturance and expressiveness as past pain is reassessed could, arguably, be considered integrative thinking. In retrospect, each of these theories provides an understandable use of deferred empathy for middle-aged adults. Changing perspective to adapt and to understand others more fully might be a beginning, preparatory stage for the integration called for in later life.

Two general benefits of deferred empathy seemed to be consistent in most of the individuals across our sample. First, most respondents mentioned the defusing of negative emotion as a result of the experience. Second, the experience of deferred empathy appeared to mobilize energy for more positive future directions. In the first case, individuals noted that they regarded a target person or group more positively than they had in the past. In addition, they implied that they felt better about themselves, either from a feeling of doing the right thing or from resolving cognitive dissonance. In the second case, all individuals reported that they changed thoughts, feelings, and/or behaviors in a more positive direction as a result of their insights. Although expressed differently, an underlying theme throughout was a resolve to approach the relevant issue differently in the future.

In examining the responses to the deferred empathy questionnaire, it became apparent that gender differences in type of response (instrumental and integrative) may exist. Subsequent analysis indicated that males gave fewer integrative responses than females. Due to the small sample size and under-representation of men in our sample, follow-up analyses could not conclusively determine whether this gender difference is primarily in the young-adult group or whether it is stable across all ages. Future research should include more equal gender representation.

This study was a testing of the first step of the model. Subsequent research on the construct of deferred empathy must certainly test other components of the model. The second stage, an attributional shift, is present by definition. However, the third stage of cognitive dissonance, the fourth of controlled empathy, and the fifth of changes in thoughts, feelings, and behavior are all stages of the model that need to be substantiated empirically.

An additional line of research would be the connection between forgiveness and deferred empathy. Intuitively, there seems to be an inherent link between the two concepts: changing, in a positive way, one's perspective and feelings about a past relationship seems to overlap closely with the phenomenon of forgiveness. Furthermore, some individuals specifically stated that their experiences with deferred empathy led to feelings of forgiveness. Worthington (1998) described a pyramid model of forgiveness in which empathy could be a key step to re-condition cognitive and emotional experiences. It is quite possible that a deliberate use of deferred empathy could be a therapeutic tool in healing hurtful events from the past. Older adults, who use deferred empathy for integrating meaning and for interpersonal understanding, may also enhance forgiveness in their lives. Additionally, they may be powerful mentors for teaching this strategy to those adults younger than themselves.

Identifying deferred empathy as a constructive intrapersonal and interpersonal tool might makes it more available for proactive benefits. Since the phenomenon of deferred empathy has been identified, named, and defined, it becomes more retrievable from memory and more usable as a coping strategy.

References

Allport, G. (1961). *Pattern and growth in personality.* New York: Holt, Rinehart, Winston.

Batson, C. D., Early, S., & Salvarani, G. (1997). Perspective taking: Imagining how another feels versus imagining how you would feel. *Personality and Social Psychology Bulletin, 23,* 751-758.

Bruun, C., & Wholeben, B. M. (2001, November). Deferred empathy: Reconsidering past relationships. Poster session presented at the annual meeting of the Gerontological Society of America, Chicago, IL.

Butler, R. N. (1963). The life review: An interpretation of reminiscence in the aged. *Psychiatry, 26,* 65-76.

Carstensen, L. L., & Turk-Charles, S. (1994). The salience of emotion across the adult life span. *Psychology and Aging, 9,* 259-264.

Davis, M. H. (1994). *Empathy: A social psychological approach.* Boulder, CO: Westview Press.

Eisenberg, N., & Okun, M. A. (1996). The relations of dispositional regulation and emotionality to elders' empathy-related responding and affect while volunteering. *Journal of Personality, 64,* 157-183.

Erikson, E. (1963). *Childhood and society.* New York: W. W. Norton.

Jenkins, J. M., & Oatley, K. (1996). Emotional episodes and emotionality through the life span. In C. Magai & S. H. McFadden (Eds.), *Handbook of emotion, adult development, and aging* (pp. 421-441). New York: Academic Press.

Jung, C. G. (1933). *Modern man in search of a soul.* New York: Harcourt, Brace, & World.

Kiecolt, K. J. (1994). Stress and the decision to change oneself: A theoretical model. *Social Psychology Quarterly, 57,* 49-63.

Kohut, H. (1977). *The restoration of the self.* New York: International Universities Press.

Labouvie-Vief, G. (1999). Emotions in adulthood. In V. L. Bengston & K. W. Schaie (Eds.), *Handbook of theories of aging* (pp. 253-267). New York: Springer.

Labouvie-Vief, G., DeVoe, M., & Bulka, D. (1989). Speaking about feelings: Conceptions about emotion across the life span. *Psychology and Aging, 4,* 425-437.

Lawton, M. P., Kleban, M. H., Rajagopal, D., & Dean, J. (1992). Dimensions of affective experience in three age groups. *Psychology and Aging, 7,* 171-184.

Levinson, D. J. (1978). *The seasons of a man's life.* New York: Ballantine.

May, B. A., & Alligood, M. R. (2000). Basic empathy in older adults: Conceptualization, measurement, and application. *Issues in Mental Health Nursing, 21,* 375-386.

McAdams, D. P. (1996). Narrating the self in adulthood. In J. E. Birren, G. M. Kenyon, J. E. Ruth, J. J. F. Shoots, & T. Swenson (Eds.), *Aging and biography: Explorations in adult development* (pp. 131-148). New York: Springer.

Mead, G. H. (1934). *Mind, self, and society.* Chicago: University of Chicago Press.

Randall, W. L. (1996). Restorying a life: Adult education and transformative learning. In J. E. Birren, G. M. Kenyon, J. E., Ruth, J .J. F. Shoots, & T. Swenson (Eds.), *Aging and biography: Explorations in adult development* (pp. 224-247). New York: Springer.

Regan, D. T., & Totten, J. (1975). Empathy and attribution: Turning observers into actors. *Journal of Personality and Social Psychology, 32,* 850-856.

Rogers, C. R. (1957). The necessary and sufficient conditions of therapeutic personality change. *Journal of Consulting Psychology, 21,* 95-103.

Ryff, C. D. (1982). Self-perceived personality change in adulthood and aging. *Journal of Personality and Social Psychology, 42,* 108-115.

Ryff, C. D. (1989). In the eye of the beholder: Views of psychological well-being among middle-aged and older adults. *Psychology and Aging, 4,* 195-210.

Ryff, C. D., & Baltes, P. B. (1976). Value transition and adult development in women: The instrumentality-terminality sequence hypothesis. *Developmental Psychology, 12,* 567-568.

Ryff, C. D., & Heincke, S. G. (1983). Subjective organization of personality in adulthood and aging. *Journal of Personality and Social Psychology, 44,* 807-816.

Vaillant, G. E. (1977). *Adaptation to life.* Boston: Little, Brown.

Whitbourne, S. K. (1996). Psychosocial perspectives on emotions: The role of identity in the aging process. In C. Magai & S. H. McFadden (Eds.), *Handbook of emotion, adult development, and aging* (pp. 83-98). San Diego, CA: Academic Press.

Wong, P. T. P., & Watt, L. M. (1991). What types of reminiscence are associated with successful aging? *Psychology and Aging, 6,* 272-279.

Worthington, E. L. The pyramid model of forgiveness. In E. L. Worthington (Ed.), *Dimensions of forgiveness: Psychological research & theological perspectives* (pp. 107-137). Philadelphia: Templeton Foundation Press.

On Responsibility Inferences and the Perceived Moral Person

BERNARD WEINER

Abstract

Empirical evidence, primarily from social psychological research, is presented to illuminate the layperson's judgments of responsibility. Among the differentiations examined are effort versus ability as causes of achievement performance, causal versus outcome evaluation, a biological versus a behavioral basis of stigmas, stigma onset versus stigma offset, welfare recipients versus the poor, and retributive versus utilitarian punishment goals. Finally, the determinants of being judged a moral person are considered.

As a social psychologist, I will not focus my attention on feelings of personal responsibility, but rather on how one infers the responsibility of others and determines if another is or is not a moral person. This has great implications for personal life meaning, and self- and other-perception share many common properties. My more specific goals are to bring to your attention evidence regarding:

- Some behaviors, states, and antecedent conditions that promote responsibility judgments for others.
- Some strategies people use to mitigate these judgments.
- Some emotional and behavioral consequences of holding others responsible or not.
- More speculatively, the determinants of considering others as moral or immoral beings.

ACHIEVEMENT EVALUATION

Responsibility judgments are most frequently associated with interpersonal transgressions, which vary greatly and can include criminal encounters as well as the relatively benign act of arriving late for an appointment. But there are many situations in which responsibility beliefs are elicited even though another individual is not directly victimized (although "society" may be regarded as damaged). Achievement settings provide one such context.

In his classic book, *The Protestant Ethic and the Spirit of Capitalism*, Max Weber (1904) called attention to the association between achievement strivings and morality. He argued that it is a moral duty to put forth effort and to strive for success. In support of this line of reasoning, a large number of research studies (see review in Weiner, 1986) have documented the intuitively evident—the person who fails to put forth effort and performs poorly is held responsible for that outcome and is reprimanded or punished. This contrasts with failure caused by the absence of ability or aptitude, which is construed as not controllable by the failing person, thus abrogating judgments of responsibility and, in turn, precluding punishment. One illustrative type of research investigation that supports these conclusions asks for evaluative feedback (say, from +5 to –5) to students described, for example, as follows:

- Student A: High in ability, low in effort, failing an exam.

- Student B: Low in ability, high in effort, failing an exam.

- Student C: High in ability, low in effort, succeeding at an exam.

You might do this now. It is expected that the reader (just as the participants in this research) will recommend a harsher evaluation to Student A than to Student B. Student A is more responsible for failure and is less moral than Student B because the cause of the negative outcome is controllable and "it could have been otherwise." Controllable failure, in turn, will be punished more than uncontrollable failure.

It also is the case that the combination of lack of effort accompanied by success (Student C) is evaluated more positively (or, less negatively) than lack of effort accompanied by failure (Student A). This finding documents that outcome also is a determinant of appraisal, which is the case in nonachievement as well as in achievement contexts. Thus, for example, a fireman who risks his life and saves a child receives a hero's medal; the one who fails with the same risk merely is consoled. Similarly, although two drivers may be equally guilty of breaking the law because of fast driving, only the driver of the car that happens by chance to hit a child is severely punished. Outcome severity (degree of failure, seriousness of a transgression) thus is another determinant of morality.

Research also has documented that people believe it "fair" to punish lack of effort more harshly than lack of ability when these are specified or implied as the causes of failure (Farwell & Weiner, 1996). In these investigations, participants judge combinations of teacher evaluations such as these:

1a) Student A has high ability, did not put forth effort, and failed an exam. Evaluative feedback from the teacher was –4.

1b) Student B has low ability, put forth much effort, and failed an exam. Evaluative feedback from the teacher was –1.

How fair was the teacher? Please respond to that now.

2a) Student A has high ability, did not put forth effort, and failed an exam. Evaluative feedback from the teacher was –1.

2b) Student B has low ability, put forth much effort, and failed an exam. Evaluative feedback from the teacher was –4.

How fair was the teacher?

I feel quite sure that the responses of the reader will again be similar to those of the typical college students who serve as research participants in most of these investigations. That is, it will be regarded as "fair" or "just" if the teacher evaluated the lack of effort student more severely than the student lacking in ability, so that evaluation of Pair #1 will be judged as fairer than teacher evaluation for Pair #2.

Even given lack of effort, strategies are available that reduce inferences of personal responsibility. Excuses can be provided such as "I became ill" or "The library was closed because of an electrical outage," thus transforming not studying from a controllable to an uncontrollable act. In addition, justifications can be offered that appeal to higher moral goals as a means of reducing responsibility. For example, "I helped my hospitalized grandmother," reduces the responsibility of the pupil for failing to put forth sufficient effort (if this account is accepted), even though the lack of effort nonetheless is perceived as controllable. Individuals have as part of their arsenal of interpersonal strategies a variety of impression management techniques that are used to reduce inferences of personal responsibility and the understood consequences of these inferences (Weiner, 1995).

Not surprisingly, expected negative reactions to lack of effort also are taken into account when individuals describe the causes of their failure to others (see Juvonen, 2000). Even young children communicate different causes of failure to teachers and peers, telling teachers that they "could not" and peers that they did not try. That is, they anticipate the negative reactions of teachers to not trying, realizing that this results in a judgment of responsibility and harsh punishment.

STIGMAS

Now I will turn my attention from achievement striving to an entirely different domain, that of stigmatization, but again examining judgments of responsibility and beliefs about morality. A stigma embraces any mark or sign for an undesirable perceived deviation from a norm. That is, the stigma typically defines the person as not only deviant, but in some way flawed or "spoiled." Stigmas differ on many characteristics, including their visibility or concealability, the danger posed by the person, the difficulty of normal social interaction with that individual and on and on. In addition, and most pertinent in this context, stigmas differ in the perceived responsibility of the person for having this plight. Here again moral judgments are rendered although no personal transgression has been reported.

Simple experimental procedures illustrate the differential beliefs about the personal responsibility of the stigmatized for their condition (see Weiner, Perry, & Magnusson, 1988). Participants may, for example, be given a list of stigma labels, with no other information, and then merely asked how responsible are the individuals for having this state or condition (on a scale ranging, say, from "not at all" to "entirely"). In addition, other ratings might be obtained, including the amount of sympathy they experience for these individuals and the extent to which they would be willing to provide them with help.

In such investigations, it has been consistently found that stigmas having a biological (somatic, genetic) source give rise to inferences of nonresponsibility. For example, Alzheimer's disease, blindness, cancer, heart disease, paraplegia, and so on elicit beliefs of nonresponsibility. On the other hand, stigmas with a behavioral component that is regarded as causal, including AIDS, alcoholism, drug use, and obesity, give rise to judgments of personal responsibility. The former stigmas are construed as "sickness," whereas the latter are markers of "sin"—there is a moral failure. Given a biologically-based stigma, the person is regarded as having no choice or volitional control over the plight, whereas among the behaviorally-based stigmas, it is presumed that volitional alteration in behavior (e.g., do not engage in permissive sex, eat less, etc.) could have prevented the onset of and/or eliminated the aversive condition (see review in Weiner, 1995). Note that contrasting a biological versus a behavioral basis of stigmas is conceptually similar to the distinction between ability and effort as causes of failure in the achievement domain. That is, lack of ability, like Alzheimer's disease, is regarded as uncontrollable, whereas drug use is considered similar to lack of effort in that both are regarded by the layperson as controllable. Hence, they bring about similar reactions and share conceptual or genotypic similarity.

In this context, a distinction between responsibility for the onset versus the offset of the stigma also is of value (Brickman et al., 1982). For example, one may be responsible for the onset of AIDS, but then not responsible for its offset. Alcoholics Anonymous makes this same assumption regarding excessive drinking (although, in the eyes of the lay public, the person also is responsible for drinking offset. After all, there are Mothers Against Drunk Driving, but not Mothers against Alzheimer's Patients). Given either onset or offset responsibility, the stigmatized person is reacted to as a "sinner."

Many (but not all) of these responsibility inferences can be altered with specific information that contradicts the a priori beliefs regarding the cause of the stigma (Weiner et al., 1988). For example, AIDS can be described as due to a blood transfusion, as opposed to the typical construal of transmission through sexual behavior. This results in great changes not only in responsibility beliefs, but also in reported sympathy, intentions to help, and other judgments as well. In a similar manner, cancer traced to smoking as opposed to living in a polluted environment, or heart disease attributed to an unhealthy life style as opposed to a genetic predisposition, produces quite disparate psychological reactions. Thus, even biological or somatic stigmas can be perceived as subject to volitional control and the person is then regarded as responsible for this condition. However, it should be recognized that causal change might not alter all reactions to the stigmatized person. For example, children can be taught to attribute obesity to uncontrollable rather than to controllable factors (a thyroid dysfunction rather than overeating), yet they still do not want overweight others as their friends (Ansbury & Tiggeman, 2000).

For some conditions, however, changing responsibility and moral judgments is difficult, or perhaps impossible, to accomplish (see Weiner et al., 1988). For example, a person with Alzheimer's disease is unlikely to be blamed (given the public understanding of this condition), and it is equally improbable that a child abuser will be regarded as not responsible for this deed.

Mental illnesses, which comprise one class of stigmas, also are of interest in terms of responsibility beliefs of the layperson. Depression often is regarded as controllable and the person is held responsible for continued sadness (Hooley & Licht, 1997). Schizophrenia, on the other hand, is likely to be considered uncontrollable when the symptoms are "active" or "positive" such as hallucinations, but less so when the symptoms are "passive" or "negative" such as social withdrawal (Weisman & Lopez, 1997). Parents of schizophrenics differ greatly regarding their perceptions of responsibility for this illness, with some expressing criticism toward their ill family members for not overcoming their plights, whereas others are accepting of an uncontrollable condition (Lopez, Nelson, Mintz, & Snyder, 1999).

Laypersons also make a distinction between individuals on welfare and the poor, although these are very overlapping stigmatized populations (Rasinski, 1989). Persons described as on welfare (which, at its inception, was targeted to assist widows) are reacted to much more negatively than individuals described as poor. In contrast to the poor, welfare recipients are seen as responsible for their problems. More specifically, they are perceived as not working, whereas the poor are thought to be working but not receiving sufficient wages to provide for a decent life.

Examples of these contrary stereotypes exist in political rhetoric that surrounds the welfare and poverty issues. In two different speeches, President Bush reinforced these very different images of welfare recipients and the poor. With respect to welfare, Bush warned: "Those who remain on welfare… if you refuse to help yourself, then Texas cannot help you" (Bush, 1999, Jan. 27). Regarding poverty, he stated in a later speech: "We will rally the armies of compassion in our communities to fight a very different war against poverty" (Bush, 1999, July 22). This conjures a contrasting image of the helpless poor.

Democrats also have reinforced these stereotypes. Former President Clinton strategically named his welfare reform policy the "Personal Responsibility and Work Opportunity Act," noting that, "Our welfare reform proposal will embrace two simple values: work and responsibility" (Clinton, 1995). This sentiment implies that the new American welfare policy will no longer be handouts to the lazy.

INDIVIDUAL DIFFERENCES IN RESPONSIBILITY INFERENCES

Thus far it has been implied that all persons react similarly in, for example, not holding the poor responsible for their condition but condemning those on welfare. However, this is not the case. Reactions to the stigmatized may vary, and one predictor of the differential reactions is the political ideology of the respondents (in spite of the similarity in the Bush and Clinton quotes given above). Considering poverty, conservatives tend to attribute this state to causes such as self-indulgence (drinking and drugs) and laziness, beliefs implicating personal responsibility. On the other hand, liberals are more likely to view the poor as victims of society (no job opportunities, inadequate education, etc.; Skitka & Tetlock, 1993). Indeed, for a wide variety of negative situations or conditions, conservatives tend to perceive the cause as more controllable than do liberals, thereby ascribing greater responsibility and immorality to the person in need. For example, research has documented that conservatives are more likely to hold the obese responsible for their weight problem than are liberals (Crandall & Martinez, 1996). Overweight female children even receive less financial support from conservative as opposed to liberal parents (Crandall, 1995).

CONSEQUENCES OF RESPONSIBILITY JUDGMENTS

I have thus far addressed some of the antecedents that promote responsibility judgments, such as perceptions of control, stigma label, and type of mental illness.

I next consider the consequences of these judgments, for examining the results of responsibility inferences provides the opportunity to present a more complete meaning of this construct. Consequences were frequently alluded to in the prior discussion, but they were not explicitly examined. Let me first turn to emotional consequences, followed by a discussion of punishment for transgressions.

There is high agreement among emotion theorists that a number of affects are linked with judgments of personal responsibility, with two of the most prominent being anger and sympathy (Roseman, Spindel, & Jose, 1990). Anger is an accusation or a value judgment that follows from the belief that another person "could and should have done otherwise" (Averill, 1982). When persons report instances of anger, they most often include accusations of voluntary and unjust behavior, such as another telling a lie, or unintended behavior that nonetheless is perceived as controllable, such as coming late for an appointment because of oversleeping. Lack of effort elicits anger among teachers and parents, as does obesity when the related other is overeating. Sympathy, on the other hand, follows when the plight of another is uncontrollable. Thus, athletic failure because of a physical handicap, school failure because of a lack of aptitude, and obesity because of an overactive thyroid, are prototypical predicaments that elicit sympathy.

It also is known that, in addition to emotions, both prosocial behavior (help giving) and antisocial behavior (aggression) are greatly influenced by perceptions of responsibility although, of course, there are many determinants of these actions. For example, we are more likely to give charity to the blind than to those having AIDS, to paraplegics rather than to alcoholics, and the like. That is, we support sickness but not sin. Sickness is associated with nonresponsibility and sympathy, whereas sin is linked to responsibility and anger.

PHILOSOPHIES OF PUNISHMENT

In addition to emotions and broad behavioral domains, such as helping and aggression, responsibility judgments are directly linked to beliefs about punishment. Philosophers have pointed out that two types of goals guide punishment: utilitarian and retributive. Utilitarian goals consider the costs and the benefits of the punishment; the focus is on the future, with aims reached through a reduction in the likelihood of a misdeed by the perpetrator and/or by others in society. The second major category of punishment is retribution, which pertains to avenging a past wrong rather than being concerned with the subsequent consequences of the punishment.

How might the utilitarian-retribution distinction be related to inferences of responsibility? It appears that social transactions deemed controllable by the actor, that is, those negative actions that result in inferences of personal responsibility and immorality, elicit anger and retributive responses. On the other hand, uncontrollable transgressions do not give rise to judgments of responsibility and therefore elicit sympathy and utilitarian concerns. Of course, punishment can (and does) serve both goals, but nonetheless it is important to know which of the aims is more salient in any given situation. There is specificity concerning which goal of punishment is predominant, with the aim dependent on aspects of the situation, and specifically a function of perception of responsibility for the transgression.

THE MORAL PERSON

Now I want to briefly examine one final issue—whether moral judgments should be linked solely with positive thoughts and/or positive actions, or might such judgments have greater complexity. In the discussion of achievement motivation it was argued that when students do not try, evaluation is affected by task outcome, so that the failing person is evaluated more harshly than is the student who succeeded. Taking actions and outcomes into account in moral evaluation is evident in nonachievement-related contexts as well. Imagine the following three individuals:

- Person A thinks benevolent thoughts about others. However, she does not act upon these thoughts.

- Person B thinks benevolent thoughts about others. She is known to help others in distress.

- Person C does not think benevolent thoughts about others. Nevertheless, she has been known to help others in distress.

If you are asked which of these three individuals is most moral, my intuition is that certainly Person B and perhaps even Person C would receive more votes than Person A. Good thoughts without correspondent actions may not qualify one as (very) moral, whereas neutral thoughts with prosocial actions may well define one as a moral person.

Now let us consider the case of evil thoughts and transgressions (as contrasted with the prior comparison of "good" thoughts and prosocial behaviors). Compare the following two individuals:

- Person A has strong inner desires to engage in sexual behavior with children. He calls these his "demons" and says he lives life "one day at a time" fighting these demons. He has never engaged in such behavior.

- Person B has no desire to engage in sexual acts with children. He never has engaged in such behavior.

Which of these individuals do you regard as more moral? That is intuitively less clear and in need of empirical study. There are some hints in the literature, however. Persons who overcome behavioral stigmas, such as the recovered alcoholic, the model citizen who formerly was a drug addict, the long-distance runner who at one time was obese because of overeating, and the previously lazy person who now employs many in her firm, are very admired and often are perceived as "cultural heroes" (particularly by conservatives; see Sniderman, Piazza, Tetlock, & Kendrick, 1991). These reformed persons are perceived as fully responsible for the offset of their immoral ways.

These data suggest that the person fighting demons and not acting immorally might be regarded as a very moral being, in spite of (or because of) having evil thoughts. That is, the inhibition of immoral desires, just as the overcoming of prior immoral actions, may enhance inferences of morality, indicating that morality cannot be solely tied to positive thoughts and beneficial actions. In sum, there are complex and subtle antecedents associated with responsibility beliefs, inferences of morality, and perceived life meaning.

References

Anesbury, T., & Tiggemann, M. (2000). An attempt to reduce negative stereotyping of obesity in children by changing controllability beliefs. *Health Education Research, 15*, 145-152.

Averill, J. R. (1982). *Anger and aggression: An essay on emotion.* New York: Springer.

Brickman, P. Rabinowitz, V. C., Karuza, J., Coates, D., Cohn, E., & Kidder, L. (1982). Models of helping and coping. *American Psychologist, 37*, 368-384.

Bush, G. W. (1999, January 27). *State of the union address.* Retrieved July 17, 2002, from http://www.georgebush.com/speeches/1-27-99sos.html

Bush, G. W. (1999, July 22). *The duty of hope.* Retrieved July 17, 2002, from http://www.georgebush.com/speeches/72299_duty_of_hope.htm

Clinton, W. J. (1996). Address before a joint session of the Congress on the state of the union: January 24, 1995. In Public Papers of the Presidents of the United States: William J. Clinton, 1995, Book 1 (pp. 75-86). Washington, DC: U.S. Government Printing Office.

Crandall, C. C. (1995). Do parents discriminate against their heavyweight daughters? *Personality and Social Psychology Bulletin, 21*, 724-735.

Crandall, C. C., & Martinez, R. (1996). Culture, ideology, and antifat attitudes. *Personality and Social Psychology Bulletin, 22*, 1165-1176.

Dodge, K. A. (1980). Social cognition and children's aggressive behavior. *Child Development, 51*, 162-170.

Farwell, L., & Weiner, B. (1996). Self-perceptions of fairness in individual and group contexts. *Personality and Social Psychology Bulletin, 22,* 868-881.

Hooley, J. M., & Licht, D. M. (1997). Expressed emotion and causal attributions in the spouses of depressed patients. *Journal of Abnormal Psychology, 106,* 298-306.

Juvonen, J. (2000). The social functions of attributional face-saving tactics among early adolescents. *Educational Psychology Review, 12,* 15-32.

Lopez, S. R., Nelson, K. A., Mintz, J., & Snyder, K. S. (1999). Attributions and affective reactions to family members and the course of schizophrenia. *Journal of Abnormal Psychology, 108,* 307-314.

Rasinski, K. A. (1989). The effect of question wording on public support for government spending. *Public Opinion Quarterly, 53,* 388-394.

Roseman, I. J., Spindel, M. S., & Jose, P. E. (1990). Appraisals of emotion-eliciting events: Testing a theory of discrete emotions. *Journal of Personality and Social Psychology, 59,* 899-915.

Skitka, L. J., & Tetlock, P. E. (1993). Providing public assistance: Cognitive and motivational processes underlying liberal and conservative policy preferences. *Journal of Personality and Social Psychology, 65,* 1205-1223.

Sniderman, P. M., Piazza, T., Tetlock, P. E., & Kendrick, A. (1991). The new racism. *American Journal of Political Science, 35,* 423-447.

Weber, M. (1958). *The Protestant ethic and the spirit of capitalism* (T. Parsons, Trans.). New York: Scribner's Sons. (Original work published 1904)

Weiner, B. (1986). *An attributional theory of motivation and emotion.* New York: Springer.

Weiner, B. (1995). *Judgments of responsibility: A foundation for a theory of social conduct.* New York: The Guilford Press.

Weiner, B. (2001). An attributional approach to perceived responsibility for transgressions: Extensions to child abuse, punishment goals and political ideology. In A. E. Auhagen & H-W. Bierhoff (Eds.), *Responsibility: The many faces of a social phenomenon* (pp. 49-60). London: Routeledge.

Weiner, B., Graham, S., & Reyna, C. (1997). An attributional examination of retributive versus utilitarian philosophies of punishment. *Social Justice Research, 10,* 431-452.

Weiner, B., Perry, R. P., & Magnusson, J. (1988). An attribution analysis of reactions to stigmas. *Journal of Personality and Social Psychology, 55,* 738-748.

CPSIA information can be obtained at www.ICGtesting.com
Printed in the USA
LVOW08s1713020815

448551LV00001B/247/P